Immunology and Immunopathology

Basic Concepts

Immunology and Immunopathology

Basic Concepts

Yoshitsugi Hokama, Ph.D.

Professor of Pathology,
University of Hawaii John A. Burns School of Medicine;
Director, Clinical Research Laboratory,
Clinical Program, Cancer Center of Hawaii,
University of Hawaii at Manoa

Robert M. Nakamura, M.D.

Adjunct Professor of Pathology,
University of California, San Diego, School of Medicine;
Chairman, Department of Pathology,
Cecil H. and Ida M. Green Hospital of the Scripps Clinic,
Scripps Clinic and Research Foundation,
La Jolla, California

Little, Brown and Company : Boston

Library of Congress Catalog Card No. 81-82895

ISBN 0-316-36932-2

Printed in the United States of America

HAL

Contents

Contributing Authors

Lucille H. Kimura, Ph.D.
Associate Researcher in Immunology,
Clinical Program, Cancer Center of Hawaii,
University of Hawaii at Manoa

W. Stephen Nichols, Jr., M.D.
Associate Clinical Member,
Department of Pathology,
Cecil H. and Ida M. Green Hospital of the Scripps Clinic,
Scripps Clinic and Research Foundation,
La Jolla, California

Preface

This book represents the authors' views of the essential elements necessary for the understanding of clinical immunology and immunopathology. We have used many diagrams to explain the complex concepts of immunology and immunopathology. In some instances the illustrations may have been oversimplified, and for this we are entirely responsible. Other immunologists and immunopathologists may disagree with our selection of information and references. The authors take full responsibility for any errors or omissions.

This book is intended for students in both medical school and the biological sciences, including medical technology and veterinary medicine. It should also be helpful to medical professionals and others interested in immunology and immunopathology.

We acknowledge with many thanks our appreciation to the individuals who have contributed to make this text possible. They include Drs. Nichols and Kimura for their contributions in Chapters 7, 15, and 17, respectively; Mr. Allen Perreira for his detailed illustrations in Chapters 1, 2, 5, 10, 11, and 12; Mr. Jeffrey Teraoka for the drawings in Chapters 3, 7, 8, and 13, and Mr. Glenn Kimura for the illustrations in Chapters 14 and 17; Drs. Eugene Yanagihara and Hong-Yi Yang for the H&E histological tissues in Chapters 1 and 12, and Drs. Takuji Hayashi and Joiner Cartwright for the electron microscopic photographs in Chapters 1 and 8; Mrs. Haruko Hazama, Mrs. Cleo-Mae Mrozek, and Miss Mary Lam for their meticulous typing; Mr. Bert Weeks, Mr. Jeffrey Teraoka, and Miss Katherine Shiraki for the photographic work; and to Mrs. Haru Hokama for proofreading the drafts of Chapters 1 through 6 and 8 through 13.

We are also indebted to Ms. Gretchen Dietz Denton of Little, Brown and Company for her critical review of the entire textbook and for her many suggestions.

We wish to thank Ms. Helane Manditch-Prottas, Book Editor, Ms. Nancy Mimeles Carey, Editorial Assistant, and Mr. Curtis Vouwie, Medical Editor, of Little, Brown and Company for their patience, support, encouragement, and faith in the authors.

Y. H.
R. M. N.

Immunology and Immunopathology

Basic Concepts

1 : The Immune System: Cellular Basis

Humans normally possess numerous complex defense mechanisms to protect themselves against pathogenic microorganisms and harmful foreign substances, such as bacteria, viruses, parasites, and toxins, to which they are constantly exposed. This capacity to withstand the deleterious agents within the environment is *native* or *innate* immunity. For the most part native immunity is genetically determined within a species with respect to a particular agent or *antigen* (Ag). *Antigen* is a term given to substances (see Chapter 4) that stimulate an immune response when administered to a host: substances that are generally foreign in molecular structure to the host, which recognizes them as *non-self*. This inherited capacity may vary within species and between individuals. Specifically *acquired immunity,* on the other hand, is an individual property dependent on a person's previous experience with an antigen, a particular harmful agent, or a toxin.

Native Immunity

Native immunity can be considered under two broad general areas: (1) *active* and (2) *passive* immunity. The active defense mechanisms of the host involve the tissues and structures of the body and those components of them that are in part or wholly functionally directed for active resistance to harmful external or opportunistic endogenous microorganisms and their toxins. The passive defense mechanism, or nonsusceptibility, involves no specific tissues or structures but is, rather, an environmental situation within the host that fortuitously is unsuited for initiation of a disease process by a particular pathogenic microorganism.

Active Defense

EPITHELIAL SURFACES. The outer covering of the body (the skin), together with the mucous membranes, composed of specialized epithelial cells lining the respiratory and gastrointestinal tracts, serve as the first line of defense against infection. These surfaces act primarily as mechanical barriers to invasive and pathogenic microorganisms. In addition, substances such as fatty acids found on the surface of the skin are bactericidal to certain pathogenic microorganisms. An example of this is the bactericidal effect of lactic acid against some species of the genus *Salmonella*. The specialized epithelial cells of the mucous membranes secrete mucus (protein-carbohydrate complexes), enzymes, and other bactericidal factors that contribute to the host's ability to resist

Table 1-1 : Antimicrobial Substances in Tissue and Body Fluids

Molecular Substance	Major Source	Chemical Type	Type of Bacteria Affected
Group I			
Fatty acids	Ubiquitous	Short- and long-chain fatty acids	Gram-negative
Bile salts	Gall bladder, liver, intestines	Steroids	Gram-positive
Heme	Red blood cells, white blood cells	Porphyrins	Gram-positive
Group II			
Polylysine, polyarginine	Thymus, tissues rich in histones	Low molecular weight basic peptides	Mainly gram-positive
Protamine	Sperm	Low molecular weight basic peptide	Gram-positive
Spermine, spermidine	Pancreas, prostate	Basic polyamines	Gram-positive
Group III			
Lysozyme	Ubiquitous	Low molecular weight basic protein (enzyme)	Mainly gram-positive
Phagocytin	Leukocytes	Globulin	Gram-negative
Beta lysin	Serum	Multiple enzymatic system; protein	Gram-positive
Properdin	Serum	Serum proteins (see Chapter 9)	Gram-negative
Opsonin	Serum	Globulins (natural antibodies?)	Gram-negative
Complement	Serum	Complex group of serum proteins consisting of 15 components	Gram-negative

attack by pathogenic microorganisms and harmful agents. Figures 1-1 and 1-8 illustrate those tissues and cells of the skin and mucous membrane that are associated with active defense of the host.

TISSUE AND BODY FLUIDS. When microorganisms enter the host after trauma or injury to the epithelial surfaces, they are immediately confronted by secondary defense substances found in body fluids: some in serum and others in tissue fluids. When isolated from animal tissue and body fluids, these compounds show antimicrobial activity. Characteristics of some of these chemical substances are summarized in Table 1-1. Information as to whether all these materials exert antimicrobial activity in the body itself is as yet incomplete. Nonetheless, since these molecular compounds are found distributed throughout the tissues, their potential function as bactericidal agents cannot be excluded.

The antimicrobial effect, in the laboratory, of short-chain and long-chain fatty acids has long been known. Short-chain fatty acids may act as metabolic inhibitors against microorganisms and in this manner exert their killing effect, whereas long-chain

Fig. 1-1 : A. The human skin, showing the epidermal and dermal layers and the major tissues. B. Histological section (X125) of normal human skin tissue.

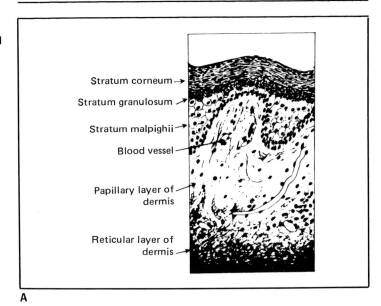

Stratum corneum →

Stratum granulosum →

Stratum malpighii →

Blood vessel →

Papillary layer of dermis →

Reticular layer of dermis →

A

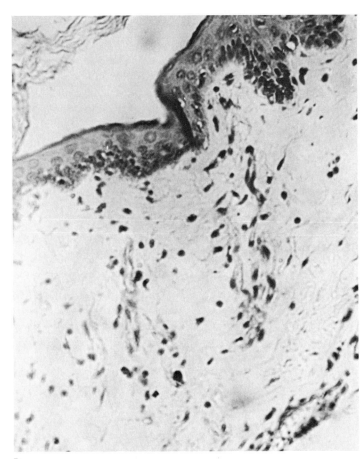

B

fatty acids appear to exert antibacterial effects by their action as surfactants (surface-acting agents). Sterols (lipids), such as bile salts (cholates and desoxycholates of bile), also act as surface-acting agents, killing and lysing particularly the gram-positive capsulated pneumococci, but with an exception: the related *Streptococcus faecalis* proliferates in media containing bile salts and in this way appears to be similar to some gram-negative organisms of the *Enterobacteriaceae.* This explains its presence in the intestinal flora.

Free porphyrins exert a high degree of bactericidal activity in vitro against gram-positive microorganisms. Porphyrins occurring in nature, however, are normally bound to proteins to form hemoproteins, which appear to have no antimicrobial activity. The hemoproteins are found in tissues as enzymes, such as catalases of the liver and red blood cells, myeloperoxidases of the leukocytes, and hemoglobin of the erythrocytes. These body fluids are indicated in Table 1-1 as Group I compounds.

Numerous basic polypeptides containing high levels of basic amino acids have shown various degrees of antimicrobial activity in vitro and are found in a variety of highly specialized tissues. They affect primarily the gram-positive microorganisms. Their bactericidal power seems to reside in their ability to complex or bind with the surfaces of the microorganisms. Studies have shown that, in vitro, the bactericidal activity of basic polypeptides can be neutralized by the addition of acid mucopolysaccharide, deoxyribonucleic acid (DNA), and ribonucleic acid (RNA) to the medium, thus nullifying the ability of the basic compounds to bind to the cell surface of the microorganisms. The fact that the basic polypeptides react with acidic compounds would suggest that the target on the bacterial cell may be an acidic residue, such as a terminal sialic acid residue. These compounds are listed under Group II in Table 1-1.

The chemically complex group of antimicrobial substances of body fluids are listed under Group III and include the following:

1. Lysozyme, a thermostabile, low molecular weight basic protein found in saliva, tears, leukocytes, macrophages, and many other sources. It primarily acts on gram-positive microorganisms in vitro. As an enzyme, it hydrolyzes the complex acetylaminopolysaccharide (muramic acid). Thus, microorganisms that possess muramic acid in their wall structure would be readily lysed by lysozyme. The microorganism *Micrococcus lysodeikticus* is extremely sensitive to lysozyme action and thus is readily lysed by it. The antimicrobial action of lysozyme is chiefly effective within narrow pH ranges near neutrality. The cytoplasm of alveolar macrophages and leukocytes of the blood is especially rich in lysozyme.

2. Phagocytin, a cytoplasmic protein yielded by extraction of leukocytes (white cells) of blood with acid solution. In the test tube, phagocytin appears to have a wide range of antimicrobial action on both gram-negative and gram-positive microorganisms. Its bactericidal effect is greater on gram-negative than on gram-positive microorganisms, however.

3. Beta-lysin, which probably functions as an enzyme.

4. Properdin, a serum protein that acts via the alternative complement pathway. The complement system (see Chapter 9) comprises a complex group of serum proteins, some of which are heat labile. Bactericidal activity has been exhibited against gram-negative bacteria in the presence of the complement proteins and magnesium ions (Mg^{++}). Properdin, complement, and Mg^{++} ions constitute the components in the alternative pathway of C activation (to be discussed in Chapter 9). The system has also been implicated in the inactivation of a number of viruses.

5. Opsonins, proteins that exist in normal fresh serum of animals and that enhance the phagocytosis by leukocytes of bacteria and inert particles. Opsonins are natural antibodies. Opsonin has no specificity and in this respect differs from a specific antibody (Ab), but it does appear to have predilection for gram-negative microorganisms and inert particles such as carbon. Like properdin, opsonin activates complement. A nonimmunoglobulin, α-globulin, has been shown to have opsonic properties also. Opsonin is measured or titrated by determining the number of microorganisms ingested per phagocyte (phagocytic index) in normal fresh serum and then comparing this with the number of microorganisms ingested per phagocyte in fresh serum of a patient. This gives the opsonic index:

$$\text{Opsonic index} = \frac{\text{Patient's phagocytic index}}{\text{Normal phagocytic index}}$$

6. Complement (C) made up of a group of several distinct functionally interrelated protein entities. Complement is found in the blood serum of animals and occurs in a variety of species. It generally decreases or increases in concentration during some disease processes. Differences in complement activity among various species are attributable to variations in proportion of the constituents of the C components. Details of the complement system are presented in Chapter 9.

CELLULAR ELEMENTS IN INNATE IMMUNITY. The phagocytes, or eating cells, of the blood and reticuloendothelial system are one of the most important active defense mechanisms in native resistance to pathogenic microbes. They act by ingesting bacteria or other foreign particles. Metchnikoff recognized this significance of leukocytes as an outgrowth of his earlier observation of intracellular digestion by cells of the water flea.

In the animal body there are two main varieties of phagocytic cells, microphages and macrophages. The microphages include the polymorphonuclear leukocytes, which make up more than half the white cells of the blood. Of these the neutrophils exhibit the greatest phagocytic activity and constitute the major cells in the acute inflammatory response to infection; the number and proportion rises rapidly in a case of acute appendicitis, for example. Eosinophils and basophils exhibit less phagocytic activity.

The cells of the reticuloendothelial system are composed of macrophages, either sessile or wandering. *Sessile,* or *fixed,* macrophages are found lining the capillary endothelium and sinuses of the liver (Kupffer's cells), spleen, bone marrow, lymph nodes, and other organs. They phagocytize foreign bodies from the blood as they flow past. The wandering macrophages, also known as *histiocytes,* include the blood monocytes that migrate through the endothelium and tissues and assist in the repair of damaged tissue by ingesting dead tissue materials and inert particles and further aid in the disposal of inactive erythrocytes and leukocytes that have passed through into the injured areas of the tissues. The characteristics and biochemical mode of action of these cells are discussed in Chapter 8.

Passive Defense

A variety of conditions that may be closely synonymous with innate resistance create an indifference or passivity on the part of animal tissue such that the tissue fails to offer a nurturing environment for the ubiquitous pathogens. Some of the more significant conditions include body temperature, tissue metabolites, oxygen tension, and nonsusceptibility to toxins.

It is known that animals of different species have different body temperatures. It is to be expected that animals with different body temperatures will exhibit different inhibition of microbes. An instance of such a phenomenon was shown by Pasteur, who demonstrated that chickens, which have high body temperatures, are normally resistant to *Bacillus anthracis.* They became susceptible when their body temperature was lowered by immersion in cold water. On the other hand, the *Bacillus* is highly infectious for mammals in general. Viruses and bacteria require certain specific basic chemical compounds or metabolites in order to grow. Thus animals with tissues deficient in the necessary metabolites would selectively inhibit growth of microbes requiring such metabolites. High oxygen tension in normal tissues prevents proliferation of anaerobic microbes and in this way maintains passive resistance. Finally, certain species of animals possess tissues that are indifferent to bacterial exotoxins. For example, frogs are entirely resistant to diphtheria and tetanus toxins. Whereas these toxins are lethal to most mammals.

Acquired Immunity

As already indicated, acquired immunity is an individual property, dependent on the host's previous exposure to or experience with the foreign agent. Nevertheless, the ability to respond immunologically is an inherent property and is genetically endowed within a given species.

Individuals may acquire immunity by either active or passive means. Natural active immunity may be acquired by a previous infection with a pathogenic microbe or by active immunization with bacterial and viral antigens (vaccination). Subsequent to these experiences, the individual develops antibodies specifically for the microorganism and thus acquires an active immune or resistant state to the microbe. This immune state may be of short or long duration, its length generally dictated by the inciting agent. For example, immunity to virus infections such as smallpox and yellow fever viruses may persist for years, whereas resistance developed against pneumococci or typhoid organisms is generally of short duration. The host response is dependent on the nature of the antigen and whether T or B cells or both have been activated (see Chapter 5).

Passive acquired immunity (borrowed immunity) may result from the transfer of human or animal serum that contains antibodies protective against a specific agent to another individual who has no protective antibodies. An example of this is the transfusion of neutralizing antibodies against measles virus to expectant mothers who have been exposed to the viruses in early pregnancy. Passive transfer to individuals of serum containing specific antibodies to certain infectious microbes was common practice prior to antibiotic therapy. It is generally no longer used for infectious diseases, but passive transfer of antivenoms or antitoxins is still employed against snakebites and other toxins. Transfer of immune cells is termed *adoptive immunity.* This type of passive transfer has been used therapeutically in immune deficiency diseases and in cancer patients (Chapters 15 and 16).

In the remainder of this text we shall discuss the details of the systems associated with innate and acquired immunity in man and animals.

Cellular Basis

Present immunology texts based on traditional teaching generally begin with antigens or immunogens. This is understandable since much information has been available regarding the nature of the immunogens. Early concepts of immunology and the study of immunity relied on the premise that the inoculation of a foreign substance (bacterial proteins, etc.) into an animal resulted in the production and release of various kinds of antibodies into the serum of the host. Understandably, the physical and chemical analyses of these foreign substances, called *antigens* progressed far more rapidly than the analysis of the underlying biological response of the animals to the antigens. Thus, it was to be expected that the teaching of immunology emphasized and began with the antigens.

With the astounding advances due to new developments such as the use of radioisotopes, improved tissue culture techniques, and sophisticated assay procedures (see Chapters 4, 5, and 6), the nature of the responses of animals, including man, especially at the cellular and molecular levels, are better understood today. Therefore our emphasis will be on the host — the response of the host's tissues, cells, organelles, and macromolecules to the antigen (immunity). This section encompasses the description, characteristics, distribution, and ontogeny of the cellular system associated with the host defense or surveillance against deleterious agents, especially those leading to pathological processes. The tissues and cells to be described constitute the members of the two-component lymphoid system, the *T* and *B lymphocytes.*

Central Lymphoid System

Tissues associated with the lymphoid system are characterized as *central* or *peripheral.* Within these lymphoid tissues are distributed the lymphocytes that constitute the thymus-dependent (cell-mediated) and the thymus-independent or bursa-equivalent (humoral) systems. Unlike birds, which have an organ (*bursa of Fabricius*) consisting of B lymphocytes that is situated near the rectal region of the gastrointestinal tract (Figure 1–2), man has no such specific organ. An equivalent organ in mammals has not been found but the B lymphocytes in man are considered as *bursa-equivalent* or *thymus-independent* (Ti). Since the mammalian B lymphocytes perform the same functions as do the bursal lymphocytes of birds, the term *B cells* or *B lymphocytes* is retained. The bone marrow, liver, and the gut-associated lymphoid tissues (GALT), which include the appendix, tonsils, and lymphoid tissues of the intestine, have been implicated as likely candidates for bursa-equivalency in mammals. Thus the central lymphoid system comprises the *thymus* and *bursa of Fabricius* in birds and the *thymus* and *bursa-equivalent* tissues in mammals.

Ontogeny, Immune System

The genesis and development of immunocompetent T and B lymphocytes and their relationship to each other and to various lymphoid tissues of the body are shown in Figure 1-3. As indicated in the figure, T and B lymphocytes originate from the same sources (although not illustrated, both the yolk sac and embryonic liver in addition to bone marrow have been implicated as stem cell sources, especially during embryogenesis).

Fig. 1-2 : A. An avian bursa of Fabricius with plicae containing the lymphoid follicles. B. Cellular details of the lymphoid follicle found in the plicae.

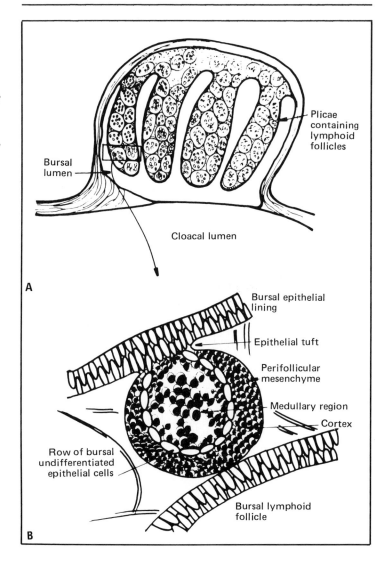

A

Plicae containing lymphoid follicles

Bursal lumen

Cloacal lumen

Bursal epithelial lining

Epithelial tuft

Perifollicular mesenchyme

Medullary region

Cortex

Row of bursal undifferentiated epithelial cells

Bursal lymphoid follicle

B

THYMUS: CENTRAL LYMPHOID SYSTEM (T CELL). The thymus (Figure 1-4) is formed from the III and IV pharyngeal pouches (Figure 1-3), which contribute the mesenchymal (epithelial) cells, and from the stem cells of the bone marrow, which contribute the prethymocytes (pre-T cells).

Earlier literature on the morphology of the thymus stated that the thymus showed atrophy with age, and the immunological functions associated with the T cells are now known to be related to these morphological changes. The thymus consists of the cortex and medulla with (interspersed) connective tissues. There are no fixed germinal centers or plasma cells.

Fig. 1-3 : The
dichotomy in the
development,
source, and dis-
tribution of the
immune cells in
man.

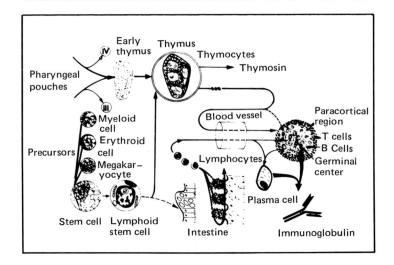

Fig. 1-3 : The dichotomy in the development, source, and distribution of the immune cells in man.

Changes in thymic cell mass, related to age and area of the thymus, have been recognized for many years. The thymus's relationship to immune processes, however, has been recognized, and evidence for it obtained, only in the past two decades. Atrophy begins soon after birth, but the greatest changes start at age 12. One of the identifying marks of the thymus is Hassall's corpuscle (Figure 1-4A), presumably consisting of atrophied thymic cells. Most of the Hassall's bodies are found in the medulla. Hassall's bodies are missing in some immunodeficiency syndromes (see Chapter 15). These bodies are also used to identify thymic tissues.

The epithelial cells are the source of the hormone *thymosin,* which is necessary for the maturation of thymocytes to T lymphocytes of the peripheral lymphoid system. *Thymosin,* a protein, has been isolated from thymus tissue. The congenital occurrence of rare thymic abnormalities (aplasia) in newborns with T cell immunodeficiency disorders (see Chapter 15) has led to the suggestion that the thymus is related to the development of the immune system. Additional evidence from neonatal thymectomy in the mouse has shown the following: (1) a decrease in circulating lymphocytes (lymphopenia); (2) severe impairment of the animals' ability to reject graft; (3) reduced humoral antibody responses to some (those antigens requiring T helper cells, i.e., T-dependent antigens) but not all antigens; (4) wasting disease at 1 to 3 months after thymectomy, probably the result of inability to combat infections effectively, since a germ-free environment or use of antibiotics can minimize or prevent *wasting* disease; and (5) loss of cell-mediated immunity.

The deficit initiated by neonate thymectomy can be restored with transplant of whole thymus, crude extracts of thymus, or with the purified hormone *thymosin.*

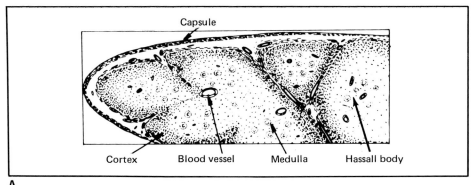

A

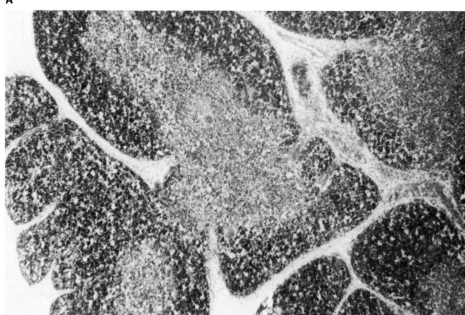

B

Fig. 1-4 : A. Diagram and B. microscopic section (X 125) of the thymus, with details of the major areas and cells. (Histological section courtesy of Dr. E. Yanagihara).

Impairment of the immune system can also be demonstrated in the adult thymectomized mouse. In this case impairment is attributed to loss of *thymosin,* which is synthesized by the residual epithelial cells of the hypertrophied adult thymus. The changes observed in the *adult* thymectomized mouse can be divided into two phases, early and late.

Early changes are the loss of E-rosette-forming T cells, due to deletion of or membrane changes in, surgace receptors; loss of RNA synthesis; loss of serum thymosin; and decrease in T suppressor cell. Hence there is a tendency toward formation of autoantibodies and an increase in autoimmune diseases, especially in the older thymectomized animals.

Late changes include loss of surface antigens (θ-antigens in mouse T cell) or a decrease in number of these cells (due to loss of thymosin); loss of mixed lymphocyte cytotoxicity (MLC) and mitogen responses; and loss of phytohemagglutinin (PHA), concanavalin A (Con A), and graft-versus-host response (GVHR). Humoral immune responses to antigens dependent on T helper cells tend to decrease in thymectomized animals.

T LYMPHOCYTES. T lymphocyte precursors from the bone marrow (Figure 1-5), known as prethymic cells, seed the thymus. There they become thymocytes and initiate the development of the thymus. The thymocytes proliferate from the cortex of the thymus at a rapid rate and move inward to the medullary region, where they undergo maturation. When these *mature thymocytes* enter the circulating pool of lymphocytes, they are called *T lymphocytes.* They have a relatively long half-life. In addition to composing 70 to 80 percent of the circulating lymphocytes of the blood, T cells are found in the perivascular region of the white matter of the spleen (Malpighian corpuscles) (Figure 1-6), the perifollicular and deep cortical regions of the lymph node (Figure 1-7), the thoracic duct, and the bone marrow (Figure 1-5). The T lymphocytes are a heterogeneous group of cells with diverse functions. They differ in turnover rates, circulating routes, and surface antigenic markers. There are two populations of small lymphocytes in the blood and the thoracic duct lymph. One population is formed at a slower rate, is long-lived (having a half-life of 100 to 200 days), and moves back and forth between blood and lymph. The other is produced rapidly (two to three mitotic divisions per day) and has a circulating life span of less than two weeks ($T_{1/2}$ of 3 to 4 days). Although the thymus and bone marrow are the major sites for these short-lived lymphocytes, other lymphoid centers can also produce them (Peyer's patches).

As indicated earlier, an organ equivalent to the bursa of Fabricius of birds has not been found in man. The embryonic liver, bone marrow, spleen, and gut-associated lymphoid tissues have all been implicated. Neither has a hormone equivalent to thymosin been defined or found. The embryonic liver and especially the bone marrow (Figure 1-5A), however, are sources of stem cells. This is true for the bone marrow. In addition to stem cells of lymphoid T and B cells the bone marrow contains precursor cells of the myeloid, megakaryocytic, erythroid, and monocytic series. Whether all these cells originate from a single pluripotential cell (monophyletic theory) or each of these cells originate from individual (polyphyletic theory) remains a controversial question. According to the monophyletic concept, presumably a single undifferentiated and uncommitted bone marrow stem cell may become committed through the poietins. For example, stem cell conversion to the erythroid series is via erythropoietin. The

Fig. 1-5 : A.
Diagrammatic
illustration and B.
microscopic section
(X 125) of human
bone marrow
demonstrating the
major cells of this
tissue.

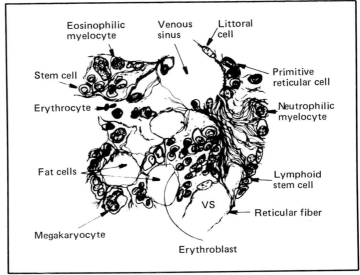

A

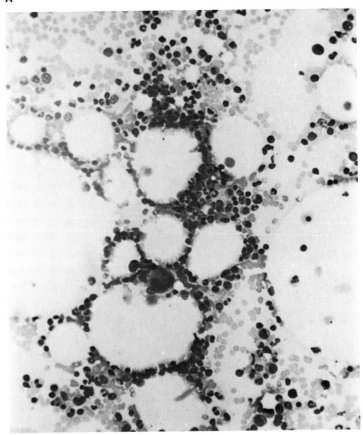

B

Fig. 1-6 : A. Diagrammatic illustration and B. microscopic section of the human spleen with description of the major structural areas and cellular distribution.

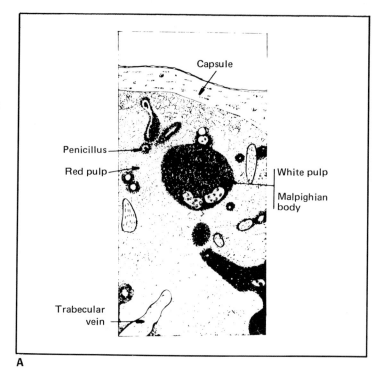

Capsule

Penicillus

Red pulp

White pulp

Malpighian body

Trabecular vein

A

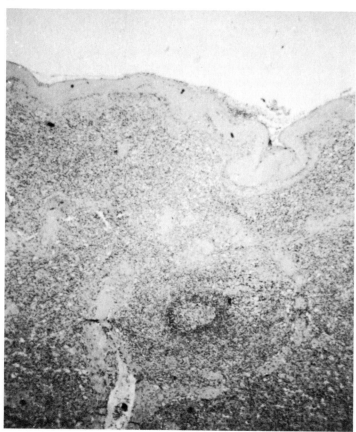

B

Fig. 1-7 : A. Schematic illustration and B. microscopic section (X 125) of a lymph node demonstrating the important cells of the immune system.

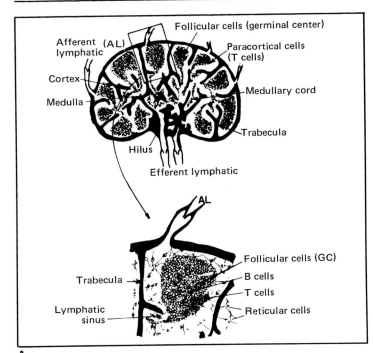

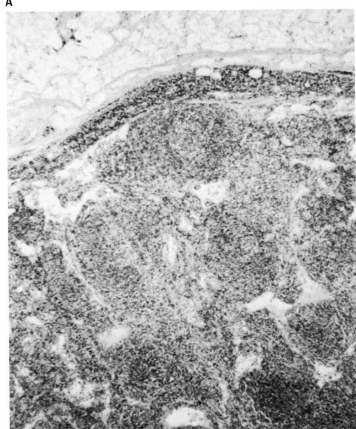

A

B

latter is a low molecular weight glycoprotein synthesized by the kidney when erythrocyte levels in peripheral blood drop below a critical level. Similarly a granulopoietin and thrombopoietin have been designated for conversion or stimulation of bone marrow stem cells to production of the myeloid and thrombocytic series, respectively. A *lymphopoietin* or a poietin for the lymphoid series has not been described or reported as yet.

BURSA-EQUIVALENT: B LYMPHOCYTES. B lymphocyte precursors are also of bone marrow origin. They may be distributed directly to spleen, lymph nodes, and other lymphoid tissues or may first traverse or be regulated by the liver, bone marrow, appendix, intestines (GALT), or tonsils in order to become functional B lymphocytes. Evidence for B cell control similar to that shown for birds is not as convincing in the mammalian system as yet, although the intestine, appendix, tonsils, liver, and bone marrow have been suggested as possible bursa-equivalent tissues. As well as being found in the peripheral blood (20 to 30 percent of circulating lymphocytes of varying sizes), B cells also exist in the germinal centers of lymph nodes and spleen (Figures 1-6 and 1-7), the lamina propria of the gastrointestinal tract, the secretory glands, bone marrow (Figure 1-5), the appendix (Figure 1-8), and other lymphoid tissues associated with the reticuloendothelial system.

Peripheral Lymphoid System

The peripheral lymphoid system that is associated with the immune system in the mature individual (capable of immune responses) resides primarily in the peripheral lymphoid tissues. These consist of the lymphatics, spleen, lymph nodes, lymphoid tissues of the gastrointestinal tract, respiratory tract, secretory glands, and lymphocytes of the blood.

B lymphocytes

B lymphocytes, as indicated earlier, are found in the germinal centers of lymphoid follicles within the lymph nodes and spleen. The plasma cells are found in the medullary regions of the lymph nodes and red pulp of the spleen. The distribution of B and T cells within the lymph node, spleen, and appendix is shown in Figures 1-6, 1-7, and 1-8. Plasma cells, the final cellular product of B lymphocyte development, are involved in antibody (Ab) synthesis that is elaborated into blood and serous fluids. These cells may be found scattered throughout the lymphoid systems, including the bone marrow. The sequence of B cell transformation to plasma cells via lymphoblast, following antigenic stimulation, is shown later (see Chapter 5). Plasma cells found in endothelial areas of the respiratory tract, nasal cavities, secretory glands, and gastrointestinal tract are associated generally with the synthesis of IgA and IgE. These immunoglobulins are consequently referred to as *secretory immunoglobulins.* The structure

Fig. 1-8 : A. Diagrammatic representation and B. microscopic illustration (X 125) of a human appendix showing the important cells of the immune system.

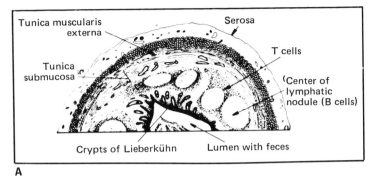

A

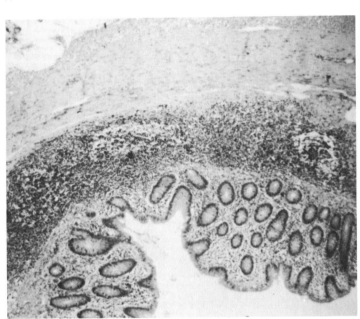

B

of organelles of a typical plasma cell is shown in Figure 1-9. B lymphocytes and the process of their conversion to plasma cells play a significant role in humoral immunity. B lymphocytes contain the light chain and the V_H and C_H regions of the Fab domain of the immunoglobulins on their membrane surfaces, while the plasma cells ultimately secrete the immunoglobulin. This system provides defenses against viral and bacterial infections by synthesis of specific antibodies (immunoglobulins) against the antigen (Ag) of the infectious agents.

The B lymphocytes of the lymph nodes of mammals and the peripheral blood of man can be functionally differentiated from T lymphocytes by their response to nonspecific mitogens (substances that induce blastogenesis) (summarized in Table 1-2).

Fig. 1-9 : A. Dia-
grammatic illustra-
tion and B. electron
micrograph
(X 8000) of a
plasma cell showing
typical eccentric
nucleus and numer-
ous endoplasmic
reticulum charac-
teristic of this cell.
(Courtesy of Dr.
T. Hayashi).

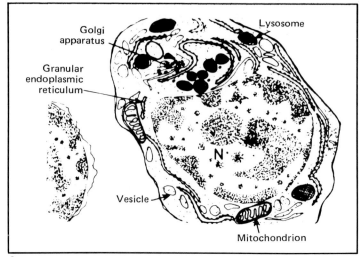

A

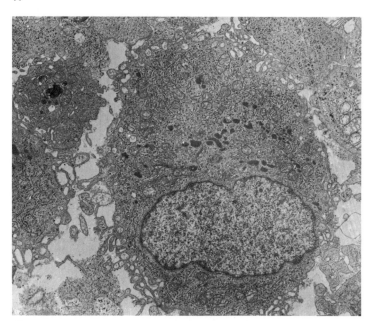

B

A positive response (indicated by a +) consists of an increased rate of mitosis and, consequently, of DNA synthesis.

T lymphocytes respond to phytohemagglutinin (PHA) (enhanced by adherent cells or macrophages) and concanavalin A (Con A) but give no response to lipopolysaccharide (LPS) and pokeweed mitogen (PWM). B lymphocytes respond only to PWM, LPS (of mouse B cells), and possibly to PHA stimulation. B lymphocytes

Table 1-2 : Mitogenic Responses by T and B Lymphocytes

Mitogens (Soluble)		B Lymphocytes	T Lymphocytes
Pokeweed mitogen	(PWM)	+	—
Phytohemagglutinin	(PHA)	±	+
Concanavalin A	(Con A)	—	+
Purified lipo-polysaccharide	(LPS)	+ (mouse) (No response in man)	—

of man show no responses to LPS. Both T and B lymphocytes respond to insoluble PHA, PWM, and Con A. These responses are generally assayed by determining the amount of ^{3}H-thymidine incorporated into the new DNA synthesized in the lymphocyte culture following stimulation by the mitogen in question. This is done using cells in short-term cultures (generally 2 to 7 days). The ^{3}H-thymidine uptake is determined in the scintillation spectrometer following precipitation of the cellular material with trichloroacetic acid, appropriate washing with alcohol and ethyl ether, and solubilization of the precipitate in the scintillation solution.

T lymphocytes

T lymphocyte function is associated with cell-mediated immunity (CMI) (see Chapter 3). The distribution of these cells has been discussed in earlier paragraphs. They have been implicated in primary transplantation rejection, delayed hypersensitivity, surveillance against neoplastic transformation, and protection against viruses and bacterial infections. T lymphocytes do not transform to plasma cells nor do they elaborate immunoglobulins, but they do have specific antigens on their membrane surfaces (the antigens of mouse T lymphocytes, for example) and in man, MHC (major histocompatibility complex) antigens. Both T suppressor and T helper functions have been attributed to T lymphocytes. The T suppressor cells regulate antibody synthesis by B cells. T suppressor cells regulating T cells have also been demonstrated. T helper cells, on the other hand, are required for B cell synthesis of antibody to T-dependent antigens.

Sensitized T lymphocytes must be in direct contact with target antigens for their activation. This interaction initiates the release of a variety of factors that affect macrophages, polymorphonuclear leukocytes, lymphocytes, and other cells. These factors, called *lymphokines,* will be discussed in Chapter 3.

Fig. 1-10 : A. Dia-grammatic illustra-tion and B. electron micrograph (X 5600) of a small peripheral lymphocyte, show-ing its major organelles. (Electron micrograph courtesy of Dr. T. Hayashi.)

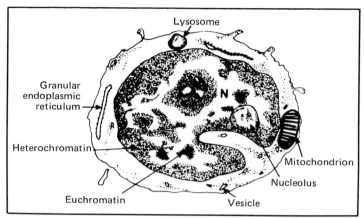

A

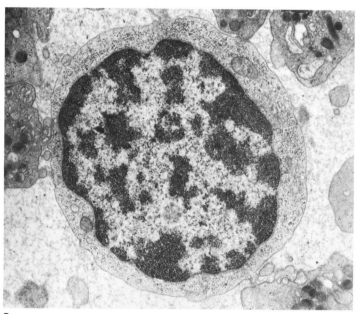

B

Lymphocytes and Plasma Cells: Characteristics and Properties

A normal mature peripheral lymphocyte is shown in Figure 1-10. Morphologically it is difficult to differentiate T from B cells.

The lymphocytes of the peripheral blood comprise nearly 40 to 50 percent of circulating leukocytes and are the major immuno-logical cells. They are a heterogeneous population in both size and function. Both B cells and T cells can be found in the circu-lation. The T cells constitute the major group of lymphocytes in a normal individual (70 to 80 percent of the circulating lympho-cytes) (see Table 1-3). B cell lymphocytes constitute the re-mainder of the lymphocytes (15 to 20 percent). Lymphocytes

Table 1-3 : Membrane Characteristics of T and B Cells and Their Distribution in Various Tissues and Blood

Cell Type	Membrane Receptors
T cells	For sheep RBC (E-rosettes), (immunoglobulins?), Clq, FcμR, FcγR
B cells	For (immunoglobulins), Fc, C3d, C4b, Clq, C3b (EAC-rosette–binding site)

T and B cells are distributed in the tissues and blood in the following percentages.

Tissue	T Cells	B Cells
Thymus	>75	<25
Bone marrow	≪25	>75
Tonsil	50	50
Spleen	50	50
Lymph node	75	25
Lymph	>75	<25
Blood, peripheral	55–75	15–20
Thoracic duct	>90	<10

Table 1-4 : Enzymes Associated with the Cytoplasmic Granules of Lymphocytes

Organelle	Enzymes
Peroxisome-related organelles	D-amino acid oxidase L-α-hydroxy acid peroxidase; catalase
Lysosomes	Arylsulfatase, β-glucuronidase, β-glucosaminidase, α-mannosidase, α-arabinosidase, β-xylosidase, β-cellobiosidase, β-furosidase, cathepsin D

vary in size from 8 to 12 μ in diameter. Their functions have been discussed in earlier sections. Lymphocytes are the pivotal cells in immunology. The intracellular enzyme profile, which is limited, of lymphocytes is shown in Table 1–4. The major morphological characteristics of lymphocytes are their large, homogeneous, nonlobed nucleus, and light-staining, nongranular cytoplasm. The membrane receptors (R) attributable to T and B cells and their distribution in various tissue and blood are summarized in Table 1-3 and illustrated in Figure 1–11. FcμR and FcγR refer to receptors (R) for the Fc portion (H-chain) of immunoglobulins M and G, respectively.

Plasma cells are rarely found in peripheral blood in normal individuals. These cells, as indicated earlier, are associated with antibody synthesis and secretion and are the end cells of B

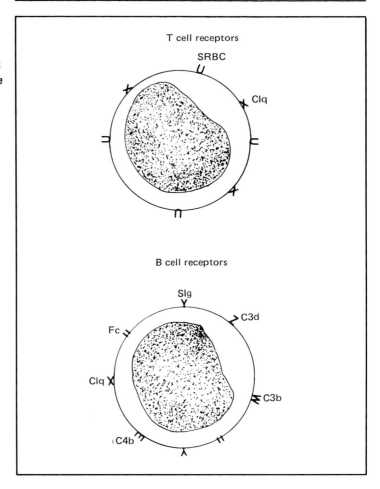

Fig. 1-11 : Schematic representation of receptors summarized in Table 1-3 on membrane surface of T and B lymphocytes. FcμR and FcγR have also been demonstrated in some T cell subsets (see Chapter 3).

lymphocyte development. Their major morphological characteristics are their eccentric cartwheel-like nuclei. The cytoplasmic area is much larger and stains much more intensely with basic dyes (grayish blue) than does that of a lymphocyte. Electron micrographs show numerous channels of endoplasmic reticulum lined with polyribosomes in the cytoplasm (Figure 1-9). Few or no granules characteristic of granulocytes are evident.

Functions

The major functions and participations of the T and B cell lymphocytes, the cell-mediated and humoral systems respectively, are summarized in Table 1-5.

Circulation of Lymphocytes

In man, the peripheral blood contains hemopoietic stem cells, designated *null cells,* which are progenitor cells of the various blood cell classes. Furthermore, the hemopoietic populations in the spleen, lymph node, and to a lesser extent the thymus are

Table 1-5 : Major Functions of the Plasma Cells Derived from the B Cells and of the T Cells (the Members of the Two-Component Lymphoid System)

B and Plasma Cells	T Cells
Humoral immunity	Cell-mediated immunity
Immunoglobulin synthesis	Homograft rejection
Production of the wide diversity of antibodies (immunoglobulins)	Delayed hypersensitivity reactions
Immediate hypersensitivity reactions	Graft-versus-host response (GVHR) reactions
Production of lymphokines	Helper activity for T-dependent antigens
	Suppressor cell production of lymphokines
	Production of lymphokines

Fig. 1-12 : A schematic pattern of lymphocyte circulation in the lymphatic and blood vessel systems and the relationships of the major tissues associated with the immune system.

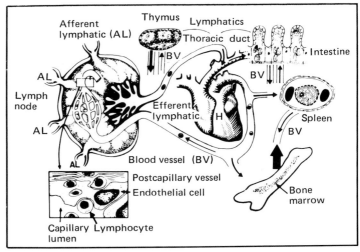

continually replaced in adult life by an inflow of circulating stem and progenitor cells. Hemopoiesis in adult life essentially occurs only in the bone marrow and thus is not dependent on an inflow of stem cells; rather, the bone marrow is the source of these stem cells for the other lymphoid tissues. Figure 1-12 diagrams the circulation of lymphocytes in man. The low levels of circulating stem cells essentially follow similar circulatory pathways. The lymphocytes circulate in blood and between blood and the lymphatic system. Lymphocytes in the lymph drift through connective tissues, particularly beneath exposed epithelial surfaces (gastrointestinal and respiratory tracts) and are engaged in a continuous mission of immunological surveillance. The entry of the blood lymphocytes into the lymphatics occurs primarily in the deep paracortical region of the postcapillary venules of the lymph nodes. Unlike macrophages and polymorphonuclear cells, lymphocytes penetrate the endothelial cells and traverse through and exit into the lymphatic sinusoids of the lymph node. These lymphocytes and those from the afferent lymphatics pass through the medullary region of the lymph node, exit via the efferent lymphatics into the thoracic duct, and reenter the blood circulation in the region of the major veins in the proximity of the heart (left brachiocephalic vein), which empties into the superior vena cava and then into the right atrium. Lymphocytes also enter the lymphatics from the lymphoid tissues of the intestines and the thymus, from the latter organ especially during the early stages of development and growth.

Evolution of the Lymphoid System

The most significant characteristics of immunological responses are *specificity* and *anamnesis* (see Chapter 5). These two criteria must be considered in distinguishing true immunity from para-immunological phenomena in the study of the evolution of the immune system. The examination of invertebrate tissues shows no lymphoid system or cells comparable to those found for vertebrates, although the ability to reject allografts has been demonstrated in all phyla of the invertebrates examined thus far (the protozoa through the protochordata). Nevertheless, these graft rejections showed *no specificity.* The earthworm of the phylum *Annelida,* however, demonstrated some specificity in the graft rejection as well as anamnesis of short duration. In addition to the annelids the sea urchin *Lytechinus pictus* has been shown to mount an immune response to grafted tissue similar to that of the vertebrates. Both primary and secondary set responses were reported in the *sea urchin* graft studies. In addition, accelerated second set rejections were demonstrated, thus fulfilling the criteria of anamnesis. No specific inducible antibodies have been demonstrated in all invertebrates. Humoral factors that react with the ABO antigens of erythrocytes (Chapter 11) comparable to plant lectins have been found in nearly all invertebrates.

All vertebrates have shown distinct lymphocytes including the class *Agnatha* (lamprey, hagfish, dipnoi). In these animals specific antibodies and cell-mediated functions are demonstrable: a beginning of the dichotomy of the immune system that is characteristic of all vertebrates. Nevertheless, the *Agnatha* (jawless fishes), which include the cyclostomes, hagfish, and lamprey, have primitive thymuses and spleen, but lack plasma cells.

In the development of the lymphoid system the T cell system appears to have occurred initially, with the B cell system arising from the first primordial lymphoid cell. The μ-chain containing immunoglobulin and its primitive counterpart appear to be the

Table 1-6 : Immunological Characteristics of the Vertebrates

Class	Lympho-cytes	Plasma Cells	Thymus	Bursa	Spleen	Lymph Nodes	Specific Antibodies	Allograft Rejection
Agnatha (jawless fish)	+	−	Primitive	−	Primitive	−	+	+
Chondrichthyes								
Primitive	+	−	+	−	+	−	+	+
Advanced	+	+	+	−	+	−	+	+
Osteichthyes (bony fish)	+	+	+	−	+	−	+	+
Reptilia	+	+	+	+?*	+	+?*	+	+
Aves	+	+	+	+	+	+?*	+	+
Mammalia	+	+	+	+?*	+	+	+	+

*? indicates some question of their existence, although equivalent lymphoid functional cells have been reported.

first immunoglobulins (see Chapter 2). These are found in the *Agnatha.* The immunological characteristics of the vertebrates from *Agnatha* to *Mammalia* are summarized in Table 1-6.

Summary

1. Native immunity encompasses both active and passive host defense mechanisms. Active immunity is associated with the tissues and organs of the host, which are functionally directed for active resistance to harmful agents. Passive immunity is related to the environment of the host, which is unsuitable for deleterious agents to act. Acquired immunity is an individual property dependent on the host's previous exposure to or experience with the foreign agent. Acquired immunity may also be active or passive.

2. The cellular elements of peripheral blood (erythrocytes, platelets, neutrophils, eosinophils, basophils, monocytes, and lymphocytes) are derived from a common ancestral cell. This cell is referred to as the *pluripotent hemopoietic stem cell.*

3. The pluripotent hemopoietic stem cell differentiates into an active progenitor cell via the action of hemopoietins (hormones) such as erythropoietin, thrombopoietin, and granulopoietin. The lymphoid progenitor cell is responsive to hormone-like factors (thymosin and bursa-equivalent factors) that induce the progenitor cell to begin to differentiate into functional cells.

4. The thymus is the central lymphoid organ for the T cell or cell-mediated immune system and produces the hormone *thymosin.*

5. The *bursa of Fabricius* in birds and the bursa-equivalent tissues in mammals (bone marrow or GALT) are the central lymphoid system for the B cells, and they regulate the maturation and development of the B cell or humoral immune system.

6. Lymphocytes leave the primary lymphoid organs and migrate to the peripheral (secondary lymphoid organs) lymphoid tissues. These are the spleen and lymph nodes. The T cells are found in the paracortical regions, and the B cells are found in the germinal centers of the lymphoid follicles of the spleen and lymph node.
7. Lymphocytes in the primary lymphoid organ (thymus) are not able to respond to antigen. Lymphocytes in the secondary organs are capable of participating in the immune response.
8. The T cell or cell-mediated system is associated with delayed type hypersensitivity (DTH), graft-versus-host response (GVHR), allograft rejection, cell-mediated lympholysis (CML), mixed lymphocyte reaction (MLR), T helper and T suppressor functions, and production of lymphocytes.
9. The B cell or humoral-mediated system is associated with antibodies, neutralization of toxins, immediate hypersensitivity, production of lymphokines, and immunoglobulin synthesis.
10. Lymphocytes circulate in peripheral blood and between blood and the lymphatic system. There are three times more T cells than B cells in peripheral blood. The lymphocytes constitute approximately 20 to 50 percent of the total leukocytes in the peripheral blood.
11. In the evolution of the lymphoid system, all vertebrates have shown distinct lymphocytes, including the class *Agnatha.* Specific antibodies and cell-mediated immunity functions have been demonstrated in the lower forms of vertebrates, which however, lack plasma cells.

Bibliography

General

Fudenberg, H. H., Stiles, D. P., Caldwell, J. L., and Wells, J. V. *Basic and Clinical Immunology* (2nd ed.). Los Altos, Calif.: Lange, 1978.

Hokama, Y. Immunochemistry. In N. Bhagavan (Ed.), *A Comprehensive Review of Biochemistry.* Philadelphia: Lippincott, 1978.

Marchalonis, J. J. Phylogenetic Origins of Antibodies and Immune Recognition. In L. Brent and J. Holborow (Eds.), *Progress in Immunology* II, Vol. 2. North Holland: Elsevier, New York:American Elsevier, 1974.

Origins of Lymphocyte Diversity. Cold Spring Harbor Symposia on Quantitative Biology, XLI. Cold Spring Harbor Laboratory of Quantitative Biology, Cold Spring Harbor, L.I., New York, 1977.

Yoffey, J. M., and Courtice, F. C. (Eds.). *Lymphatics, Lymph and the Lymphomyeloid Complex.* New York: Academic 1970.

Cellular Basis

Barr, R. D., and Whang-Peng, J. Hemopoietic stem cells in human peripheral blood. *Science* 190:284, 1975.

Boyd, E. The weight of the thymus gland in health and disease. *Am. J. Dis. Child.* 43:162, 1932.

Goldstein, A. L., Thurman, G. B., Cohen, G. H., and Hooper, J. A. The Role of Thymosin and the Endocrine Thymus on the Ontogenesis and Function of T Cells. In E. E. Smith, and D. W. Robbins (Eds) *Molecular Approaches to Immunology.* New York: Academic, 1975. Pp. 243-262.

Goldwasser, E. Erythropoietin and the differentiation of red blood cells. *Fed. Proc.* 34:2285, 1975.

Miller, R. G., and Phillips, R. A. Development of B lymphocytes. *Fed. Proc.* 34:145, 1975.

Mosier, D. E., and Cohen, P. L. Ontogeny of mouse T lymphocyte function. *Fed. Proc.* 34:137, 1975.

Owen, J. J. T., Cooper, M. D., and Raff, M. C. *In vitro* generation of B lymphocytes in mouse fetal liver, a mammalian "bursa equivalent." *Nature* 249:361, 1974.

Function, Evolution, and Circulation

Altman, L. C., Chassy, B., and Mackler, B. F. Physiochemical characterization of chemotactic lymphokines produced by human T and B lymphocytes. *J. Immunol.* 115:18, 1975.

Coffaro, K. A., and Hinegardner, R. T. Immune response in the sea urchin *Lytechinus pictus. Science* 197:1389, 1977.

Cohn, S. The Role of cell-mediated immunity in the induction of inflammatory responses. *Am. J. Pathol.* 88:502, 1977.

Hokama, Y. Host Responses to Pathogenic Microorganisms and Other Foreign Agents. In D. A. Anderson (Ed.), *Introduction to Microbiology.* St. Louis: Mosby, 1973.

Kierszenbaum, F., and Budzko, B. D. Cytotoxic effects of normal sera on lymphoid cells. I. Antibody-independent killing of heterologous thymocytes by guinea pig, rabbit, and human sera: Role of the alternate pathway of complement activation. *Cell. Immunol.* 29:137, 1977.

Mackler, B. F., Altman, L. C., Rosenstreich, D. L., and Oppenheim, J. J. Induction of lymphokine production by EAC and of blastogenesis by soluble mitogens during human B cell activation. *Nature* 249:834, 1974.

Metcalf, D., and Moore, M. A. S. (Eds.) *Haemopoietic Cells.* North Holland: Elsevier, New York: American Elsevier, 1971.

Metchnikoff, E. *L'immunité dans les Maladies infectieuses.* Paris: Masson, 1901.

Siskind, G. W., and Goidl, E. A. Ontogeny of B lymphocyte function with respect to the heterogenicity of antibody affinity. *Fed. Proc.* 34:151, 1975.

Weissman, I. L., Small, M., Fathman, C. G., and Herzenberg, L. A. Differentiation of thymus cells. *Fed. Proc.* 34:141, 1975.

2 : Immunoglobulins: Humoral-Mediated System

Immunoglobulins are elaborated by plasma cells following the transformation of antigen-stimulated B lymphocytes. (A typical plasma cell appears in Figure 1-9.) This elaboration constitutes the humoral immune system. The genesis of the humoral immune system and the lymphoid tissues involved in this development were presented in Chapter 1. Discussions here will be confined to (1) nomenclature and classification based on the recommendations of the World Health Organization (WHO), (2) the structure of immunoglobulins and the theories that account for antibody diversity, and (3) their biological function.

Classification and Basic Structure of Immunoglobulins (Ig)

Classification

Five major classes of immunoglobulins have been recognized (IgG, IgA, IgM, IgD, and IgE), with four subclasses in immunoglobulin G (IgG), (IgG1, IgG2, IgG3, and IgG4) and two each in immunoglobulin A (IgA) and immunoglobulin M (IgM). Prior to 1964, immunoglobulin designations were a conglomerate of names based primarily on physicochemical properties (see Table 2-3 for the common synonyms). Immunoglobulin D (IgD) and immunoglobulin E (IgE) lack synonyms, since they were discovered after 1964 and their original naming followed the standardized procedure for classification established by WHO. Each class can also be referred to as a member of the kappa (κ) or lambda (λ) type, according to the nature of its L-chain constituent. Thus, the designation of the immunoglobulin depends upon the antigenicity and nature of the polypeptide chains that constitute the complete molecule.

Immunoglobulins are composed of four peptide chains: two light chains (L-chains) and two heavy chains (H-chains) per molecule. These chains are linked by disulfide bonds. There are two classes of light chains, κ and λ, thus creating two series of immunoglobulin molecules. Each class of immunoglobulin contains a unique type of heavy chain: γ, α, μ, δ, or ϵ. The immunoglobulins and their chemical formulas are represented in Table 2-1.

Table 2-1 : Chemical Formulas of the Five Classes of Immunoglobulins

	H-chain	κ-Type	λ-Type
IgG	γ	$\kappa_2\gamma_2$	$\lambda_2\gamma_2$
IgA	α	$\kappa_2\alpha_2$	$\lambda_2\alpha_2$
IgM	μ	$\kappa_2\mu_2$	$\lambda_2\mu_2$
IgD	δ	$\kappa_2\delta_2$	$\lambda_2\delta_2$
IgE	ϵ	$\kappa_2\epsilon_2$	$\lambda_2\epsilon_2$

Structure

The structural analysis of immunoglobulins began with Porter's early studies using the proteolytic enzyme papain on rabbit immunoglobulin. Since then, in addition to papain, pepsin (another proteolytic enzyme) and the reducing agents mercaptoethanol and dithiothreitol have been widely used for structural analysis of immunoglobulins. The reducing agents are necessary for the reduction of the disulfide linkages. Immunoglobulin fragments obtained by proteolysis or reduction have been analyzed and separated by adsorption and gel filtration chromatography and by zonal electrophoresis on starch or polyacrylamide gel supports. Figure 2-1 shows the fragments obtained following cleavage with papain and pepsin. Papain hydrolysis, under proper pH and time conditions, cleaves IgG into three fragments. Two of these fragments are similar and are each designated Fab, each contains an antigen-binding site. The third fragment is called Fc, because it is crystallizable, being obtained as flat, rhomboid crystals from aqueous solution. Pepsin, on the other hand, produces one large fragment (designated F[ab']$_2$), which contains *both* antigen-binding sites, and eight smaller peptides (four per chain). The small peptides are derived from the region corresponding to the Fc fragment of papain digestion. The principal site of both papain and pepsin action is in the "hinge" region of the molecule (see Figure 2-1). This is a segment of the heavy chain peptides that is linear (or randomly coiled) due to the presence of three proline residues, which prevent helical folding. This "openness" makes the hinge region susceptible to enzymatic attack.

Polypeptide Chains

Reduction of immunoglobulins with mercaptoethanol or dithiothreitol, followed by alkylation of the exposed sulfhydryls, results in the cleavage of the interchain disulfide linkages. Two L-chains and two H-chains are obtained by gel filtration chromatography on Sephadex G-100. Alkylation and the cleavage points and reduction of the interchain -S-S- bonds are illustrated in Figure 2-2. Under mild conditions, the intrachain -S-S- bonds remain intact and retain the configuration and biological properties of the chains.

Fig. 2-1 : Effect of the enzymes papain and pepsin in the cleavage of IgG. A solid line between chains indicates an inter-chain disulfide bond, while "SS" represents an intra-chain disulfide group.

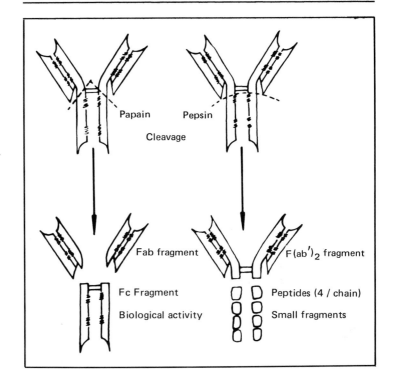

Fig. 2-2 : Mild treatment of immunoglobulin with mercaptoethanol or dithiothreitol and other reducing agents followed by alkylation results in the formation of two H- and two L-chains.

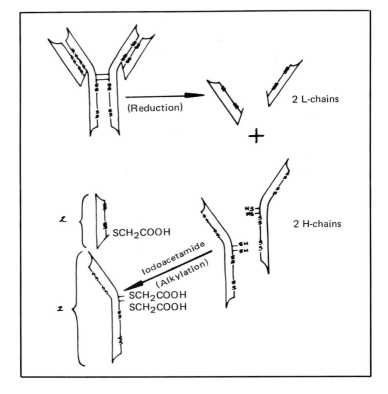

Table 2-2 : Properties of the Subunits and Major Enzymatic Fragments of Human Immunoglobulin G

Property	Subunits		Enzymatic Fragments			
	H-Chain	L-Chain	Fab	Fc	Fd	F(ab')$_2$*
Mode of production	Reduction of interchain	Reduction of interchain	Papain digestion	Papain digestion	Reduction of Fab	Pepsin digestion
	Disulfide bonds	Disulfide bonds				
Molecular weight	50-55,000	20-25,000	42,000	48,000	25,000	90,700
Sedimentation coefficient	3.0S	1.5S	3.5S	3.5S	1.5S	5.0S
Electrophoretic mobility	Heterogeneous	Heterogeneous	Slow	Fast	Hetero-geneous	Slow
Presence of carbohydrate	+	0	0(?)	+	0?	0?
Antigenic determinants						
Specific for IgG	+	0	0	+	+	0
Specific for Kan	0	+	+	0	0	+
Genetic factors						
6m	+	0	±	+	±	±
InV	0	+	+	0	0	+
Antibody activity / number of binding sites	—	—	+/1	0/0	—	+/2
Antibody specificity	+	0	—	—	—	—
Placental transport	+	0	±	+	±	±
Skin sensitization (fixation)	+	0	0	+	0	0
Complement binding	+	0	0	+	0	0
Reacts with rheumatoid factor	+	0	0	+	0	0

*Reduction of F(ab')$_2$ will give Fab'.

Table 2-2 summarizes the physicochemical properties and functions of the subunits and the major enzymatic fragments of human immunoglobulin G.

These enzymatic cleavages and chemical reductions have led to the understanding of the spatial orientation of the subunits and the structure-function relationships of immunoglobulins, which will be discussed in later paragraphs. In addition, amino acid sequence studies and immunological analysis have contributed much to the elucidation of the heterogeneity, genetics, antibody diversity, and configurational arrangement of the five

Fig. 2-3 : The five known classes and subclasses of immunoglobulins.

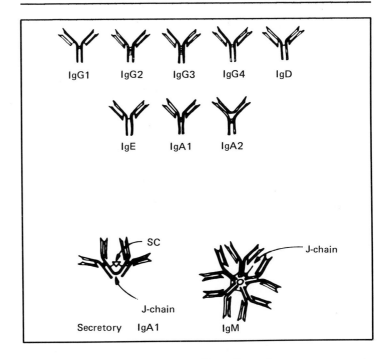

IgG1   IgG2   IgG3   IgG4   IgD

IgE   IgA1   IgA2

— SC

J-chain

J-chain

Secretory   IgA1   IgM

major classes of immunoglobulins. To reiterate, monomeric immunoglobulins are composed of four polypeptide chains (two H-chains and two L-chains), which loop and twist to form the three-dimensional configuration. The configuration of each Ig is of extreme importance for its ultimate biological function. The three-dimensional structure is maintained by two major physical bonding forces: (1) noncovalent bonds (non-electron-sharing); and (2) disulfide bonds formed by two neighboring cysteine (half-cystine) residues. The interchain disulfide bridge connecting the light and heavy chains in the molecules of subclass IgG is closer to the bridges between the two heavy chains than it is in the other immunoglobulins. This is reflected in schematic diagrams by drawing the L-H bond as a line *perpendicular* to both chains in IgG1, but *angled* to both chains in the other immuno-globulins, as shown in Figure 2–3 for IgG1 and IgG2.

IgA2 has no disulfide linkages between the L- and H-chains, and the orientation of the L-chains relative to the H-chains is opposite to that normally seen (see Figure 2–3). In this instance, the H-L bridges are attributable to hydrogen bonding, salt linkages, and van der Waals forces. Individually these are weak bonds, but collectively they constitute strong bonding forces.

The light chain consists of about 214 amino acids. The NH_2-terminal region, about 107 to 115 amino acids long, is called the L-chain *variable (V_L) region.* The remaining (carboxyl)

Fig. 2-4 : Structure
of IgG, showing the
domains and
homology units.
CHO represents car-
bohydrate attached
to the heavy chain
constant regions.

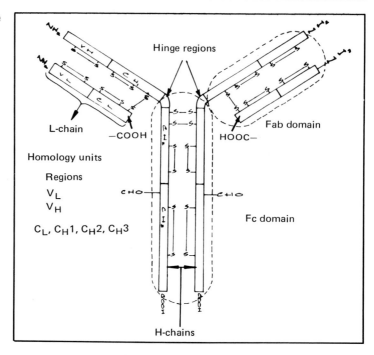

Fig. 2-4 : Structure of IgG, showing the domains and homology units. CHO represents carbohydrate attached to the heavy chain constant regions.

portion of the L-chain has about 107 to 111 amino acids and is termed the L-chain *constant (C_L) region.* The heavy (H) chain has about 450 amino acid residues. As in the L-chain, the 107 to 115 NH_2-terminal residues compose the variable H-chain (V_H) region, while the remaining (310 to 330) COOH-terminal residues make up the H-chain constant (C_H) region. The C_H region can be further subdivided, on the basis of sequence homologies, into the C_H1, C_H2, and C_H3 sequences, as shown in Figure 2-4. The constant regions of the heavy chain (C_H1, C_H2, and C_H3) are those portions whose amino acid sequence is relatively unchanging from one member of a particular class (γ, μ, etc.) of heavy chain to another member of the same class. Likewise, the C_L regions of all κ-chains are closely similar, as are those of the λ-chains. The *variable* regions (V_L and V_H) have sequences that depend on the immunological specificity of the immunoglobulin. As might be expected, the antigen-binding site is located in the variable sequences. IgG and IgA consist of four domains, one variable (V) and three constant. The L-chain consists of a V (V_L) and a C (C_L) domain while the H-chain is made of one V (V_H) and three C (C_H1, C_H2, C_H3) domains. IgM and IgE, on the other hand, consist of five domains; one V (V_L, V_H) and four C (C_L, C_H1, C_H2, C_H3, C_H4) regions.

In part, the amino acid sequence regulates the three-dimensional configuration of the immunoglobulins. In some cases the substitution of a single amino acid at a key position may have a significant effect on the immunogenicity of the molecule without affecting the biological function. A classic example is the observation that the immunogenicity of pig and human insulin is not precisely the same. This difference is accounted for by residue 30 of the β-chain, which is alanine in the human hormone and threonine in the porcine material. Part of this antigenic variance may be attributable to the three-dimensional configuration differences between pig and human insulin, which would be difficult to assess. Another familiar case in which the difference of a single amino acid profoundly affects the biological function of a molecule is the substitution of valine for glutamate in the 6 position of the β-chain of hemoglobin. This substitution is the only difference in amino acid sequence between normal hemoglobin A and hemoglobin S (sickle cell trait). In this respect, immunoglobulins are similar in behavior to insulin, since amino acid substitution creates antigenic differences without altering biological function.

Physicochemical and Biological Properties of the Immunoglobulins

Some of the major physicochemical and biological properties of the five major classes and several subclasses of immunoglobulins are compiled in Tables 2–3 and 2–4.

Immunoglobulin G (IgG)

IgG comprises 80 to 85 percent of the circulating immunoglobulins in the blood. Prior to the standardization of nomenclature of immunoglobulins in 1964 by WHO, these globulins were designated by a variety of names, such as γ, $7s\gamma$, $\gamma\gamma$, 6.6γ, and γss. These designations were derived from electrophoretic mobilities and ultracentrifugal studies. Approximate molecular weights, sedimentation, extinction and diffusion coefficients, isoelectric points, and partial specific volume were obtained for IgG without reference to subclass distinction. This may account for the range found in different studies, especially in the sedimentation coefficient and isoelectric points. Subclasses IgG1, IgG2, and IgG3 have similar mobilities in agar immunoelectrophoresis, migrating with the globulins, while IgG4 appears to have a slightly faster mobility (moving with the IgG1 fraction). This may, in part, have caused the variation in the isoelectric points. The valence or binding capacity (number of binding sites per molecule) for IgG is 2, although in some instances a valence of 1 has been reported. This may be attributable to a weaker binding capacity rather than a true valence of 1, since this so-called univalent antibody has been shown to have all four polypeptide chains (two H- and two L-chains). Molecules in all four of the IgG subclasses contain γ H-chains and either κ or λ L-chains. The total carbohydrate content of IgG molecules is approximately one-fourth that of the other immunoglobulin classes.

Table 2-3 : Physicochemical Properties and Other Biochemical Characteristics of the Immunoglobulins of Man

Immunoglobulin Class	IgG				IgA		IgM		IgD	IgE
Immunoglobulin Subclasses	γ_1	γ_2	γ_3	γ_4	α_1	α_2	μ_1	μ_2	—	—
1. Synonyms	γ, 7Sγ, 6.6γ, γ_2, γSS				β_2A, γ_1A		γ_1M, β_2M, 19Sγ, γ-macroglobulin		None	None
2. Approximate MW*	149,000–153,000				150,000–600,000		900,000		180,000	188,000–209,000
3. Approximate S$_{20,w}$*	616-7.2				7, 9, 11, 13		18-32		7	7-8.2
4. Diffusion coefficient (1 X 10^{-7} cm^2/sec)	4.0				3.0-3.6		1.71-1.75		—	3.71
5. Extinction coefficient (E$^{1\%}_{280nm}$)	13.8				13.4-13.9		13.3		—	15.3
6. Partial specific volume ($\bar{V}_{20}$, cm^3/gm)	0.739				0.729-0.723		0.723		—	0.713
7. Isoelectric point (in pH units)	5.8-7.3				—		5.1-7.8		—	—
8. Valence (Ag-binding sites)	2				2		5		2	2
9. Total carbohydrate content (wt. %)	3.0				12.0		12.0		13.0	12.0
10. Mean survival in serum (T/2 in days)	11-12	11-12	6-7	20-21	5-6	4.5	5		2.8	1.5
11. Mean concentration in serum: (mg/dl) (range in parentheses)	Total for IgG: 1240 (900–2000); 820, 286, 90, 50				280 (200-350)		120 (75-150)		3.0 (<0.3-40)	0.03 (0.007-0.18)

	γ (50,000)	α (65,000)	μ (65,000–70,000)	δ	ε (72,500)
12. Heavy chain class (MW)	γ (50,000)	α (65,000)	μ (65,000–70,000)	δ	ε (72,500)
13. Light chain	κ or λ	κ or λ	κ or λ	κ or λ	κ or λ
14. κ to λ ratio (range)	1.42 to 2.41 / 0.96 to 1.10 / 1.25 to 1.12 / 7 to 5	1 / 2	1 / 1–4	1/20	—
15. Number of interchain disulfide-bonds	4 6 6 4	5? 5?	15	3	3?
16. Allotypes H-chain Gm	+ — ++ ++	— — ++ ++	—	—	—
Am₂	+ — ++ ++	— — ++ ++	—	—	—
L-chain InV	+ — ++ ++	— +++ +++ +++	— ++ ++	— ++ ++	— ++ ++
Oz	0 — ++ ++	5? +++ +++			3?
17. Electrophoretic mobility in agar	γ₂ γ₂ γ₂ γ₁	γ₁–β	γ₂–β₂	γ–β	γ₁
18. Intrinsic viscosity	0.06	— ++	0.162	—	—
J-chain	— — —	+	+	—	—
Secretory piece	— — —	+ (secretory) IgM			

*MW = molecular weight; $S_{20}w$ = sedimentation coefficient corrected to water at 20°C; blank spaces = data unknown. In some cases, data are given for each *subclass*; in others, *average* values for the *class* are indicated.

Table 2-4 : The Biological Properties of Human Immunoglobulins

Immunoglobulin Class Immunoglobulin Subclasses	IgG				IgA		IgM	IgD	IgE
	IgG₁	IgG₂	IgG₃	IgG₄	IgA₁	IgA₂	IgM	IgD	IgE
1. mg/ml (serum)	5-12	2-6	0.5-1	0.2-1	0.5-2	0-0.2	0.5-2	0-0.4	0-0.002
2. Specific antibodies									
a. anti-RH	+				+		+		+
b. anti-dextran		+							
c. anti-levan		+							
d. anti-Factor VIII				+					
3. In secretions	0	0	0	0	+++	+++	++	0	+
4. Complement fixation									
Classical pathway	+	±ʷ	+	0	0		+	0	0
Alternate pathway	0	0	0	+	+	+	0	+	+
5. Passive cutaneous anaphylaxis (PCA)	+	0	+	+	0		0	0	0
6. Placental transfer (Pt)	+	+	+	+	0		0	0	0
7. Reacts with rheumatoid factor (antigen)	+++	+++	0	+++	+		+		+
8. Rheumatoid factor (antibody)	+	+	+	+	+	+	+	0	0
9. Reacts with *Staphylococcus* protein A	+	+	0	+					0
10. Fc receptor on									
(Macrophage)	+	0	+	+	0		0	0	0
Basophils	0	0	0	0	0		0	0	++
Neutrophils	+++	0+	+++	0+	0		0	0	0
Platelets	+	+	+	±	0	0	0	0	0
Lymphocytes	±	±	±		0		0	0	0
11. Prausnitz-Küstner (P-K) reaction	0	0	0	0	0		0	0	++ (0-1.0 ng (AbN/ml))
12. Isohemagglutinin	(positive, (+) in hyper-immunized individuals)				+		+	0	0
13. Synthesis: mg/kg/day	25	3.4			24	21.3	7	0.4	0.02
14. Cryoglobulins		+			+ (rare)		+		
15. Reverse P. C. K.	+	0	+	+	0	0	0	0	0

+ = reacts (antibody present); 0 = does not react; w = weakly; AbN = antibody nitrogen; ± = possible reaction. Blanks indicate data not known.

κ/λ ratios in the subclasses increase in the order IgG2 < IgG3 < IgG1 < IgG4, while serum concentrations of the subclasses decrease in the order IgG1 > IgG2 > IgG3 > IgG4. The mean total serum concentration of IgG is 1240 mg/dl, with a normal range of 900 to 2,000 mg/dl. The mean half-life of the IgG subclasses varies from a low of 6 to 7 days for IgG3 to a high of 20 to 21 days for IgG4. IgG1 and IgG2 have a half-live of 11 to 12 days. A mean of 23 days has been indicated for total IgG. IgG1 and IgG4 have four inter-chain disulfide bridges, two between L- and H-chains and two between the two H-chains. IgG2 and IgG3 have six interchain disulfide covalent bonds with four bonds between the two H-chains rather than the two demonstrated for IgG1 and IgG4.

Human immunoglobulins are excellent antigens or immunogens (see Chapter 4) and antisera to them can be raised in a variety of animals (monkey, horse, sheep, donkey, goat, and rabbit). By using these antisera, specific antigenic sites on the immunoglobulins can be correlated with structural features and with specific amino acids in the polypeptide chain. The antigens are conveniently cat-egorized into three major groups: (1) *isotypic* antigens, which are present in all normal sera and can be differentiated into the five major classes and their subgroups (types); (2) *allotypic* antigens, which are present in some (but not all) normal sera and are governed by allelic genes; and (3) *idiotypic* antigens, which are unique to one particular antibody molecule, and hence, by inference, are related to the V region or antigen-binding site. The isotypic and allotypic antigens are related to the C region of the H-chains.

The class-specific antigens of the C region represent one group of isotypes. Cross-reactions between the major immunoglobulin classes have not been demonstrated, although regions of homology based on sequence studies have been shown. Within subclasses, however, many shared antigens have been found through precipitation and hemagglutination inhibition tests. Antibodies to some subclass antigens are difficult to raise in animals. The allotypic antigens for the H-chains are referred to as Gm (gamma markers). The Gm markers are restricted to the C_H region of the H-chains of IgG and IgA (see IgA section). Gm (1), (22), (4), and (17) are restricted to IgG1; Gm(24) is specific for IgG2; and Gm(3), (5), (6), (13), (14), (15), (16), and (21) are specific for IgG3. No regular Gm for IgG4 has been demonstrated as yet. IgG4 has a nonmarker, Gm-variant antigen designated (4a) and (4b) on the C_H3 homology region. Other Gm antigens are shared between the subclasses. There are at present a total of 27 Gm antigens. The allotypic marker InV is found on the κ-chain. Valine at residue position 191 on the κ-chain represents a positive test for InV (b^+), whereas substitution at this position with leucine results in InV (a^+). Amino acid substitution at position 190 in the λ-chain controls the presence or absence of the isotype Oz.

The biological activities attributed to the IgG subclasses are shown in Table 2-4. The major subclass associated with specific antibodies is IgG1. Specific antibodies to dextran, levan, Rh, and Factor VIII reside in the different subclasses of IgG. IgG4 does not fix complement, while IgG2 does so, weakly in the classic pathway, but not the alternate pathway. Passive cutaneous anaphylaxis (PCA) in guinea pigs is negative for IgG2. IgG3 does not react with rheumatoid factor and staphylococcal protein A. No reaction with macrophage receptor has been shown for IgG2 and IgG4. Isohemagglutinin related to IgG antibody is found following hyperimmunization with ABO antigens. IgG antibodies are generally related to the later-occurring antibodies following antigenic stimulation. IgG antibodies do not participate in the P-K (Prausnitz-Küstner) reaction. Cryoglobulins and rheumatoid factor (antibody) in some diseases may be associated with IgG. With the exception of IgG3, all IgG's can act as the antigen for rheumatoid factor (antibody).

Immunoglobulin A
(IgA)

IgA has two subclasses, IgA1 and IgA2. There are two major differences between these subclasses: (1) the allotype Am_2 is present in the C region of the H-chain of IgA2 (Am_2^+) and is absent in IgA1 (Am_2^-), and (2) the L-chains in IgA2 are not linked to the H-chains by disulfide bonds. In addition, as was indicated earlier, the orientation of the L-chains in IgA2 is opposite to that of the L-chains in the other immunoglobulins (Figure 2-4). The significant physicochemical and biological properties of IgA are listed in Tables 2-3 and 2-4. Some of these properties belong to secretory IgA, which is a dimer of IgA1 held together by a secretory piece or component (SP or SC) and a polypeptide J (juncture)-chain. Properties of both SC and J-chain are shown in Table 2-5.

Note that this polymeric IgA contains subunits in addition to H- and L-chains. The secretory piece and J-chain have also been noted in IgM. Skeletal diagrams of each of the major classes and subclasses of immunoglobulins with interchain disulfide (S–S) linkages are shown in Figure 2-3. The location of the J-chain and SC in IgM and secretory IgA1 is still speculative, although it is postulated to be, as shown, somewhere near the carboxyl termini of the heavy chains. The secretory component is antigenic and is present in its free form in bodily secretions. In IgA1, IgA2, and IgE the numbers of disulfide bonds connecting the two heavy chains are not known for certain.

It appears that there are no chemical differences between the forms of IgG, IgD, and IgE that circulate in peripheral blood and those that are found in the secretions of mucous membrane cells. However, a portion of IgM and almost all of IgA have a

Table 2-5 : Properties of Secretory Component and J-Chain

Properties	SC	J-Chain
Molecular weight	70,000	15,000
Carbohydrate	9.5-15.0%	8.0%
Sedimentation coefficient, S_{20w}	4.20	1.28
Partial specific volume (cm^3/gm)	0.726	—
$E^{1\%}_{280}$	12.7	6.3-7.0
Electrophoresis (relative mobility)	β-globulin	Fast-moving component in gel
Associated with H-chains	α and μ	α and μ

Fig. 2-5 : The formation and secretion of the secretory immunoglobulin A dimer, containing a secretory component and a J-chain. IgA, (IgA)$_2$, and (IgA)$_2$ + SC have sedimentation coefficients of 7S, 10S, and 11S, respectively.

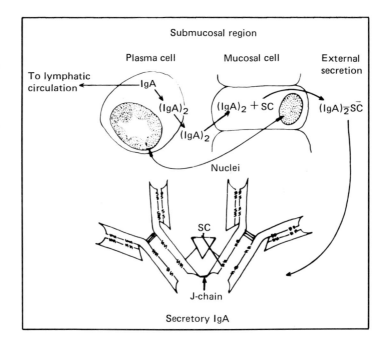

secretory component (SC) attached to them when they occur in external secretions.

A question arises as to the need for the SC that is synthesized and attached to IgA dimers in the mucosal cells (see Figure 2-5). It has been suggested that SC may facilitate transport of the dimer through the mucosal cell by protecting the molecule from intracellular degradative processes (e.g., proteolysis). It may also participate in the functioning of IgA as an antibody in an external environment. A similar mechanism for synthesis of secretory IgM containing SC seems likely.

The primary function of IgA has not been elucidated. Recent studies in orally vaccinated or spontaneously infected human subjects appear to confirm the protective value of exocrine IgA antibodies. Previous reports on the absence of complement fixation by IgA antibodies may have to be revised, since it has been observed that colostral-type IgA to *Escherichia coli* was able to lyse this bacterium in the combined presence of lysozyme and complement (see Adinolfi, et al, 1966). The tendency of IgA to polymerize probably accounts for the various sedimentation coefficients and molecular weights observed. It is likely that this tendency also contributes to the activation of complement via the alternative complement activation route. This will be discussed later (see Chapter 9).

It has also been reported that porcine milk IgA enhances the ability of phagocytes to destroy certain types of encapsulated bacteria, such as *Pneumococcus*. This is known as *opsonization,* and substances, such as IgA, that have this ability are known as *opsonins.* It has also been suggested that one of the major functions of IgA is to react with various antigens to form unabsorbable antibody-antigen complexes. This would prevent entrance of these deleterious materials via the gut and other endothelial surfaces, such as the respiratory tract. This tendency is compatible with the high circulating antibody titers to food antigens found in individual with IgA deficiency. IgA deficiency also can be correlated with a high incidence of autoimmune disease. Nonetheless, complete absence of IgA is not incompatible with good health, since in many instances of secretory IgA deficiency, IgM appears to assume IgA functions. IgA is negative for passive cutaneous anaphylaxis (PCA), placental transfer, and P-K reaction, and several naturally occurring serum isohemagglutinins are IgA molecules. Some IgA cryoglobulins are found, but rarely, in certain diseases.

Other possible functions of secretory immunoglobulins (in particular IgA) follow: (1) prevention of viral and bacterial infections that may have access to the external secretions, as for example, in the lungs, mouth, intestines, and ear canals, and (2) participation as opsonins in the phagocytic process (involving principally monocytes in the submucosal region) when the infective agent has penetrated the mucosal barriers. In diseases produced by respiratory viruses, such as influenza, local immunization appears to augment the effectiveness of immunization by parenteral routes. In fact, in those viral infections affecting primarily the mucosal regions, local immunization may be the preferred method. The local immunization obtained, for example, by administration of a vaccine via the alimentary route may have an additional advantage in control of viruses that produce systematic infections. This advantage is the elimination of the carrier state. For example, a person immunized against poliomyelitis by the Salk method (systemic introduction of killed viral antigens) may develop neutralizing antibodies systemically but not in the secretory IgA. Such individuals may be immune to the disease but may become carriers by harboring the virus in their intestinal tract. On the other hand, the Sabin method of immunization (attenuated live virus by oral route) produces not only systemic antibodies but also secretory antibodies. The latter may prevent local infection by neutralizing the virus particles.

Within the intestinal tract the committed B cells associated with synthesis of dimeric IgA are situated in the lamina propria. The dimeric IgA (J-chain-attached) molecules enter the epithelial cells where the secretory components are attached and the dimeric secretory IgA elaborated into the mucous layer of the epithelial cells in touch with the lumen of the intestinal tract (see Figure 2-5 for SC attachment).

Immunoglobulin M (IgM)

The largest immunoglobulins are those of the IgM class, with molecular weights of 900,000 or greater. The existence of subclasses of different allotypes has been suggested. The significant physicochemical properties of IgM are indicated in Table 2-3. The valence number is of particular interest. Although 10 would be anticipated from structural analysis, only 5 binding sites have been shown in reactions with antigens. This may in part be due to steric interferences at binding sites and thus may not represent the true potential valence. Like IgA and IgE, the total carbohydrate content of the molecule is four times that of IgG. Because of its size, its intrinsic viscosity and diffusion coefficients are strikingly different from those of other immunoglobulins.

The significant biological characteristics of IgM are shown in Table 2-4. IgM fixes complement (C1q in the $C_\mu 4$ region), and it is probably the major isohemagglutinin (anti-A or anti-B). One of the cardinal features of IgM is its early appearance following antigenic stimulation. It possesses strong agglutination or precipitation properties, perhaps due to its pentavalency. It can react with other Ig as a rheumatoid factor, and it is considered to be one of the factors itself. Rheumatoid factors in both antigenic and antibody roles have also been associated with IgG and IgA. It has been suggested that IgM is one of the more primitive of the immunoglobulins, since it is synthesized early in neonatal life and even in some species by the fetus in utero. IgM does not traverse the placental barrier under normal conditions. A J-chain is also a part of the IgM molecule, probably bound to some region at or near the carboxyl termini of the H-chains. IgM also participates as a secretory immunoglobulin containing a secretory piece. It is one of the major immunoglobulins on the surface of B cells, especially in the newborn.

Immunoglobulin D (IgD)

Information on IgD is limited, and no significant biological function has been attributed to these molecules. Of interest is its low level in serum (only IgE is lower) and its high λ/κ ratio. It is not a secretory Ig like IgA or IgE and its P-K response is negative. The study of surface IgD as receptors on B cells has been of interest in the immune response. It is one of the major immunoglobulins on the surface of B cells (10 to 14 percent), especially in the newborn. In general the biological activity of IgD appears to be limited. The alternative pathway of C activation seems to be initiated by IgD. The available physicochemical and biological data for IgD are shown in Tables 2-3 and 2-4.

Immunoglobulin E (IgE)

The physicochemical and biological properties of IgE are summarized in Tables 2-3 and 2-4. It is the least concentrated and has the shortest survival time in serum of any of the immunoglobulins. The affinity of IgE for mast cells and its relationship to immediate hypersensitivity and to the homocytotropic antibodies of other animals are among the most studied aspects of this immunoglobulin. IgE has been equated with the reaginic antibody of man associated with the release of histamine, SRS-A (slow-reacting substance of anaphylaxis), eosinophil chemotactic factor (ECF), and platelet-activating factor (PAF) following interaction with specific antigens. The term *reagin* is used in man to refer to cytotropic antibodies. These antibodies are bound to target cells (e.g., mast cells)in individuals sensitized to an antigen. When the antigen presents itself again, the cytotropic antibodies bind it, thereby triggering the release of vasoactive amines from the target cells (mast cells). IgE does not bind complement in the classic pathway but activates C via the alternative pathway. IgE can passively sensitize monkey and human skin (P-K reaction) and leukocytes, but gives no PCA response in the guinea pig. Addition of specific antigen to IgE-sensitized leukocytes induces release of histamine and SRS-A. This has been utilized as a means of detecting allergies (type I) in man: the antigen is added, and the subsequent morphological changes in the leukocytes are studied or the histamine release is measured. Similar changes, with release of histamine and SRS-A, occur with monkey lung tissues. The Fc region of the IgE molecule contains the site for binding to basophilic leukocyte and mast cells.

Although much is known of the role of IgE in allergic manifestation of the atopic variety, there is little knowledge of its real

Table 2-6 : Five Possible Covalent Pathway Assemblies of the Four Chains of Immunoglobulin Biosynthesis

1. $H + L \rightarrow HL + HL \leftarrow H + L$

   $\downarrow$

   H_2L_2

2. $H + L \rightarrow HL + H \rightarrow H_2L + L = H_2L_2$

3. $H + L \rightarrow HL + L \rightarrow HL_2 + H = H_2L_2$

4. $H + H \rightarrow H_2 + L \rightarrow H_2L + L = H_2L_2$

5. $L + L \rightarrow L_2 + H \rightarrow HL_2 + H = H_2L_2$

function in normal metabolic processes. IgE is considered a secretory immunoglobulin with a distribution similar to that of IgA in areas such as the respiratory and gastrointestinal tract mucosal tissues. However, IgE does not have secretory component or a J-chain. IgE as an important antihelminth antibody has been recently demonstrated against some parasites. IgE in hypersensitivity states will be discussed in Chapter 13.

Diversity of Antibodies

Multivalent antigens, such as bacteria, have many antigenic determinants. Since each determinant can, theoretically, induce the synthesis of a different immunoglobulin molecule, the response of the humoral system to even the simplest antigen can be quite heterogeneous. When a B cell transforms to a plasma cell, each member of the clone that develops from that cell is capable of producing only one molecular species of immunoglobulin. Thus the number of different Ig molecules reflects the number of B lymphocyte clones that synthesized them.

The biochemistry of antibody protein synthesis, transcription, and translation using DNA, mRNA, tRNA, polyribosomes, and the appropriate enzymes is carried out by the B and plasma cells. Like albumin and hemoglobin, immunoglobulins have a constant rate of degradation and de novo synthesis. This rate depends on the nature of the immunoglobulins. Specific immunoglobulin (antibody) synthesis occurs when the appropriate clone is stimulated by a specific antigenic determinant, as was indicated earlier. Although much is known of the fundamentals of protein synthesis and of immunoglobulin structure, the manner in which H-chains and L-chains are put together to form the tetrapeptide has not been completely elucidated. The five suggested pathway sequences of the four-chain polypeptide biosynthesis of immunoglobulins are shown in Table 2-6. Of interest also is the manner in which a single B cell switches from IgM to IgG synthesis (See

Chapter 5). Some mechanism of feedback inhibition by IgG has been suggested, but information in these areas is limited.

The basic structure of human immunoglobulin is given in Figure 2-4. The important features of this molecule are as follows: (1) Two identical L-chains (about 22,500 daltons each) and two identical H-chains (approximately 53,000 to 70,000 daltons each) are present, linked by disulfide bonds and noncovalent interactions; (2) the molecule is folded into three regions (two Fab and one Fc), which are separated by the H-chain region; (3) the polypeptide chains of both H and L can be divided into an NH_2-terminal (variable) region and a COOH-terminal (constant) region. The V and C regions are defined by amino acid sequence homology; for example, in the C region of the predominant L-chain, only one amino acid substitution occurs, and it behaves as a single mendelian allele. In the V region of the same L-chain, as many as 15 to 40 amino acid substitutions can occur. The V regions of H- and L-chains from the same immunoglobulin show striking sequence homologies with one another. Such homologies would also be anticipated between the V region of the H- and L-chains of antibodies from different species following stimulation of both species by the same antigenic determinant (i.e., the binding site sequence is relatively independent of species when the immunoglobulins are formed against the same antigen). Sequence homologies are also found in the C regions of H- and L-chains.

Present evidence strongly supports the concept of a single immunoglobulin polypeptide chain encoded by two germline (heritable) genes, a V-gene and a C-gene, which are joined somatically. On the basis of amino acid sequence homology and genetic linkage studies, three major families of immunoglobulin in polypeptides could be envisioned: the families of the H-chain and the two L-chains (κ and λ). The constant regions of some of these families can be further divided into classes and subclasses. Classes and subclasses of C_H chains are $C_{\gamma 1}$, $C_{\gamma 2}$, $C_{\gamma 3}$, $C_{\gamma 4}$, $C_{\alpha 1}$, $C_{\alpha 2}$, $C_{\mu 1}$, $C_{\mu 2}$, C_δ, and C_ϵ. Classes and subclasses of C_L chains are C_{arg}, C_{lys} for γ and C_K for κ. Each of these is encoded by a germline gene. V regions are also divided into subgroups controlled by separate genes, but these regions are of a more complex nature.

The structural features of the immunoglobulins are intimately associated with their biological features. Thus, antibody diversity is encoded in the V regions, while the general functions of antibody molecules (placental transfer, complement and macrophage binding) are mediated by the various C regions of the H-chain (Fc portion).

Theories of Antibody Diversity

Numerous theories have been advanced to explain antibody production. With the tremendous advances over the past decade in the knowledge of antibody molecules, immunologists now generally accept a modified version of Burnet's clonal selection theory. This theory postulates that clones of potential immunologically competent cells, each containing the genetic codes (C-gene and V-gene, one of each for H- and L-chains) of the immunoglobulin complementary to one antigenic determinant, are present from birth. A sufficient number of different clones would provide an immune potential against all existing antigens that an individual might encounter. The immunogen thus selects or affects its specific complementary clone, which is provided with the appropriate, specific, receptor site, and stimulates it to proliferate and synthesize the corresponding specific antibody. This concept stresses the role of the immune cells. Since antibody diversity reflects a corresponding immune cell gene diversity, there is the question of how this gene diversity arose in the immune cell population in the first place. Three generally acceptable theories have been formulated: (1) The *somatic mutation theory* postulates that antibody diversity results from hypermutation during somatic differentiation of the immune cells; (2) the *germline theory* proposes that antibody diversity is encoded by a large number of germline genes (i.e., multiple genes encode the V regions, while a separate gene encodes the C region in a given immune cell); and (3) the *somatic recombination theory* suggests that somatic recombinations occur in a limited number of antibody genes.

Of these three hypotheses, the germline and somatic mutation theories have greatest support from amino acid sequence analysis of the immunoglobulins for various species.

Biosynthetic Pathway of Immunoglobulin Synthesis

The major assembly point of immunoglobulins is within the cisternae of endoplasmic reticulum following the synthesis of the H- and L-chains by the ribosomes. The factors that can affect the assembly are (1) the concentration of the H- and L-chains, (2) the complementary fit between the H- and L-chains, (3) the rate of disulfide formation, which is dependent on the proximity of the chains and the presence of the disulfide enzymes, and (4) the relative number of chains.

The disulfide linkage between H- and L-chains appears to occur more readily than linkage between two H-chains. Table 2–6 lists five possible sequential pathways of assemblage of the four-chain polypeptide immunoglobulin in the cisternae of the endoplasmic reticulum. The first three equations are probably the more common pathways. However, all these biosynthetic pathways have been shown, some of them demonstrated in multiple myeloma cells.

The complete assemblage of the final immunoglobulin is achieved following attachment of the carbohydrate residue in the Golgi complex. The attachment of the oligosaccharide residue generally occurs by means of an N-glycosidic linkage between the N-acetylglucosamine residue and an asparagine residue of the C region of the heavy chain (usually the C_H3 region). Other linkages have been observed. For example, an O-glycosidic linkage between the carbohydrate side chain and the serine residue of the heavy chain has been reported. The carbohydrate residues of immunoglobulin have been found linked primarily to C heavy chain regions, the secretory piece, and the J-chain. However, in multiple myeloma (lymphoproliferative disorder—malignancy of the bone marrow) carbohydrate residues have been found in the V_L or V_H regions, but in small amounts. The functions of the carbohydrate residues in immunoglobulins have not been delineated. It has been suggested that these residues serve as umbilical cords for attachment to the membrane surface of the vesicle carriers and help to resist proteolytic digestion in the region of the Fc fragment. That they alter the physico-chemical properties such as electrophoretic mobility, solubility, and configurational changes of the immunoglobulin have been established.

The complete immunoglobulin following the attachment of the oligosaccharide is transported from the Golgi complex via a secretory vesicle to the membrane (attachment to B cell membrane) or is secreted through the plasma cell wall (plasma cells). This sequence of biosynthesis of immunoglobulin and release is shown in Figure 2-6.

Evolution of the Immunoglobulins

The ability to mount immunological responses of a humoral nature has been examined in many animals. The presence of agglutinins has been shown in body fluids of the invertebrates, such as the coelomic fluid of earthworms, the serum of the horseshoe crab (*Limulus polyphemus*) and coconut crab (*Birgus latro*), the hemolymphs of snails (*Biomphalaria glabrata*), and of the American oyster (*Crassotrea virginica*); and proteins isolated from the coelomocytes of the sea star (*Asterias forbesi*); and several insect species. These agglutinins are primarily directed toward mammalian erythrocytes. Like plant lectins their body fluids tend to have anti-A and anti-B activity. (A and B refer to the hemagglutinogen or antigens of the human erythrocytes, as explained in Chapter 11). The agglutinins responsible for this reaction with erythrocytes do not resemble mammalian immunoglobulins in their physical and chemical properties. Lower vertebrates have been shown to mount molecules with specificity and inducibility comparable to that of mammalian immunoglobulins.

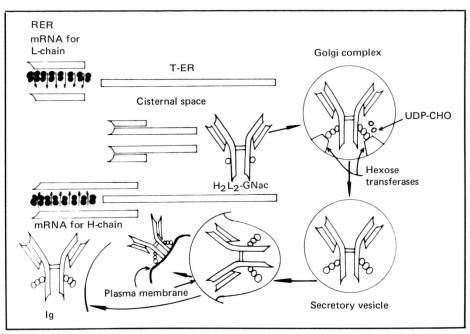

Fig. 2-6 : Sequential representation of the formation of immunoglobulins following syntheses of L- and H-chains in the rough or granular endoplasmic reticulum (RER) by ribosomes (<u>dark circles</u>). Formation of the four-chain polypeptide (H_2L_2-GNac) occurs in the transitional endoplasmic reticulum (T-ER), and the subsequent attachment of the polysaccharide residue takes place in the Golgi complex. Immunoglobulin either remains on the plasma membrane surface or is secreted, essentially by plasma cells.

Table 2-7 summarizes the hypothetical evolutionary development of the immunoglobulin genes that are expressed in present-day vertebrates. It is postulated that, sometime after the paleozoic period and prior to the appearance of the vertebrates, the primordial gene of 110 residues, through detached duplication, formed the ancestral genes specifying the C and V regions. The ancestral genes for C_L, C_H, V_L, and V_H arose sometime during the period of the emergence of the lower vertebrates. The lower vertebrates such as the lamprey and dipnoi (lung fish) have both two L-chains and two H-chains and the characteristic four-chain polypeptide structure. Both the 6.6S and 14S molecules have been shown for the lamprey. The molecular weight of the L-chain is about 25,000 daltons, and of the H-chain, about 70,000 daltons. The H-chain appears to be similar to that of the human μ-chain. Other immunoglobulins containing four polypeptide chains, but unlike mammalian chains, have also been demonstrated.

C_κ and C_λ and V_H, V_κ, and V_λ appeared subsequently, during the period of emergence of the amphibians. Amphibian immuno-

Table 2-7 : Evolution of Genes from Primordial Ancestor of 110 Residue Coding for Immunoglobulin Polypeptide Chains and β_2-M-G.

Paleozoic Era	Primordial gene (110 residues) $>500 \times 10^6$	Ancestral Genes — Emergence of Vertebrates (400×10^6 years)	Emergence of Amphibians (200×10^6 years) Genes	Mammals Genes	C region Genes
C region {		C_L	C_κ	C_κ	(each = one gene)
			C_λ	$C_\lambda 03^+$, $C_\lambda 02 - C_\lambda vern^+$, $C_\lambda vern^-$, $C_\lambda mcg^+$, $C_\lambda mcg^-$	
		C_H (μ-like)		$\gamma_1, \gamma_2, \gamma_3, \gamma_4, \delta_1, \delta_2, \mu_1, \mu_2, \epsilon, \alpha$	
		$G_2M\text{-}G$		β_2-Microglobulin and HL antigen C_H homology	(See Chapter 13)
V region {		V_H region	V_H	$V_{H}1, V_{H}2, V_{H}3, V_{H}4$	V region
			V_κ	$V_\kappa 1, V_\kappa 2, V_\kappa 3, V_\kappa 4$	
		V_L region	V_λ	$V_\lambda 1, V_\lambda 2, V_\lambda 3, V_\lambda 4, V_\lambda 5, V_\lambda 6$	Genes (no. unknown)

globulins have been shown to be comparable to those of mammals. The symbols (C_L and C_H) in the C region given for both L- and H-chains of mammals represent a single known gene and have all been reported. The number of variable H- and L-chain regions is unknown. Those shown in Table 2–7 have been characterized. The β_2-microglobulin has been shown to have homology with the C_H3 of IgG. Further discussion of this protein will be presented in Chapter 12. Detached duplication and point mutation of genes have been suggested as fundamental processes leading to diversification of the polypeptide chains at each stage in evolutionary development.

Functions of Immunoglobulins

The major functions of immunoglobulins were presented in Table 1–5 of Chapter 1. In addition, the specific known biological activities of each of the immunoglobulins are summarized in Table 2–4. The significant feature is that, as part of the humoral-mediated immune system, immunoglobulins react with their specific immunogens via the NH_2 terminal amino acid variable region of the H- and L-chains (the Fab portion), while the COOH terminal of the constant region (the Fc portion of the H-chains) is associated with their biological functions.

Summary

1. The immunoglobulins comprise the humoral-mediated system.
2. Five major classes of immunoglobulins have been recognized (IgG, IgA, IgM, IgD, and IgE). There are four subclasses in IgG (IgG1, IgG2, IgG3, and IgG4). The basis for the classification is the antigenic properties of the heavy chains and the amino acid sequence of each of these chains.
3. The heavy chains are designated γ, μ, α, δ, and ϵ, for G, M, A, D, and E, respectively.
4. Immunoglobulins as antigens are categorized as: (1) *isotypes,* present in all normal sera, which can be differentiated into the five major classes and their subgroups; (2) *allotypes,* present in some, but not all, normal sera and governed by allelic genes; and (3) *idiotypes,* unique to one particular antibody molecule and related to the V region or antibody combining site.
5. The light chains are designated κ and λ.
6. Both the H- and the L-chains have a variable (NH_2-terminal) and a constant (COOH-terminal) region.
7. The antigen-binding site of the antibody is called the Fab region and consists of the variable region of the H- and L-chains. The biologically active region is the Fc portion and consists of the constant region of the H-chain.
8. The variable regions contribute to the antibody diversity and are controlled by the Ir (Immune response) genes (Chapter 10).

9. A complete molecule of the IgG, IgA, IgD, and IgE classes consists of two H- and two L-chains and is controlled by four genes. That is, for each H- or L-chain, two genes are involved; two genes for a single polypeptide, one for the C region and one for the V region of H- or L-chain.

10. Diversity of antibodies has been explained by two major theories, the *germline* and *somatic mutation* theories. The germline theory proposes that antibody diversity is encoded by a large number of germline genes and immune cells, while the somatic mutation theory postulates that diversity results from hypermutations during somatic differentiation of the immune cell. Neither theory has completely explained antibody diversity, however.

11. The major assembly area of the polypeptide chains of immunoglobulins is the endoplasmic reticulum of the immune cell. Attachment of the carbohydrate residue takes place in the Golgi complex. The immunoglobulin remains on the surface of a B cell or is elaborated into the surrounding microenvironment by the plasma cell.

Bibliography and Selected Reading

General

Antibodies. Cold Spring Harbor Symposia on Quantitative Biology, XXXII, Cold Spring Harbor Laboratory of Quantitative Biology, Cold Spring Harbor, L.I., New York, 1967.

Capra, J. D., and Kehoe, J. M. Hypervariable Regions, Idiotypy, and Antibody-Combining Site. In F. J. Dixon and H. G. Kunkel (Eds.), *Advances in Immunology,* Vol. 20. New York: Academic, 1975. Pp. 1–37.

Hokama, Y. Immunochemistry. In N. Bhagavan (Ed.), *A Comprehensive Review of Biochemistry.* Philadelphia: Lippincott, 1978.

Ishizaka, K. Cellular Events in the IgE Antibody Response. In F. J. Dixon and H. G. Kunkel (Eds.), *Advances in Immunology,* Vol. 23. New York: Academic, 1976. Pp 1–70.

Ishizaka, K., and Dayton, D. H., Jr. (Ed.). *The Biological Role of the Immunoglobulin E System.* Bethesda, Md.: National Inst. Child Health and Human Development, 1972.

Koshland, M. E. Structure and Function of the J-Chain. In F. J. Dixon and H. G. Kunkel (Eds.), *Advances in Immunology,* Vol. 20. New York: Academic, 1975. Pp. 41–67.

Nisonoff, A., Wilson, S. K., Wang, A. C., Fudenberg, H. H., and Hopper, J. E. Genetic Control of the Biosynthesis of IgG and IgM. In B. Amos (ed.) *Progress in Immunology.* New York: Academic, 1971. Pp. 61–70.

Classification and Structure of Immunoglobulin

Amzel, M. L, and Poljak, J. R. Three-dimensional structure of immunoglobulins. *Ann. Rev. Biochem.* 48:961, 1979.

Bubb, M. D., and Conradie, J. D. Isolation and identification of the $C_\mu 4$-domain of IgM. *Immunol. Commun.* 6:33, 1977.

Edelman, G. M., Cunningham, B. A., Gall, W. E., Gottlieb, P. D., Rutishauser, U., and Waxdal, M. J. The covalent structure of an entire gamma-G immunoglobulin molecule. P. N. A. S. 63: 78, 1969.

Wang, A. C., Pink, J. R. L., Fudenberg, H. H., and Ohms, J. A variable region subclass of heavy chains common to immunoglobulins G, A, and M and characterization by an unblocked amino-terminal residue. *Proc. Natl. Acad. Sci. U.S.A.* 66:657, 1970.

Wang, A. C. The structure of immunoglobulins. In H. H. Fudenberg, D. P. Stites, J. L. Caldwell, and J. V. Wells, (Eds.), *Basic and Clinical Immunology* (2nd ed.). Los Altos, Calif.: Lange, 1978. P. 23.

World Health Organization. Immunoglobulin E, a new class of human immunoglobulin. *Bull. WHO* 38:151, 1968.

Physicochemical and Biological Properties

Bubb, M. O., and Conradie, J. D. Studies on the structural and biological functions of the $C\mu3$ and $C\mu4$ domains of IgM. *Immunology* 34:449, 1978.

Poljak, R. J. X-ray diffraction studies of immunoglobulins. In F. J. Dixon and H. G. Kunkel (Eds.), *Advances in Immunology,* Vol. 21. New York: Academic, 1975. Pp. 1–30.

Uhr, J. W., and Vitetta, E. S. Synthesis, biochemistry and dynamics of cell surface immunoglobulin on lymphocytes. *Fed. Proc.* 32:35, 1973.

Walker, W. A., and Isselbacher, K. J. Intestinal antibodies. *New Engl. J. Med.* 297:767, 1977.

Diversity, Biosynthesis, Evolution, and Function of Antibody and Immunoglobulins

Adinolfi, M., Glynn, A. A., Lindsay, M., and Milne, C. M. Serological properties of YA antibodies to *Escherichia coli* present in human colostrum. *Immunol.* 10:517, 1966.

Hood, L. E. Two Genes, One Polypeptide Chain — Fact or Fiction? *Fed. Proc.* 31:177, 1972.

Hood, L., and Ein, D. Immunoglobulin lambda chain structure: Two genes, one polypeptide chain. *Nature* 220:764, 1968.

Jerne, N. K. The somatic generation of immune recognition. *Eur. J. Immunol.* 1:109, 1971.

Potter, M. Gene regulation in differentiation and development. *Fed. Proc.* 34:21, 1975.

Seidman, J. G., Leder, A., Nau, M., Norman, B., and Leder, P. Antibody diversity: The structure of clonal immunoglobulin genes suggests a mechanism for generating new sequences. *Science* 202:11, 1978.

Sherr, C. J., Schenbein, I., and Uhr, J. W. Synthesis and intracellular transport of immunoglobulin in secretory and nonsecretory cells. *Ann. N.Y. Acad. Sci.* 190:250, 1971.

Williamson, A. R. The biological origin of antibody diversity. *Ann. Rev. Biochem.* 45:467, 1976.

3 : Cell-Mediated Immunity: T Lymphocyt

This chapter will be restricted essentially to the description and biological functions of the T lymphocytes (T cells) associated with cell-mediated immunity (CMI); however, it must be emphasized that the host immune response is an interplay of B cells, macrophages, specific and nonspecific humoral factors, and T cells. The dissection in this chapter is presented for a better understanding of the complex immune processes. As indicated in Chapter 1, the CMI system is specified and regulated by the thymus (T) through its hormone *thymosin* or *thymopoietin*; hence the designation *T-dependent lymphocyte* or *T cell*. CMI is also synonymous with delayed type hypersensitivity (DTH), which will be discussed later in this chapter and in Chapter 13.

The heterogeneous nature of the effector T cells of the mouse system has been extensively examined and characterized in congenic inbred strains. The success of these studies has been facilitated by advances in procedure in the following interrelated areas: (1) the development of techniques to separate subclasses (subsets) of lymphocytes; with specific monoclonal antibodies prepared in mouse spleen hybridomas to T cell subsets membrane antigens and with sheep erythrocyte rosette formation that differentiates T from B cells, and from the natural experiments of nature (immunodeficiency diseases, see Chapter 15); (2) the identification of cell surface markers on different subclasses of human T lymphocytes by in vitro procedures; and (3) the development of in vitro techniques to assess the different functional responses, properties, and interactions of subclasses of lymphocytes and monocytes (nonlymphoid cells). Studies in the characterization of subsets of T lymphocytes of man are being conducted but lag behind the abundant information on T cells of the inbred mouse.

This chapter summarizes the pertinent findings in human and mouse effector T lymphocytes. Table 3–1 summarizes the comparative characteristic differences, similarities, and biological properties of the lymphocytes of man. Table 3-2 represents the stages of T cell maturation or differentiation in man and the membrane antigenic markers that help to differentiate the T cells in the developmental processes. Ten antigenic markers have been

Table 3-1 : The Biological Functions and Characteristics of Human Lymphocytes: T Cell Subsets; B Cells, and Null Cells*

| | Lymphocytes | | | | | | |
| | T Cell | | | | | | |
Properties*	HTLA⁺	TH₁⁺	TH₂⁻(T4⁺)	TH₁⁻	TH₂⁺(T5⁺)	B Cell	Null Cell
Antigenic markers							
HTLA	+	+	—		—	—	+ (pre-T)
HBLA	—	—	—		—	—	+ (pre-B)
SIg	—	—	—			+	—
FcR	—	+ (FcμR)			+ (FcγR)	—	—
TH₁	+	+	—			—	—
C3R	—	—	—			+	—
Biological activity							
E-rosettes	+	+			+	—	—
EAC-rosettes	—	—			—	+	—
Con A	+	+			+	—	—
PHA	+	+			+	+ (aggregated PHA)	
Soluble antigens	—	—	+	+	—	—	—
PPD	?	?	—		+		
MLC-alloantigens							
Responder	—	+		—			
Stimulator	+	+	—	+	+	++	++
Suppressor	?	?		?	+		
Lymphokines							
MIF	—	+	—			+	NT
LIF	—	+	—			—	—
LMF	—	+	—			—	—
Cytotoxic							
CML	—	+	+	—	+	—	—
ADCC	—	—(±)				—(±)	+
Mitogen-induced	—	+			—	+	+
Antibody							
Production in culture	—	—			—	+	—
PFC	—	—			—	+	—
Function							
Th	—	+	+	—	—	—	—
Tc	—	+	+	—	+	—	+ (ADCC)
TDT	—	—		+	+	—	—
Ts	—	—		+	+	—	—
Miscellaneous							
Hemopoietic stem cells	—	—			—	—	+
Pre-B and -T	—	—			—	—	+
EB virus	—	—			—	+	—
Thymocyte	+	—		—	+		
Natural killer (NK)							+

*The abbreviations, some of which are indicated in the text, are as follows: HTLA, human T lymphocyte antigen; TH₁, peripheral human T antigen 1; TH₂, peripheral human T antigen 2, also referred to as T4⁺, when antigen 2 is absent, (TH₂⁻) and T5⁺ when 2 is present (TH₂⁺); Th, T helper cell; Tc, T cytotoxic cell; TDT, T delayed hypersensitivity T cell; Ts, T suppressor cell; HBLA, human B lymphocyte antigen; SIg, surface immunoglobulin; FcR, Fc, fragment or constant region of heavy chain receptor; FcμR, IgM Fc receptor; FcγR, IgG Fc receptor; C3, complement component receptor; MLC, mixed lymphocytotoxicity; MIF, migration inhibitory factor; LIF, leukocyte (polymorphonucleocyte) inhibitory factor; LMF, lymphocyte mitogenic factor; CML, cell-mediated lympholysis; ADCC, antibody-dependent cytotoxic cell; PFC, plaque-forming cell; EB. Epstein Barr; and NT, not determined.

Table 3-2 : Stages of T Cell Differentiation in Man

Stage	Thymus	Antigen Markers*	Distribution of Cells
1	Early lymphoid cells, pre-thymocyte (2 types)	(a) $T10^+$ ↓ (b) $T9^+$, $T10^+$	10%
2	Thymocytes, immature (1 type, common from stage 1, a and b)	$T10^+$, $T6^+$, $T4^+$, $T5^+$	70%
3	Thymocytes, mature (2 types, segregate from immature stage 2)	(a) $T10^+$, $T1^+$, $T3^+$, $T4^+(TH_2^-)$ (b) $T10^+$, $T1^+$, $T3^+$, $T5^+$ (TH_2^+)	? ?
4	Peripheral blood T cells (2 types, from stage 3, a to a and b to b, minus $T10^+$)	(a) $T1^+$, $T3^+$, $T4^+$ (TH_2^-) (b) $T1^+$, $T3^+$, $T5^+(TH_2^+)$	55–65% 20–30%

*The numbers after T designate the specific antigens on the T cell (membrane) determined with monospecific antibodies.

demonstrated and designated by the numbers 1 to 10. The first three stages of maturation occur in the thymus. As differentiation progresses new antigenic markers are added and some are deleted. $T4^+$ and $T5^+$ are the important antigenic markers for the mature T cells in peripheral blood. $T4^+$ and $T5^+$ cells are associated with T helper and cytotoxic/suppressor functions, respectively. Some of the mouse T lymphocytes that show a correspondence to human T lymphocytes are included in Table 3-3.

Induction of the Cellular Immune Response

The host immune response is associated with the humoral and CMI systems in association with specific and nonspecific humoral regulators. In some situations, depending on the nature of the immunogen, cell-mediated immune response is the major expressed immune reaction independent of the humoral B cell response. Antibody is not involved in this case. This phenomenon is associated with CMI and the T cells and is characterized by sensitized T cell and target cell interaction. The common feature in this type of reaction is the destruction of tissues (target cells). Sensitized viable cells transmitted to a normal individual transfer this cell-mediated response to the recipient against the specific corresponding antigen. This is called *adoptive* immunity and is in contrast to *passive* immunity, which is transferred by antibody (involves immunoglobulins and humoral immunity). Sensitized T cells in the primary response are generally detected 1 to 2 weeks after initial exposure to the immunogen. The CMI status may persist for months (*Listeria monocytogenes* antigens) or indefinitely (exposure to *Mycobacterium tuberculosis*).

Table 3-3 : The Biological Properties and Characteristics of Mouse T Cell Subsets

Properties*	T Lymphocyte Subsets			
	Th (Helper)	TDT (DTH)	Tc (Cytotoxic)	Ts (Suppressor)
Antigen markers				
Theta (θ)	+	+	+	+
Ly	1	1	2,3	2,3
Ia	(1A–B)	(I–J)	—	(I–J)
Antigenic reactivity	Carrier LD	?	SD	SD
SIg	—	—	—	—
Biological activity				
E-rosette	+	+	+	+
MLC ⌈ responder	—	—	+	+
⌊ stimulator	+	+	+	+
LMF			+	—
MIF	—	—	+	+
CML	—	—	+	—
LIF	—	—	—	+
Cytotoxicity, mitogen-induced	—	—	+	—

*The abbreviations used in this table are defined as follows: Ly, lymphocyte; Ia, gene I of H–2 complex (Chapter 10) antigen; LD, lymphocyte-determined; SD, serologically determined; SIg, surface-bound immuno-globulins; and for LMF, MIF, CML, and LIF see Table 3.1.

Table 3-4 : Examples of Delayed Type Hypersensitivity (DTH)

1. Tuberculosis—tuberculin reaction
2. Allograft rejection (primary)
3. GVHR—Graft vs host response
4. Cell-mediated lympholysis (CML)
5. Mixed lymphocyte reaction (MLR)
6. Poison ivy
7. Skin reactions to diphtheria toxoid

Delayed Type Hypersensitivity (DTH)

Table 3-4 summarizes the types of delayed hypersensitivity triggered by a variety of immunogens. DTH will be discussed in detail in Chapter 13. The classic tuberculin reaction has been the hallmark of DTH. Minute amounts of tuberculin or purified protein derivative (PPD) isolated from *Mycobacterium tuberculosis* culture, when given intradermally to an individual previously exposed to the organism or administered bacillus of Calmette-Guérin (BCG), an attenuated strain of *Mycobacterium bovis,* will induce an inflammatory reaction at the site of the immunogenic injection. An erythematous induration due to the interaction of sensitized T cells with the PPD antigen occurs approximately

48 hours after the administration of the antigen intradermally (thus the term *delayed hypersensitivity*). Examination of the lesion on the histological and molecular levels reveals the following: the T cell–PPD interaction triggers the release of lymphokines such as (1) monocytic chemotactic factor (MCF, Table 3–5 and Figure 3–7), (2) macrophage migration inhibitory factor (MIF, Table 3–5 and Figure 3–7), and (3) macrophage activating factor (MAF, Table 3–6 and Table 3–7). The chemotactic factor attracts the peripheral blood monocytes into the area of the T cell–antigen interaction; the MAF then activates these premacrophage cells to become active macrophages; and subsequently the macrophages are immobilized by the MIF. Thus, active macrophages are concentrated in the area of injury. This would be a useful means of destroying the focus of bacterial invasion.

Such a sequence of events, involving monocytic aggregation, may be the means by which granuloma formation occurs in tuberculosis. On the other hand, DTH may be deleterious to the host, as in some DTH associated with experimental autoimmune encephalitis (EAE), in which destruction of nerve tissue results from the release of lysosomal hydrolases by the macrophages. This sequence in granuloma formation and a simple diagram of the pattern obtained for MIF analysis are illustrated in Figures 3–1 and 3–2, respectively. The skin histological patterns of DTH associated with diphtheria toxoid antigens differ from the PPD type in that tissue mast cells have also been implicated.

Biological Properties and Characteristics of T Cells

The human T lymphocyte, an E-rosette-positive cell producing the lymphokines, has been characterized as having TH_1^+ antigenic markers and is found in peripheral blood (Table 3–1 and Figure 3–5). E-rosette formation results from the direct interaction of T lymphocytes with sheep erythrocytes (SRBC) to make a rosette pattern, as shown in Figure 3–3. Thus, T cells have SRBC receptors (unlike B cells, which have C3 receptors) and interact with SRBC coated with rabbit anti-SRBC-C3 complex. Thus, the term erythrocyte-antibody-complement rosette (EAC-rosette). The comparable mouse T cell is characterized by the presence of $Ly-1^+$ membrane antigen (Table 3–3).

Figure 3–4 shows how the effector cell develops through the actions of thymosin and specific antigens in the primary CMI response. The lymphokine-producing cell (TDT–T cell, delayed type), described in the preceding discussion of response to PPD, has the TH_1^+ antigen marker but lacks HTLA (human T

Fig. 3-1 : Evolution of delayed type hypersensitivity and granuloma formation or resolution.

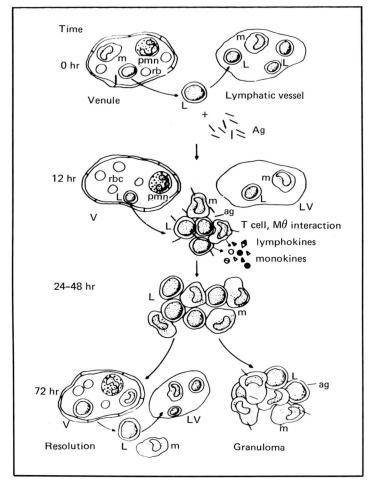

Fig 3-2 : Simplified diagram of assay for MIF in an in vitro test. A. Pattern of migration of macrophages in the absence of MIF. B. Pattern of migration inhibition of macrophages due to release of MIF following sensitized T cell interaction with specific antigen.

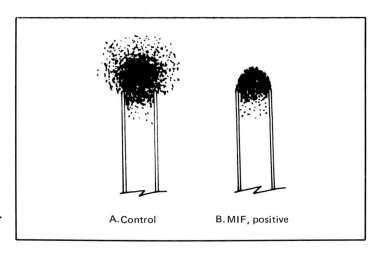

Fig. 3-3 : E-rosette formed by interaction of T cell with sheep erythrocytes.

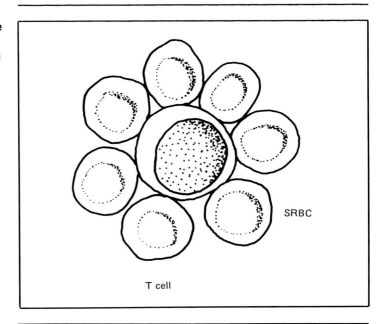

SRBC

T cell

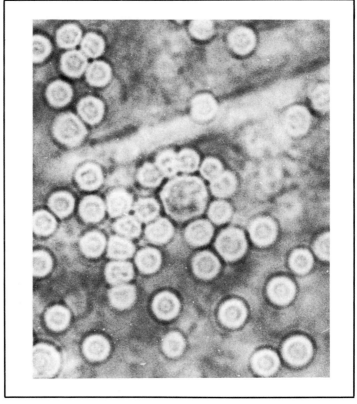

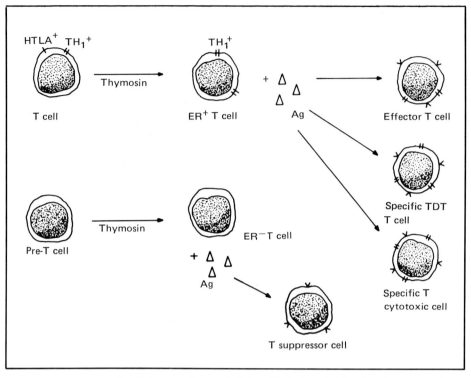

Fig. 3-4 : Development of the effector T cell following thymosin and antigen activation. HTLA$^+$ = positive for human T lymphocyte antigen; TH$_1$$^+$ = positive for human T lymphocyte antigen 1; ER$^+$ = E-rosette—positive T cell; and ER$^-$ = E-rosette—negative T cell.

lymphocyte antigen). The cell-mediated lymphocytotoxic cell (CML) is equivalent to the specific T killer cell (T cytotoxic or Tc cell, defined in the next paragraph). The Tc cell can be recognized by initially activating T cells in mixed lymphocyte culture or with mitogens (concanavalin A) for approximately 24 to 28 hours, then adding the activated Tc cells to ^{51}Cr-labeled target cells for another 24 hours, and subsequently analyzing the supernatant for ^{51}Cr released by lysed target cells. The T helper cell (Th), which also has the TH$_1$$^+$ antigenic marker, is the cell involved in the induction of humoral antibody synthesis by B cells, and it plays a significant part in the presence of T-dependent antigens (see Chapter 4). T helper cell appears to possess Fcμ receptors (receptors for the Fc portion of the IgM heavy chain) also. CML cells contain the TH$_1$$^+$ antigen μ-markers. The question as yet unresolved is whether each of these cells is an individual cell, as depicted in Figure 3-4, or whether there is a single cell with multiple functions. T suppressor cell (Ts) (Figure 3-4) differs from the effector T cells described in that it

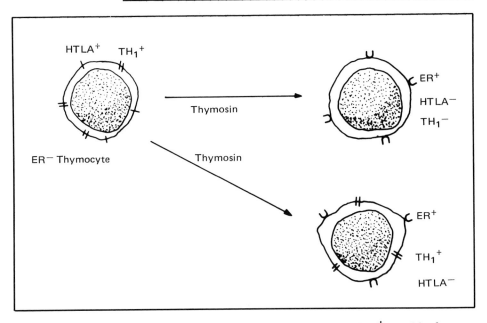

Fig. 3-5 : Antigenic markers on human T cell. $HTLA^+$ = positive for human T lymphocyte antigen; $HTLA^-$ = negative for HTLA; ER^+ and ER^- = E-rosette-positive and –negative T cells, respectively; TH_1^+ and TH_1^- = positive and negative for human T lymphocyte antigen marker 1.

has no TH_1^- antigen marker (TH_1^-) nor HTLA but has Fcγ receptors (IgG Fc receptors). Further biological properties of Ts are shown in Table 3-1, and for comparison the mouse T cells are summarized in Table 3-3. Figure 3-5 depicts the antigenic markers presently recognized for the human T cells. The thymocyte has the markers E-rosette (ER^+), $HTLA^+$ and TH_1^+; and the peripheral cells have the markers ER^+, $HTLA^-$, and TH_1, and ER^+, $HTLA^-$, and TH_1^+. The peripheral null cells, which include the hemopoietic stem cells, also have the pre-T and -B cells, containing $HTLA^+$ and $HBLA^+$ antigenic markers, respectively. However, the pre-T cell ($HTLA^+$) has no E-rosette receptor (ER^-) and thus must be activated by thymosin to become a T cell. Figure 3-4 depicts the primary response in the cellular progression of the T cell immune response. This is analogous to the B cell system, except that the humoral immunoglobulins are not produced by the T cells. The T cell–mediated immune response initiates release of lymphokines by the effector lymphocytes specified for this function. The nature of the lymphokines is discussed in the following paragraphs.

The null cells, representing 5 to 15 percent of the cells in peripheral blood, consist of hemopoietic stem cells. These include precursors of the T and B cells, myeloid, erythroid, and the

Fig. 3–6 : Mode of action of antibody-dependent cytotoxic cell. K = Killer; FcR = receptor for Fc domain of immunoglobulin.

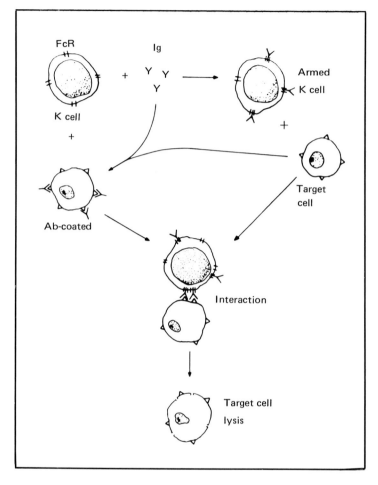

thrombocytic series. In addition, cells designated *killer* (K) cells, which possess Fc receptors, are present in the null cell population. The mode of activation of the K cell and its relationship to immunoglobulins is depicted in Figure 3–6. This cell is also called *antibody-dependent cytotoxic cell* (ADCC). Binding to the target cell is dependent on the presence of immunoglobulin (IgG or IgM).

Recent studies have shown that the peripheral T cells consist of two functional subsets as dissected by anti-TH_2^+ antiserum. Thus, peripheral T cells can be separated into TH_2^+ (TH_1^-) and TH_2^+ (TH_1^+) subsets. The TH_2^- subset appears to respond to soluble antigens, such as tetanus toxoid and mumps antigen. This response appears to be suppressed by the TH_2^+ T cells, since a greater proliferation of TH_2^- T cells has been found to occur against tetanus toxoid in the absence of TH_2^+ cells. In this regard the TH_2^+ T cells function similarly to mouse Ly-1$^+$ T cells: activated Ly-1$^+$ cells have shown suppression of the Ly-2,3$^+$ responses to soluble antigens.

CML is restricted to the TH$_2$$^+$ subset and is amplified by TH$_2$$^-$ cells (Th cells). This amplification function of TH$_2$$^-$ cells suggests that TH$_2$$^-$ may promote other immune responses (T helper cell for the B cell responses).

The TH$_2$$^+$ T cell subset is stimulated by concanavalin A to proliferate. This cell suppresses the MLC reaction. The TH$_2$$^-$ T cell subset is also induced by Con A to proliferate but shows no T suppressor effect in the MLC reaction. However, the TH$_2$$^-$ subset of T cells modulates the generation of TH$_2$$^+$ T subset to suppressor activity at 24 hours, but not at 48 hours, of exposure to Con A. Thus, the importance of T–T cell modulation in the MLC and CML reactions.

Tables 3-1, 3-2, and 3-3 summarize the various antigenic markers and some biological properties of human and mouse lymphocytes and their subsets. The properties of human B and null cells are also included in Table 3-1 for comparison with the human T cells.

Preparation of Antibody to HTLA$^+$, TH$_1$$^+$, and TH$_2$$^+$

Anti-HTLA$^+$ is raised in rabbits by immunization with E-rosette-positive lymphoblast cells from patients with acute lymphoblastic leukemia (ALL). The anti-HTLA$^+$ was rendered specific to T lymphocytes by absorption with autologous B lymphoblastoid cells. This antiserum reacts with only fetal and adult thymocytes, T cell–derived leukemia cells (blasts), and a portion of the null cell population of the peripheral blood. It does not react with mature E-rosette–positive T cells of the peripheral blood. Recognition of HTLA$^+$ with anti-HTLA$^+$ is performed by the cytotoxicity test using complement or by direct immunofluorescence. Heterologous antiserum to mature T cells of peripheral blood has been prepared. This antigen has been designated as T human 1 (TH$_1$$^+$). Evaluation of the presence (TH$_1$$^+$) and absence (TH$_1$$^-$) of this antigen has demonstrated two subsets in peripheral blood. Human TH$_1$$^+$ and TH$_1$$^-$ correspond to the defined mouse Ly-1$^+$,2$^-$,3$^-$ and Ly-1$^-$,2$^+$,3$^+$ T cells, respectively, while the HTLA$^+$ (thymocytes) antigenic marker corresponds to the TL marker of the mouse.

Preparation of Anti-TH$_2$$^+$

Anti-TH$_2$$^+$ antiserum was raised in rabbits by injection of highly purified normal human T cells. The antibody was rendered specific to T cells by absorption with AB erythrocyte, SIg$^+$ B cells, B lymphoblastoid cells, and T cells (TH$_1$$^+$ and TH$_2$$^-$) from a chronic lymphocytic leukemia patient. This antibody was designated anti-TH$_2$$^+$ and differs from anti-TH$_1$$^+$. Thus peripheral T cells can be further dissected with this anti-serum.

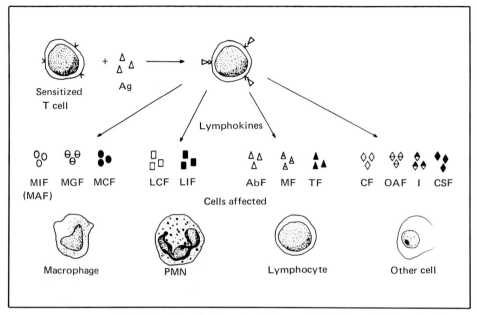

Fig. 3-7 : Lymphokine release by sensitized effector T cell, and action on target cells. I = interferon. See Tables 3-1 and 3-5 for explanation of the other abbreviations.

Purified peripheral T cells can be obtained by passage of the suspension of mononuclear cells isolated by Ficoll-Paque (mixture of Ficoll, copolymer of sucrose and epichlorohydrin, and Paque, diatrizoate sodium) density centrifugation through nylon wool columns. The nonadherent cells are further separated by treatment with sheep red blood cells. The SRBC-T cell complex is then separated from the remaining nonreacting mononuclear cells by Ficoll-Paque density centrifugation. The E-rosette-positive purified T cells are in the precipitated residue. The SRBC are removed by lysis with 0.155 M ammonium chloride solution.

Lymphokines

A sensitized T-cell, when subjected to interaction with its specific antigen, is activated and elaborates a variety of factors collectively termed *lymphokines* (Figure 3-7). Many biological functions have been attributed to these factors, and their target cells are as varied as the number of lymphokines. These factors appear to affect primarily macrophages, lymphocytes, and granulocytes, but other cells have also been affected by the lymphokines. The amounts of lymphokines produced are small, but they have a profound effect on target cells. Lymphokines play a significant role in host defense, in pathogenesis of immunological diseases, and in mobilization of uncommitted cells. Lymphokines can act specifically and nonspecifically. Table 3-5 lists the lymphokines reported in the literature and their target cells.

Table 3-5 : The Lymphokines of Human TH$_1{}^+$ T cell

Mediators Affecting

1. Macrophages

   a. Migration inhibition factor (MIF)
   b. Macrophage-activating factor (MAF)
   c. Monocyte chemotactic factor (MCF)
   d. Monocyte growth factor (MGF)

2. Polymorphonuclear leukocytes (PMN)

   a. Leukocyte chemotactic factor (LCF)
   b. Leukocyte inhibitory factor (LIF)

3. Lymphocytes

   a. Factors affecting antibody production (AbF B cell)
   b. Mitogenic factor (MF)
   c. Transfer factor (TF)

4. Other cells

   a. Lymphotoxin (cytotoxic factor—CF) and growth inhibition factor (GIF)
   b. Interferon
   c. Osteoclast-activating factor (OAF)
   d. Colony-stimulating factor (CSF)

Mediators Affecting Macrophages

Mediators affecting macrophages include migration (inhibition factor (MIF), which stabilizes or retains macrophages in the inflamed area (this observation is currently used for the in vitro determination of cell-mediated immunity); macrophage activating factor (MAF), which is indistinguishable from MIF; macrophage (monocyte) chemotactic factor (MCF), which attracts macrophages (monocytes) to the area of injury (delayed hypersensitivity); and monocyte growth factor(s) (MGF), factors demonstrated in supernatants of lymphocyte Con A cultures which induce and maintain monocytic growth in continuous culture.

Mediators Affecting PMN

The mediators affecting polymorphonuclear leukocytes (PMN) include leukocyte chemotactic factors (LCF), for neutrophils, eosinophils, and basophils, which play a role in chronic inflammation and cutaneous delayed hypersensitivity; and leukocyte inhibitory factor (LIF), which inhibits migration of polymorphonuclear leukocytes and retains PMN in the area of inflammation.

Mediators Affecting Lymphocytes

The mediators affecting lymphocytes include (1) factors affecting antibody production (B cells): a factor in mouse that triggers IgM production to sheep erythrocyte and factors inducing IgG and IgE antibody production; (2) factors associated with suppression of antibody synthesis mitogenic factors—the factors released by sensitized lymphocytes reacting with specific antigens, which stimulate other nonsensitized lymphocytes to blastogenesis; and (3) transfer factor (TF), a low molecular weight dialyzable fraction obtained from sensitized T lymphocytes, either by direct extraction or by release from cells following reaction with specific antigen, which transfers specific delayed hypersensitivity in man.

Mediators Affecting Other Cells

The mediators affecting other cells include lymphotoxin and growth inhibitory factors (cytotoxic factors, CF). Lymphotoxin is a factor released by sensitized lymphocytes that is cytotoxic to certain target cells. The growth inhibitory factor inhibits growth of cells rather than causing cell lysis. It is also referred to as *cloning inhibition factor*. The effect is only on certain target cells, such as HeLa cells. *Interferon* is a factor released in culture medium and produced by normal lymphocytes when they are stimulated with viruses, antigens, or mitogens. It is a stimulating factor that inhibits or interferes with virus proliferation by inducing the production of antiviral protein in the uninfected cells. Other factors include (1) osteoclast activating factor (OAF), which is formed by lymphocytes stimulated with specific antigens or mitogens; (2) a tissue factor (procoagulant factor activity), which acts similarly to coagulant blood Factor VIII in decreasing clotting time in blood Factor VIII deficiency plasma (this factor is produced by lymphocytes stimulated with mitogens or antigens); and (3) a colony-stimulating factor (CSF), which induces bone marrow stem cells to differentiate into granulocytes and mononuclear cells in vitro. Table 3-6 summarizes some of the physical and chemical properties of these mediators produced by lymphocytes. Figure 3-8 illustrates the possible mode of action of interferon. The major role is that of stimulating intact lymphocytes to produce an antiviral protein. Interferon can also induce and enhance release of histamine from mast cells activated by IgE-antigen complexes.

It has been demonstrated recently that partially purified interferon obtained from human leukocytes augments the activity of NK (natural killer) cells against *Herpes* virus infection. Interferon appears to play a significant role in the NK cell activity in viral infections and perhaps also in host defense in general. It has also been shown that, biochemically, interferon acts on oxidative phosphorylation (see Chapters 8 and 17).

Assay for CMI

Cell-mediated immune response in individuals can be demonstrated by in vivo and in vitro methods. Before the development of in vitro procedures the primary assay relied on the delayed type hypersensitivity skin reaction discussed in earlier paragraphs. Antigens (such as PPD), bacterial toxoids or antigens, and drugs have been employed and are presently still being routinely used for assessment of CMI in various patients clinically. The drugs generally used are dinitrochlorobenzene (DNCB) and dinitrofluorobenzene (DNFB). The bacterial antigens used in addition to PPD are streptokinase, streptolysin O and toxoids of tetanus and diptheria.

The use of in vitro procedures for assessment of CMI response has significantly advanced the understanding of the T lymphocyte

Table 3-6 : Some Physical and Chemical Characteristics of Mediators of Human T and B Lymphocytes

Mediators	Heat Stability 56° for 30 Minutes	Produce by Cell Types	MW × 10^3	Mobility in Polyacrylamide Gel Electrophoresis	Enzymes[e] A	Enzymes[e] B
MIF	Stable	T-B	25	Albumin	R	S
MCF	Stable	T-B	12-25	Albumin	—	S
MAF protein	Stable	T-B	25	Albumin	R	S
LIF	Stable	T-B	68	Albumin	R	S
LCF	—	—	24-55	Variable	—	—
LMF	—	T	20-30	—	—	—[a]
FAAP						
Enhancement	Stable	—	—	—	—	—
Suppression	—	—	25-55	—	—	—[b]
TF	Stable	T	4	—	S	—
CF protein	Stable	T	80-90	Postalbumin	S	S
Interferon	—	T-B	—	—	—	—[c]
OAF	Labile	—	13-25	—	—	S[d]
CSF glycoprotein	Stable	T	40-60	—	—	—

[a]Resistant to RNASE, DNASE and proteolytic enzymes.
[b]Resistant to RNASE and DNASE.
[c]Not affected by DNASE and RNASE but destroyed by trypsin.
[d]Inactivated by proteolytic enzymes other than chymotrypsin.
[e]A = neuraminidase, B = chymotrypsin, R = resistant, S = sensitive

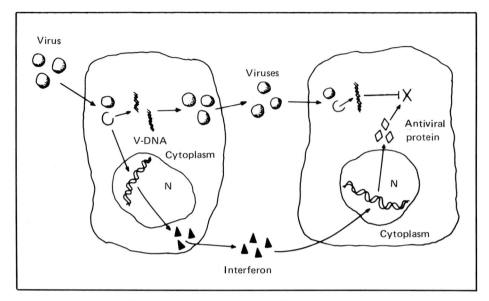

Fig. 3-8 : Schematic diagram of interferon action. N = nucleus of the cell. V = viral deoxyribonucleic acid.

system. These tests include assaying the lymphokines released following interaction of sensitized T cells with the specific antigen. Commonly measured lymphokines include MIF, MAF, MCF, LIF, and LCF. Of these, MIF has been most commonly used to assess a CMI response (see Figure 3-2).

It is of interest that the DTH response does not necessarily correlate with CMI protection. For example, it has been shown that an animal with DTH responsive to an agent such as *Cryptococcus* is not necessarily protected against the viable agent when subsequently challenged. This is also true in many instances with the humoral antibodies; a high concentration of antibody need not imply protection. In part, this is reflected in the heterogenicity of the T cells. The T cell responsible for DTH need not be the cell responsible for the cytotoxic function (see Figure 3-3).

Summary

1. The human T cells are separated into subsets and characterized by cell surface antigenic markers and cell surface receptors, which include HTLA, TH_1, TH_2, and HLA antigens and Fc and sheep erythrocyte receptors. TH_2^+ is equivalent to $T5^+$ cells and TH_2^- is the same as $T4^+$ cells.
2. Thymocytes have $HTLA^+$ and TH_1^+ antigens.
3. The peripheral T cell antigen TH_1^+ has been demonstrated in T helper, T cytotoxic, and T effector cells in delayed hypersensitivity. T suppressor cells lack TH_1 antigen (TH_1^-) but have TH_2^+ antigen.

4. The $Fc\mu$ receptor is found in the $TH_1{}^+$ lymphocyte (T helper cell.

5. The $Fc\gamma$ receptor is found in the $TH_1{}^-$ lymphocyte (T suppressor cell).

6. Lymphokines are produced by the $TH_1{}^+$ lymphocytes.

7. Lymphokines elaborated by T cells include mediators that affect macrophages (MIF, MAF, MCF, and MGF); PMN (LCF and LIF); lymphocytes (affect B cells, MF, and TF); and other cells (CF, GIF, OAF, and CSF).

8. Cell-mediated immunity can be demonstrated by in vivo and in vitro methods. In vivo methods include the delayed hypersensitivity skin reaction (classic example: tuberculin reaction). In vitro methods include analysis of lymphokines such as MIF, CSF, TF, and other factors released by a sensitized T cell against its specific antigen.

9. It is concluded that the CMI system consists of a heterogeneous population of T cells, each with its specific function in the host response.

Bibliography and Selected Reading

General

Chess, L., and Schlossman, S. F. Human Lymphocyte Population. In H. G. Kunkel and F. J. Dixon (Eds.), *Advances in Immunology,* Vol. 25. New York: Academic, 1977. Pp. 213–214.

Chess, L., and Schlossman, S. F. Functional Analysis of Distinct Human T Cell Subsets Bearing Unique Differentiation Antigens. In O. Stutman (Ed.), *Contemporary Topics in Immunobiology T Cells.* New York: Plenum, 1977. Pp. 363–379.

Fudenberg, H. H., Stites, D. P., Caldwell, J. L., and Wells, J. V. (Eds.). *Basic and Clinical Immunology* (2nd Ed.). Los Altos, Calif.: Lange, 1978.

Golub, E. S. *The Cellular Basis of the Immune Response: An Approach to Immunobiology.* Sunderland, Mass.: Sinauer, 1977. P. 269.

Greaves, M. F., Owen, J. J. T., and Raff, M. C. (eds.). *T and B Lymphocytes. Origins, Properties and Rates in Immune Responses.* New York: American Elsevier, 1974.

Miller, J. F. A. P. Introduction: Lymphocytes, Past, Present, and Future. In J. J. Marchalois (Ed.), *Lymphocytes Structure and Function,* Part 1. New York: Dekker, 1977. Pp. 1–7.

Cellular Immune Response

Cantor, H., and Gershon, R. K. Immunological circuits: Cellular composition. *Fed. Proc.* 38:2058, 1979.

Evans, R. L., Breard, J. M., Lazarus, H., Schlossmann, S. F., and Chess, L. Detection, isolation, and functional characterization of two human T cell subclasses bearing unique differentiation antigens. *J. Exp. Med.* 145:221, 1977.

Heiynen, C. J., Uytde Haag, F., Gmelig-Meyling, F. H. J., and Ballieuz, R. E. Localization of human antigen-specific helper and suppressor function in distinct T cell populations. *Cell. Immunol.* 43:282, 1979.

Kaplan, J., and W. D. Peterson, Jr., Detection of human T-lymphocyte antigens (HTLA antigens) on thymosin-inducible T cell precursors. *Clin. Immunol. Immunopathol.* 9:436, 1978.

72

Origins of Lymphocyte Diversity. Cold Spring Harbor Symposia on Quantitative Biology, XLI. Cold Spring Harbor Laboratory of Quantitative Biology, Cold Spring Harbor, L.I., New York, 1977.

Paul, W. E. Immune effector mechanisms: Duality of recognition functions. In M. E. Weksler, S. D. Litwin, R. R. Riggio, and G. W. Siskind (Eds.), *Immune Effector Mechanisms in Disease:* Proceedings of the Fourth Irwin Strasburger Memorial Seminar on Immunology. New York: Grune & Stratton, 1977. Pp. 129-144.

Reinherz, E. L., and Schlossman, S. F. Regulation of the immune response—Inducer and suppressor T-lymphocyte subsets in human beings. *New Engl. J. Med.* 303:370, 1980.

Shen, F. W., Boyse, E. A., and Cantor, H. Preparation and use of Ly antisera. *Immunogenetics* 2:591, 1975.

Lymphokines and Assay for CMI

Bloom, B. R. *In vitro* approaches to the mechanism of cell-mediated immune reactions. In F. J. Dixon, Jr., and H. G. Kunkel (Eds.), *Advances in Immunology.* New York: Academic, 1971. Pp. 102-208.

Goldstein, A. L., Thurman, G. B., Low, T. L. K., Rossio, J. L., and Trivers, G. E. Hormonal influences on the reticuloendothelial system: Current status of the role of thymosin in the regulation and modulation of immunity. *J. Reticuloendothel. Soc.* 23:253, 1978.

Klein, J. Genetics of Cell-mediated Lymphocytotoxicity in the Mouse. In *Springer Seminars in Immunopathology,* Vol. 1. New York: Springer, 1978. Pp. 31-49.

Reinherz, E. L., and Schlossman, S. F. Con A-inducible suppression of MLC: Evidence for mediation by TH+-T cell subset in man. *J. Immunol.* 122:1335, 1979.

4 : Antigens and Antigenicity

Antigens, the other half of the puzzle of immunology of which antibodies are one half, are discussed in this chapter. Antigens comprise an array of molecules which when administered to a host by various routes (by inhalation, orally, intraparentally, etc.) evoke the immune response. Both the CMI and the humoral or one or the other immune response may be stimulated. Antigens can be *complete* or *incomplete.* A complete antigen can elicit an immune response and also react with the antibody (B cell system) or the sensitized lymphocyte (T cell system). The term *immunogen* is used interchangeably with antigen to mean a complete antigen. The primary criterion of an immunogen is its ability to induce an immune response. *Tolerogen* and *hapten* are also antigens but are not immunogens. A hapten by itself cannot elicit an immune response in a host but can react with an antibody to form soluble complexes. A hapten conjugated to an appropriate immunogenic carrier (an antigen such as bovine serum albumin, BSA) can elicit an immune response, however. A *tolerogen,* generally a monomeric form of an antigen, induces unresponsiveness (see Chapter 5) in the host. Thus the term *antigen* includes immunogen, tolerogen, and hapten. Antigens can also be characterized as T-dependent or T-independent, that is, requiring or lacking the intervention of T helper cell in the formation of humoral antibody by the B cell system. Whether an antigen is T-dependent or T-independent is determined by its physical and chemical composition. The factors determining immunogenicity, tolerogenicity and haptenic properties, the classes of antigens, and the chemical and physical basis of their antigenicity will now be discussed in detail.

Factors Determining Antigenicity

The antigenicity of a molecule is determined by a variety of factors and is dependent on the condition of the host system (both experimentally and naturally occurring). The nature and dosage of the antigen, the mode of administration, the animal being immunized, and the sensitivity of the methods of detection of the immune response are of importance in the evaluation of an immunogen. The many factors that confer antigenicity on various molecules are incompletely understood. Nevertheless, a variety of factors and certain conditions must be present in order

Table 4-1 : Some General Molecular Characteristics Affecting Antigenicity

Property	Effect on Antigenicity	Examples
Size		
small $\leqslant$ 3,000 daltons	Decrease Variable	Angiotensin Insulin
large $>$ 1 X 10^6 daltons	Increase	Viruses
Shape	None	Globular and fibrous proteins
Charge		
—75% to +75% range	None	Protamines, histones
High density	Decrease	sialic acids
Tyrosine	Variable	Dependent on other factors of antigen
Metabolizability	Decrease	Gelatin readily metabolized
Particulate (aggregation)	Increase	Immunoglobulin, microorganisms
Accessibility	Increase	Synthetic polymers
Foreignness	Generally increase	Dependent on recipient
Complexity	Increase	Microorganisms, proteins, tertiary structures

for a molecule to be immunogenic (summarized in Table 4-1)

Foreignness

The immune system is capable of discriminating *self* from *nonself* in such a way that only molecules that are unrecognizable-as-self (foreign) are immunogenic. Thus, the greater the distance is in phylogenic relationship between antigen and hosts, and the more foreign the molecule, the better the resultant immunogen. For example, purified albumin obtained from a rabbit and administered to the same rabbit (autologous system) or given to another rabbit (homologous system) will not be capable of evoking an immune response (nonimmunogenic). This is true provided the albumin has not been altered in any way by the fractionation procedure. This same albumin administered to any other higher vertebrate animal is likely to elicit a substantial number of antibodies, depending on the total dose of the antigen, the frequency of injection, and the route of administration.

Complexity

An antigen must have a certain degree of chemical complexity in order to be immunogenic. The requirement of chemical complexity in immunogens has been established by studies with synthetic polypeptides and by structural information on naturally occurring compounds. For example, synthetic homopolymers

Fig. 4-1 : A. Homo-
polymer; B. copoly-
mer synthetic
polypeptide antigens.

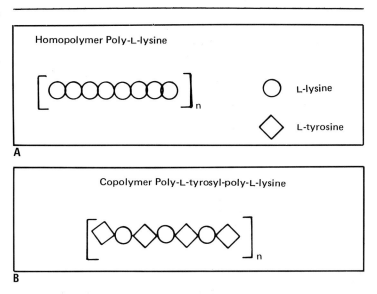

Fig. 4-1 : A. Homopolymer; B. copolymer synthetic polypeptide antigens.

consisting of repeated units of the same amino acid are poor immunogens irrespective of their molecular size. On the other hand, copolymers with repeating units of two or three different amino acids tend to be better immunogens. Figure 4-1 illustrates homopolymer and copolymer polypeptide chains. Aromatic amino acids in conjunction with other amino acids tend to increase the immunogenicity of a molecule. For example, molecules containing tyrosine are better immunogens in general than non-tyrosine-containing molecules. The generally accepted rule is that immunogenicity increases with complexity of the molecule.

Molecular Size

The size of the compound is of significance in determining the immunogenicity of the molecule. In general, macromolecular compounds are excellent immunogens (greater than 100,000 daltons). The arbitrary molecular weight threshold for immunogenicity appears to be around 100,000 daltons. Nevertheless, many compounds in the 2500 and 5000 dalton category have been shown to be immunogenic. The A- and B-chains of insulin (2500 daltons) and glucagon (3600 daltons) have each been shown to be immunogenic in guinea pigs. Low molecular weight compounds such as amino acids, fatty acids, purine and pyrimidine bases, and monosaccharides are in general incapable of inducing the immune response. These compounds, however, can act as haptens when appropriately coupled to immunogenic carriers such as macromolecular proteins and synthetic copolymers of amino acids. Some of these haptens are presented in Table 4-2. Haptenic property and immunodeterminants will be explained in the paragraphs to follow. The immunogenicity of a compound is dependent on other factors: size (molecular weight) is only one factor. Table 4-2 summarizes some of the immunogenic

**Table 4-2 : Relative Degree of Antigenicity of Compounds
on the Basis of Molecular Weight**

Compounds	Molecular MW (daltons)	Relative Antigenicity
Amino acids	$\leqslant 1 \times 10^2$	None
Fatty acids	$\leqslant 1 \times 10^2$	None
Purines and pyrimidines	$\leqslant 2 \times 10^2$	None
Monosaccharides	$\leqslant 2 \times 10^2$	None
Insulin		
A chain	2.5×10^3	Weak
B chain	2.5×10^3	Weak
Glucagon	3.6×10^3	Weak
Albumins	6.9×10^4	Good
Globulins	1.5×10^5	Good
Hemocyanins	6 to 8×10^6	Very good
Virus (tobacco mosaic virus)	7×10^7	Very good

compounds and their relative degree of immunogenicity on the basis of molecular weight.

Charge

Examination of the effect of the net charge of molecules of the antigens has revealed that charge is essentially not a significant requirement for immunogenicity. A series of studies employing synthetic copolymers (glutamic acid-lysine, and glutamic acid-lysine–tyrosine), in which the glutamic acid and lysine residues were varied and the immunization schedule and dosages kept constant, showed that the best immunogens fell in the range of -75 to $+75$ percent net charge density. Within this range the charge had no effect on the amount of antibodies formed. Polypeptides with 0 net charge elicited antibody responses comparable to the range cited (-75 to $+75$ percent). Nevertheless, excessively charged molecules tend to suppress antibody synthesis. Furthermore, excessively charged molecules, either positive or negative, tend to react with other compounds readily and thus diminish their accessibility to the immunocytes (immune cells). The naturally occurring glycoproteins with numerous neuraminic acid residues tend to be poor immunogens; however, removal of these acid residues with the enzyme neuraminidase enhances the immunogenicity of the glycoproteins. Thus, removal of neuraminic acid residues from a purified preparation of α_1 serum glycoprotein elicited an increase in anti-α_1-glycoprotein synthesis in rabbits immunized with the neuraminidase-treated serum α_1-glycoprotein.

Conformation The spatial folding of native proteins plays a significant role in the determination of their immunogenic specificity. This is aptly shown in the lack of cross-reactivity between denatured proteins and the antibodies to the same proteins in their native form. For example, antibodies to native pepsinogen have diminished reactivity to denatured pepsinogen or pepsin. Similar results can be demonstrated with albumin, immunoglobulin, myoglobulin, lysosome, hemoglobin, etc.

The *sequential* antigenic determinant consists of amino acids in sequence in a random coil, and antibodies to such a determinant are expected to react with peptides of identical or of similar sequence. A *conformational* antigenic determinant, on the other hand, is dependent on the steric conformation of the antigenic molecule and evokes antibodies that will not react with the peptides of the same sequence derived from that same region of the antigenic determinant unless the peptides have a similar conformation or coil. It appears that antibodies to native proteins are directed mostly to conformational rather than sequential determinants. Thus, the secondary, tertiary, and quaternary structures appear to be of primary importance in the immunogenic specificity of native proteins.

The significance of structural conformation in immunogenic specificity is underlined by results obtained from synthetic copolymers with defined sequence and conformation. Two copolymers with the same tripeptide determinant, although with different conformations, are shown in Figure 4–2: one copolymer has the tripeptide, L-tyrosyl-L-alanyl-L-glutamic acid, attached to the terminal residue of a multi-poly-DL-alanyl-poly-L-lysine (DL-alanine chain with short L-lysine side chains) (75,000-dalton multichain); and the other has the tripeptide in the polymerized form (100,000 daltons) as an α-helix under physiological conditions. The branched polymer in Figure 4–2A is an example of an immunogen with sequential determinants. Both polymers are good immunogens and can elicit antibodies in rabbits. There are no cross-reactions between the two immunogens and their homologous antibodies, however. The tripeptide L-tyrosyl-L-alanyl-L-glutamic acid inhibits the reaction between the branched polymer and its corresponding antibody, but not between the α-helix polymer and its homologous antibody. The immunogenic specificity of the copolymer made up of the α-helix tripeptide (Figure 4–2B) resides entirely in the region regulated by the α-helical structure of the polypeptide backbone. This is probably due to a particular juxtaposition of the amino acid chains in the rigid conformation of the α-helical macromolecule.

Antigenic molecules with β-conformational structures and with pleated-sheet configuration, like silk fibroin proteins, will con-

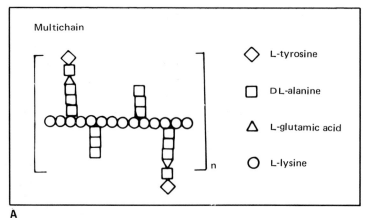

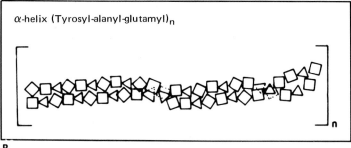

Fig. 4-2 : Synthetic multichain polypeptide. A. Sequence of tyrosyl-alanyl-glutamyl residues attached to amino terminal of DL-alanyl side chains. B. The same tripeptide as periodic copolymer. (Modified and adapted from M. Sela, Effect of Antigenic Structure on Antibody Bio-synthesis. In S. Kochwa and H. G. Kunkel (Eds.). Immunoglobulins: Biologic Aspects and Clinical Uses. Washington, D.C.: National Academy of Science, 1971.)

tribute to their immunogenic specificity. Table 4-3 presents some of the native proteins and their conformational structure.

Accessibility

Immunopotency is the capacity of a region of an antigen to serve as an antigenic determinant to evoke the formation of specific antibodies in the immunocytes. The immunopotency of the antigenic determinant site is dependent on the accessibility and charge of the antigen and on genetic factors of the host. In addition, it is a measure of the quantitative strength of an antigenic determinant.

The immunogenicity of a molecule is recognized by the host according to how accessible the antigenic determinants of the molecule are to the immunocytes involved in the immune response. Accessibility is dependent on the solubility of the

Table 4-3 : Some Antigenic Proteins and Their Structures

Proteins	Structure (Configuration/Conformation)
α-keratins	α-helix
β-keratins	β-conformation (pleated sheet)
Silk fibroins	β-conformation (pleated sheet)
Myoglobulin (sperm whale)	70% α-helix, 8 segments of polypeptide chains, no β-conformation
Lysozyme	Some α-helix
Cytochrome C	Few α-helix, some extended β-conformation
Ribonuclease	β-conformation; relatively little α-helix
Chymotrypsin	β-conformation; few α-helix

immunogen in aqueous medium. The conformation or spatial arrangement and position of the antigenic determinant in the macromolecule also plays an important role. For example, the nature and positions of the terminal residues of blood group substances, which specify ABO blood groups, are of importance in the expression of the immunochemical specificity of these molecules (see Chapter 11). Synthetic polymers provide another example. Multichain synthetic polymers with D-alanine$_n$ on the outside and tyrosine attached to the backbone on the inside (Figure 4-3B) evoke antibodies specific for anti-D-alanine; and polymers with D-alanine$_n$ attached to the backbone on the outside (Figure 4-3A) evoke antibodies specific for anti-tyrosine.

In sperm whale myoglobulin it is shown that peptides of 3 to 5 amino acids, which occupy the corners of the molecule, are important in immunochemical specificity. The three-dimensional structure of the sperm whale myoglobulin has been elucidated, and the corners are known to be the most prominently exposed (accessible) (Figure 4-4). Analysis of the structure of flagella of *Salmonella* shows that the smallest unit (flagellin, 40,000 daltons) consists of four pieces, fragments A, B, C, and D. This is demonstrated following treatment of the flagellin with cyanogen bromide.

Fragment A (18,000 daltons) contains the specific antigenic determinants and appears to be the surface exposed or accessible to the external medium.

The internal sequences of proteins and polysaccharides (masked regions) are precluded from exposure to immunocytes, since these molecules can be digested. However, antibodies elicited to the masked regions may not react with the native molecules in in vitro immunological tests unless these internal sequence regions are exposed by alteration of the native antigen.

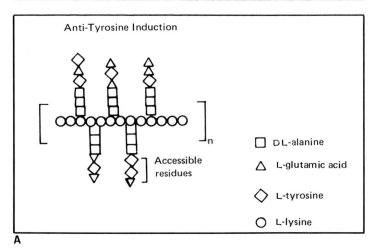

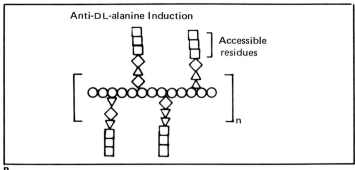

Fig. 4-3 : Examples of accessibility of antigenic determinants of copolymer synthetic polypeptides. A. The accessible dominant residue is tyrosine in the determinant. B. The accessible dominant residue is DL-alanine in the determinant. (Modified and adapted from M. Sela, Effect of Antigenic Structure on Antibody Biosynthesis. In S. Kochwa and H. G. Kunkel (Eds.). Immunoglobulins: Biologic Aspects and Clinical Uses. Washington, D.C.: National Academy of Science, 1971.)

Immunodominance and Optical Configuration

In a given antigenic determinant (generally a tetrapeptide for proteins, and having 3 to 5 residues for other molecules), the residues in the determinant will contribute unequally to the induction of an immune response and to reactivity with the antibody elicited. Thus, the quantitative degree of reactivity is a measure of the immunodominance of the residues in the antigenic determinant. Examples of the immunodominant regions of antigenic determinants are shown in Figure 4-5.

Immunodominance is dependent on the conformation, accessibility, and optical configuration of the antigenic determinant. An example of optical configuration is the remarkable display of pronounced stereospecificity of antibodies to D and L isomers. In general, antibody to D-amino acid determinants will not cross-

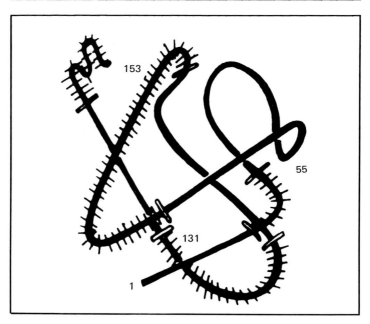

Fig. 4-4 : Schematic line drawing of sperm whale myoglobulin poly-peptide chain. Accessible immunodeterminant sites on the polypeptide are marked by lines across the schematic structure. (Modified and adapted from M. Z. Atassi and B. J. Saplin, Immunochemistry of sperm-whale myoglobulin. I. The specific interaction of some tryptic peptides and of peptides containing all the reactive regions of the antigen. Biochemistry 4:688, 1968.)

react with L-amino acid determinants. Thus, there is little or no cross-reactivity between enantiomorphic determinants. In some instances D-amino acids may be more immunodominant than their stereoisomers. Immunological stereospecificity has also been demonstrated between antigenic determinants with cis- and trans-haptenic molecules.

Soluble and Particulate Antigens

Soluble antigens can be defined as those immunogens in aqueous phase from viruses (colloidal) to small molecular weight compounds (haptens). Particulate antigens are those complex immunogens, such as bacteria, fungi, erythrocytes, viruses, and tissue cells that are chemically considered as suspensions in aqueous medium. Particulate immunogens are complex and consist of proteins, polysaccharides, lipids, and nucleic acids. For example, *Pneumococcus* has been shown to elicit antibodies in rabbits to capsular polysaccharides (type-specific), C polysaccharides (somatic), nucleoproteins, proteins, and glycolipids. Similarly, the number of antigens in erythrocytes is enormous.

The lipids and nucleic acids in particulate antigens, when extracted and purified, are unable by themselves to evoke immune

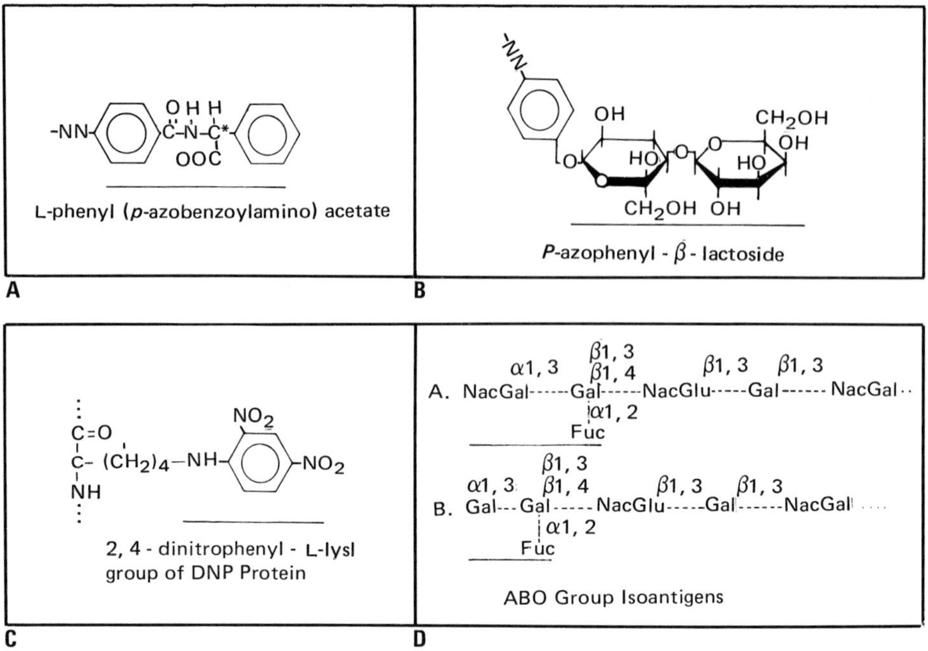

L-phenyl (p-azobenzoylamino) acetate

A

P-azophenyl - β - lactoside

B

2, 4 - dinitrophenyl - L-lysl
group of DNP Protein

C

A. NacGal------Gal------NacGlu------Gal------NacGal··
   α1, 3 β1, 3 / β1, 4   β1, 3   β1, 3
                α1, 2
                Fuc

B. Gal---Gal-----NacGlu-----Gal------NacGal ....
   α1, 3 β1, 3 / β1, 4   β1, 3   β1, 3
              α1, 2
              Fuc

ABO Group Isoantigens

D

Fig. 4-5 : Examples of the immunodominant region of haptenic molecules. The structural elements of the hapten or an amino acid of the determinant group that project distally from the central mass of the antigen are immunodominant (underlined).

responses but can act as antigenic determinants as part of the fragment from the original cells. Thus, purified lipids and nucleic acids have been shown to inhibit immunological agglutination or precipitin reactions between the antibodies and the original particulate antigens from which they were derived. These purified low molecular weight compounds can act as haptens.

Metabolizability

The ability of the host to remove and metabolize a given antigen plays an important part in determining whether the antigen becomes immunogenic, tolerogenic, or nonimmunogenic. Obviously all the properties discussed in the preceding paragraphs will contribute to the ultimate fate of an antigen. Some antigens can be readily and rapidly metabolized by normal bodily processes and hence require no intervention of the immune system. Other antigens, due to their physicochemical properties (molecular size, conformation, solubility, accessibility, etc.), persist in the circulation—either as nonmetabolizable entities or through slow metabolization behaving as self antigens and thus acting as tolerogens. These tolerogens bind to immunocytes and through appropriate receptors on B or T cells render these cells inactive. One way to test for metabolizability is to label the antigen with ^{125}I or other radioisotopes and measure the half-life and clearance

Table 4-4 : Examples of T-Independent Antigens

Antigen	Molecular Weight Rendering Antigenicity	Responsive Species
Pneumococcal polysaccharides	$>18,000$ $>75,000$	Mouse Man
Dextrans	$>90,000$	Man
Polyvinylpyrrolidone (PVP)	$24,000 - 360,000$ $\cong 1 \times 10^6$	Mouse Man
Lipopolysaccharide (LPS: gram-negative bacteria)	$1 \times 10^6 - 1 \times 10^7$	Mouse, man

rate from the blood circulation of the experimental animal. Various aspects of ^{125}I-labeled antigens in circulation, their fate, and immune responses to them are discussed in Chapter 5.

Classes of Antigens   This section discusses the various aspects of the naturally occurring chemical compounds and their ability (or lack of it) to elicit an immune response, either humoral or cell-mediated, in an appropriate host. Since the revelation of the dichotomy of the immune system and of the necessary interaction of macrophages, T cells, and B cells in the immune response (see chapter 5), immunogens have been separated into T-independent and T-dependent antigens. T-independent immunogens can activate B cells directly via appropriate receptors and messages and induce the cells to undergo transformation to blast cells and thence to plasma cells for synthesis and elaboration of humoral antibodies—this, presumably, without the intervention of the T cells. In contrast, T-dependent immunogens require the intervention of T cells (T helper cell)—possibly for transmission of a second message to the B cell through stimulation of appropriate T cell receptors. The B cell is also activated through its receptor (Ig) to the T-dependent antigen. The B cell receiving the signal from the T cell then undergoes blast transformation to a plasma cell for antibody synthesis and elaboration. Thus, in the absence of the T helper cells, humoral antibody synthesis by B cells will not occur with T-dependent immunogens. However, in some instances, polynucleotides have shown helper function. Examples of T-independent antigens are present in Table 4-4. These immunogens include polyvinylpyrrolidone (PVP), pneumococcal polysaccharides, and the lipopolysaccharides of gram-negative bacteria.

Chemical Classes and   The chemical classes considered here include both small and
Antigenicity   macromolecular naturally occurring compounds (proteins, poly-

saccharides, lipids, nucleic acids [including polynucleotides] , and drugs).

PROTEINS. Proteins were recognized as antigens early in the history of immunology and thus have been used extensively in the study of the immune response, especially the serum proteins and their fractionated components. Investigations of the chemical basis of immunogenicity were among the earliest studies carried out on proteins. On the basis of these studies some of the chemical characteristics that affect the antibody response were delineated. The chemical complexity of proteins, however, has prevented the delineation of the finer details of antigenicity in the immune response.

A variety of proteins have been examined for their immunogenicity. For example, gelatin has been examined extensively, since it was shown to be essentially nonimmunogenic and contained no tyrosine residue. The chemical coupling of a tyrosine residue to gelatin transformed it to an immunogenic compound. Therefore it was assumed that the aromatic rings were of importance in the immunogenicity of proteins. This, however, is not necessarily true, since addition of phenylisocyanate or benzoic acid to gelatin does not convert it to an immunogen. Gelatin's lack of immunogenicity may be attributable to metabolizability. Furthermore a compound such as insulin, with 12 percent tyrosine residues, is not a good immunogen but is rather weak or, in some hosts, nonimmunogenic. Some proteins retain their immunogenicity following removal of tyrosine residues, while others lose it. Thus, the immunogenicity of proteins is complex and is governed by a number of physicochemical considerations (see Table 4-1). The difficulty of manipulating the discrete portions of protein structures has contributed to our inability to understand the specific structural immunogenicity requirements of proteins. Attempts at chemical manipulation, particularly removal of the specific functional groups such as NH_2, SH, OH, and COOH, generally alter the molecular properties of the protein so drastically that immunogenicity is no longer retained. One approach has been to add functional groups to a poor immunogen, such as gelatin. Such studies have been attempted by many investigators; the results are summarized in Table 4-5. Attachment of carbohydrate residues had no effect on the immunogenicity of gelatin. The aromatic residues alone and in combination with the sugar residues increased the gelatin's immunogenic quality. However, the aromatics phenylisocyanate and benzoate had no effect. Enhancement was not restricted to aromatics alone, since aromatic amino acids and combinations of these also increased the immunogenic capacity

Table 4-5 : Effect on the Antigenicity of Gelatin of Chemical Modification with Various Compounds

Increase	No Effect
Arabinose-tyrosine	Arabinose
Cellulose-glycol-tyrosine	Cellulose-glycol
Aromatic ring–diazonium	Benzoic acid
D- and L-tyrosine	Phenylisocyanate
Tyrosine–glutamic acid	Glutamic acid
Phenylalanine	Alanine
Methionine	Serine
Lysine–glutamic acid	Lysine

of gelatin. The major factor governing immunogenicity in proteins is their conformation. Thus, the antigenic determinants of proteins are regulated to a large extent by their secondary, tertiary, and quaternary structures.

CARBOHYDRATES. The term *carbohydrate* encompasses all the sugars and saccharides including the monosaccharides and the polysaccharides (the homo- and heteropolysaccharides). Our discussions will be concerned primarily with the polysaccharides. The mono- and disaccharides will be touched on in discussion of haptens and the immunogenic determinants of carbohydrates. As immunogens, polysaccharides (like PVP, endotoxins, and lipopolysaccharides) of gram-negative microorganisms are considered T-independent antigens, requiring essentially no T helper cell intervention. Polysaccharides as immunogens evoke the synthesis of the IgM class of antibodies.

Unlike the case with proteins, the molecular weight or size of carbohydrates appears to be of significance to their immunogenic properties. Carbohydrate immunogenicity in man has been associated with carbohydrates of molecular weights of 75,000 to 100,000 or greater. Studies with dextrans given to humans have shown a lack of immunogenic consistency at molecular weights of less than 51,000. Hence monosaccharides and disaccharides are nonimmunogenic. The question of immunogenicity is based on the analysis of antibodies by standard conventional immunological procedures and is essentially not based on the more sensitive radioimmunoassay or enzyme-linked immunoadsorbent assays.

The natural heavy molecular weight polysaccharides studied in great detail are the pneumococcal type-specific capsular materials. They have been shown to elicit humoral immune responses in humans, rabbits, and mice when given in small amounts. The

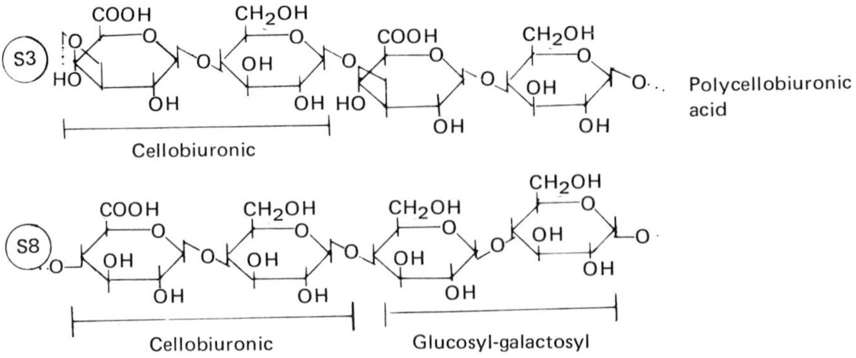

Fig. 4–6 : Antigenic residues of pneumococcal polysaccharides S3 and S8. The S3 residue is polymeric cellobiuronic acid and the S8 residues are alternating cellobiuronic and glucose-galactose.

concentration of pneumococcal polysaccharide administered to rabbits and mice is critical. Excessive amounts generally lead to immunological paralysis (see Chapter 10). Highly purified pneumococcal polysaccharides and penicilloylated dextran have induced delayed hypersensitivity in random-bred guinea pigs. Enhanced antibody synthesis in rabbits to pneumococcal polysaccharides per se can be evoked by complexing it to serum albumins. In this regard pneumococcal polysaccharides are similar to D-amino acid and vinyl polymers.

Highly purified mixtures of fourteen types of pneumococcal polysaccharides are being used for vaccination, particularly in sickle cell anemia patients, who are highly susceptible to pneumonia caused by pneumococcus. The vaccine is also used in areas of potentially antibiotic-resistant variants of *Streptococcus pneumoniae.*

Purified blood group substances, primarily with specific blood group polysaccharide antigens (see Chapter 11), are immunogenic in man and rabbit. Other purified carbohydrates known to be immunogenic in man and animals include dextran, levan, teichoic acid, and the high molecular weight meningococcal group A and somatic group C polysaccharides. Figure 4–6 illustrates the structural segment of two immunogenic pneumococcal polysaccharides.

LIPIDS. Lipids are low molecular weight compounds with high flexibility and thus have been found generally to be nonimmunogenic. Exceptions may be found in glycolipids, that is, natural compounds containing lipids covalently linked to polysaccharides. An example of this is the purified glycolipid from *Mycoplasma pneumoniae,* which appears to be a weak immunogen. In most lipopolysaccharides, such as endotoxin, the antibody elicited invariably reacts with the core carbohydrate or monosaccharide residues rather than with the lipids. Antibodies to low molecular weight lipids are generally obtained when the lipids are complexed with serum proteins or red blood cells. Thus antibodies to cytolipin H (from human epidermoid carcinoma) and to globosides of human erythrocytes have been obtained by conjugation to synthetic polypeptide in the former and by complexing to bovine serum in the latter case. The antibody to cytolipin H was directed primarily against the lactose portion of the molecule. Similarly, the antibodies to globoside were directed primarily against the carbohydrate portion. Nevertheless, in both cases antibodies to part of the lipid moieties were also present. As in the case of proteins, enhanced immunological reactivity can be shown when the lipid portion of globoside is aggregated into larger micelles. The lack of immunogenicity of purified low molecular weight lipids is also reflected by their predilection to bind to a wide variety of other molecules and their resultant inability to react independently to stimulate the immunocytes.

No phospholipid has as yet been shown to be immunogenic. It is of interest, however, that the phosphorylcholine residue associated with phosphatidylcholine (lecithin) is an antigenic determinant for IgA myeloma proteins, as demonstrated in mice. Whether phospholipids are immunogenic in these animals has not been resolved. Phosphorylcholine residue is also a common constituent of pneumococcal somatic C polysaccharide. The haptenic characteristic of lipids has been determined. The lipids include phosphatidylinositol, ceramide lactoside, ganglioside, prostaglandins, bile salts, and steroids and are conjugated to synthetic copolymer or protein carriers through covalent conjugation or by complexing with methylated bovine serum albumin. Such conjugations have been the basis for the development of radioimmunoassay (RIA) for detection of low concentration of lipids in tissues and serum. Prostaglandins and steroids have been examined by these RIA procedures in clinical medicine.

NUCLEIC ACIDS AND POLYNUCLEOTIDES. In the serum of patients with systemic lupus erythematosus (SLE) significant levels of antibodies to double-stranded DNA and RNA may be found. The levels of antibodies will vary according to the severity and nature of the disease. The anti-DNA antibody can be demonstrated by counterelectrophoresis or by a more sensitive radioimmunoassay using labeled DNA. The anti-DNA antibody can react with both native and denatured DNA. The anti-RNA antibody has been shown to react with RNA, double-stranded viral RNA, ribosomes, and the single-stranded polynucleotides of inosine, adenosine, and guanosine. These antibodies (anti-DNA and anti-RNA) in SLE patients have been identified by indirect immunofluorescence using heterologous tissue nucleus as substrates. By the nature of the immunofluorescent patterns the anti-DNA may be differentiated from anti-RNA. Similar spontaneous anti-DNA and anti-RNA antibodies have been found in NZB/NZW mice.

In spite of these findings in SLE patients, neither purified nucleic acids nor purified polynucleotides have been shown to evoke antibody responses in experimental animals. However, denatured DNA and oligonucleotides complexed with methylated bovine serum albumin (MeBSA) have been reported to elicit antibodies. In addition, double-stranded polynucleotides complexed with MeBSA have elicited antibodies in experimental animals. These antibodies reacted with homologous double-stranded polynucleotides or nucleic acids and with single-stranded polynucleotides or nucleic acids. Anti-RNA antibodies can be elicited by immunization with ribosomes. Through appropriate coupling to carriers, proteins, or synthetic copolymers, antibodies to small oligonucleotides or nucleotide bases can be produced. These antinucleotide antibodies will react with single-stranded polynucleotides and with heat-denatured nucleic acids.

Thus the purified nucleic acids and polynucleotides by themselves appear to be nonimmunogenic, but when complexed with MeBSA or coupled covalently to protein or synthetic copolymer carriers, they elicit antibody synthesis in experimental animals. In SLE the initiation of anti-DNA and anti-RNA antibodies remains an enigma, although the formation of denatured nucleic acid or DNA and their complexing with autologous proteins is a likely explanation for the elicitation of increased antibodies. In many respects the immunogenicity of nucleic acids and polynucleotides resembles that of lipids. Additionally, the degradation of DNA and RNA by serum and tissue nucleases may contribute to its lack of immunogenic properties.

DRUGS AND CHEMICALS. Small molecular weight compounds and drugs have demonstrated their ability to evoke an immune response in man and animals (guinea pig and rabbit). Table 4-6 summarizes some of the compounds reported. Arsphenamine and neoarsphenamine were used earlier in the treatment of syphilis. Patients on therapy with these drugs have demonstrated typical allergic symptoms, including serum sickness type symptoms (see Chapter 13), exfoliative dermatitis, skin eruptions, and

Table 4-6 : Chemicals and Drugs Shown to Have Antigenicity

Compound	MW (daltons)	Type of Cell Involved and Responsive Animal
Arsphenamine	367	B and T cells, guinea pig
Neoarsphenamine	466	B and T cells, guinea pig
Aminopyrine	231	B cell, man
Penicillin	350	B cell, man
Aspirin	180	B and T cells, guinea pig B cell, man
Sedormid (allylisopropylacetylurea)	184	B cell, man
Poison ivy (3-N-pentadecylcatechol)	320	T cell, man
Catechols	120–320	T cell, man
Picric acid	229	T cell, man
Picryl chloride	248	T cell, man
Quinine	324	T cell, man

systemic anaphylaxis. Neoarsphenamine appears to be immuno-genic per se, since conjugation to proteins and subsequent administration to rabbits elicited no immune response. Neoarsphenamine appears to behave similarly to that of N-2,4–dinitro-phenyl-L-tyrosine-AZO benzine-p-arsonate (DNP-RAT). The latter, a synthetic compound, elicits an humoral response to DNP, the hapten, while the RAT residue, containing arsenate, stimulates the T cells. Increasing the distance between the DNP molecule and the arsenic molecule by addition of single or triple 6-aminocaproic acid residues (DNP-SAC-RAT) had no effect on the antigenicity. However, the anti-DNP response was weaker when the determinants were joined without spacers. Figure 4–7 gives the structures of the arsenic compounds and of DNP-RAT.

Other drugs stimulating the humoral responses are aspirin, penicillin, aminopyrine, and Sedormid. Sedormid binds to platelet and acts as a hapten to elicit antibody synthesis. It also interferes with the synthesis of the enzyme catalase in liver and red cell precursors. The antibody agglutinates only platelets complexed with Sedormid, since removal of the drug shows no aggregation of platelets with the antibody. Patients receiving Sedormid tend to develop thrombocytopenia. Contact with poison ivy evokes a delayed type of skin hypersensitivity. Individuals susceptible to the reactive compound 3-N-pentadecyl-catechol in poison ivy should avoid contact with the plant. A severe pruritic reaction can be unbearable. The catechols, which are oxidized to quinones, readily complex with proteins; this

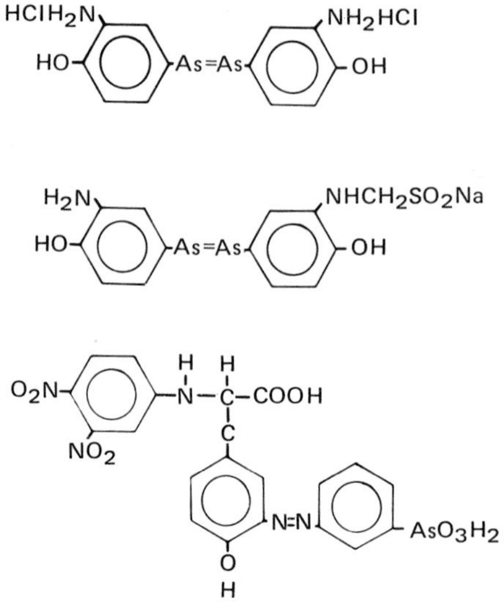

4,4′-Arseno-bis-(2 aminophenol), dihydrochloride

[5-[(3-amino-4-hydroxyphenyl) arseno]-2-hydroxyanilino 1 methanol] sulfoxylate, sodium

N-2, 4-Dinitrophenyl-L-tyrosine azobenzene-*p*-arsonate

Fig. 4-7 : Haptens of arsenic compounds and DNP-RAT. DNP-RAT demonstrates the effect on antibody induction by separation of the DNP (reacts with B cell) and arsenic (reacts with T cell) groups with L-tyrosine.

might account for their immunogenicity. A similar mechanism probably occurs with picric acid, picryl chloride, quinine, and quinidine.

Chemical Basis of Antigenicity

The delineation of the immunogenicity of proteins, carbohydrates, viruses, bacteria, etc., has been greatly helped by two major areas of study: 1) the early work of Landsteiner, who used chemical covalent coupling of compounds to carrier proteins and thus altered the immunogenicity of the carrier and demonstrated the immunogenicity of the low molecular weight chemical—a hapten (a term introduced by Landsteiner in 1921); (2) recent studies with synthetic immunogens, which have extensively increased our understanding of what makes a compound immunogenic.

Covalent Coupling Studies

HAPTENS. Since the development of coupling procedures, the importance of haptens in the analysis of antigenicity has been immeasurable. Haptens are low molecular weight free compounds isolated from animals and microbes or may be synthetic low-dalton (MW) chemicals. Although active in the in vitro immunological tests, they elicit no humoral or CMI responses when administered by the usual immunization procedures. Thus a hapten can be any substance, small or large, that does not induce an immunological response by itself but that can induce a response when coupled chemically to an appropriate carrier immunogenic protein or synthetic polymer. A hapten can also

Table 4-7 : Representative Haptens, Molecular Weights, and Method of Conjugation to Carriers

Hapten	MW (daltons)	Method of Conjugation
Hormones: peptide		
Adrenocorticotropic		
hormone (ACTH)	3,500	Carbodiimide
Angiotensins	1,019 and 1,295	Carbodiimide or toluene
I and II		diisothiocyanate
Gastrin	12,514	''
Bradykinin	1,060	''
Hormones: nonpeptide		
Histamine	111	Nucleophilic substitution
		and diazo-coupling
Prostaglandin E_1	334	Carbodiimide
Cyclic AMP	347	Succinylation and
		carbodiimide
Cyclic GMP	363	''
Folic acid	441	Carbodiimide
Barbiturates	124-184	''
Digoxin	781	Periodate oxidation
Methotrexate	454	Carbodiimide
Sulfonamide	172	Diazo-coupling
Toxins		
Arsphenamide	377	Diazo-coupling
Aminofluorene	181	Isocyanate derivative and
		coupled via carbamido linkage
DDT (1, 1, 1-trichloro-2, 2-bis-	355	Anhydride and acyl
[p-chlorophenyl] ethane)		chloride reactions
C-peptide	3,000	Carbodiimide
Galactose, glucone	180	Azophenyl or azobenzyl
Epinephrine	183	Diazo-coupling
Phosphatidyl-inositol	~1,500	Complexing with methylated
		bovine serum albumin
Oligonucleotides	700-1,500	''
Gibberellic acid	346	Carbodiimide

react with a B cell or T cell sensitized system when stimulated by a complete antigen onto which it was previously attached. The range and number of haptens examined are phenomenal and encompass diverse compounds as simple as monosaccharides, peptides, aromatic chemicals, steroids, drugs, purine and pyrimidine bases, toxins, plant and animal hormones, lipids, and nucleic acids (Table 4-7).

METHODS OF COUPLING. The methods used in coupling haptens experimentally are dependent on the functional groups on the hapten as well as on the carrier protein. The functional groups of the carrier molecules to which haptens may be attached are summarized in Table 4-8. Some of the methods employed are discussed here and the chemical reactions are illustrated in Figure 4-8.

**Table 4-8 : Functional Groups of Carrier Molecules
to Which Haptens May Be Conjugated**

Functional Group		Amino Residue on Carrier
Amino	$-NH_2$	N-terminal AA, lysine
Carboxyl	$-COOH$	C-terminal AA, aspartic and glutamic acids
Guanidino	H₂N-C-N-R with H and NH	Arginine
Imidazo	HC=C-R, N, NH, C, H ring	Histidine
Indolyl	indole ring with R	Tryptophan
Phenolyic	R-⬡-OH	Tyrosine
Sulfhydryl	$-SH$	Cysteine

The study of haptens in immunology has contributed to our understanding of antigenic determinants, structural requirements for immunogenicity, the nature of antigen-antibody reactions (see chapter 7), and the chemical, physical, and biological properties of the antibody.

Diazotization. Diazotization (Figure 4-8A) of aromatic amines containing an NH_2 group is carried out with cold dilute nitrous acid. The diazonium salt formed is conjugated to the carrier protein in an alkaline solution. The most likely site of diazo bond formation to the carrier is the aromatic ring of tyrosine and histidine and the ε-group of lysine. Either a monosubstitution or a disubstitution may occur, depending on the diazonium salt concentration used. Diazo bonds may possibly be formed on tryptophan and arginine residues also. In the final analysis, however, the nature of diazo bond conjugation is dependent on the accessibility of the reactive groups. Preferentially at low diazo salt concentrations, tyrosine and histidine are generally the active sites of binding. Diazotization has been used to couple glycosides to aromatic-containing rings. For example, *p*-amino-phenylglycoside, following diazotization, was coupled to protein carriers and antiserum prepared to the oligosaccharide protein conjugate. Thus, the diazotization procedure is applicable to a wide variety of small molecular weight compounds for which derivatives of aromatic amines can be prepared.

Fig. 4-8 : Various chemical reactions for covalent coupling of haptenic groups to carriers. A. Diazotization. B. Nucleophilic substitution. C. Carbodiimide coupling. D. Azide coupling.

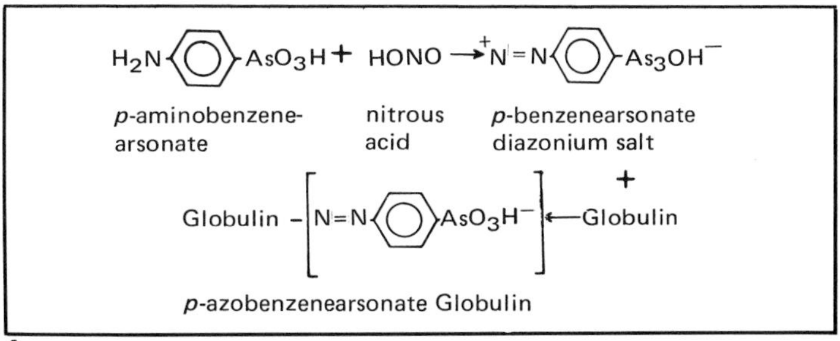

A

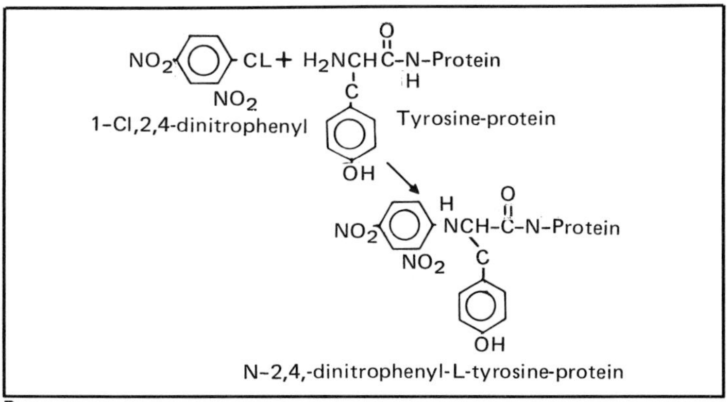

B

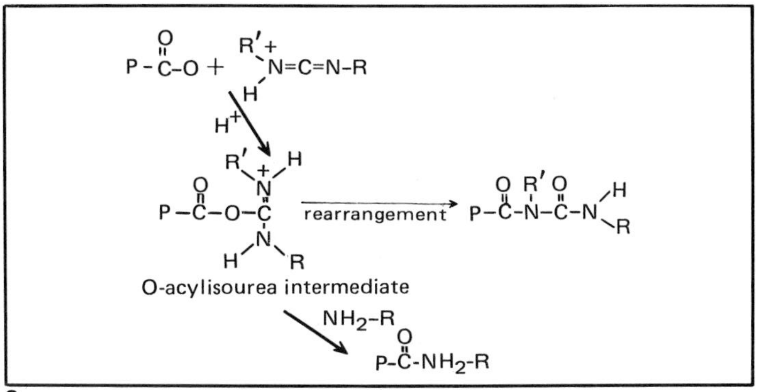

C

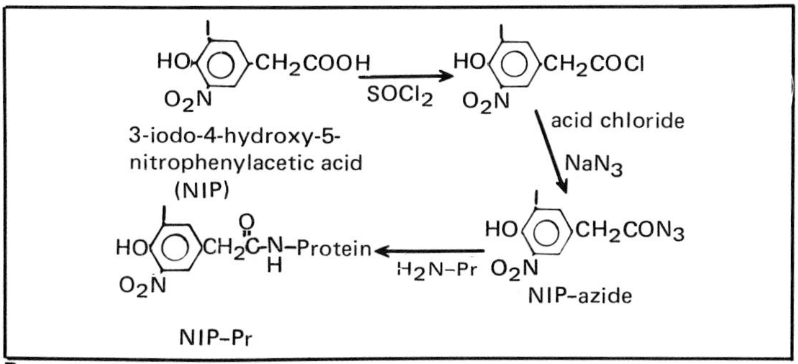

D

Nucleophilic Substitution. Among the haptens most widely used for examination of the chemical basis of immunogenicity, the sites and energy of antibody binding, and the receptor activation of B cell and T cell are the dinitrophenyl compounds. These include 2, 4-dinitrophenyl (DNP) and 2, 4, 6-trinitrophenyl (TNP). These compounds have proved of great value because of their intense and easily distinguishable absorption spectra, the stability of covalent bond they form, and especially because of their immunodominant characteristics on carriers which contribute to immunogenicity. DNP is attached to protein carriers through the nucleophilic substitution reaction, in which the active chlorine or fluorine residue is in position 1 of the benzene molecule. The halogen is activated by NO_2 groups in positions 2, 4, and 6.

The halogen is readily displaced by electron-donating groups of the protein carrier, e.g., the $-NH_2$ of lysine, the $-OH$ of tyrosine, and the $-SH$ of cystine. The chemical reaction of this mode of conjugation is shown in Figure 4-8B. As with diazo coupling, the DNP haptenic determinant is heterogenic; coupling is dependent on the position, number, and accessibility of the electron-donating residues on the carrier protein. Homogenic haptenic determinant can be achieved in some cases with use of a less reactive derivative, DNP-sulfonic acid. This compound tends to react essentially with the $-NH_2$ residue of lysine in the carrier molecule, an advantage being that it is soluble in aqueous solutions. The DNP residue can be quantitated spectrophotometrically at 360 nm, using the extinction coefficient of ϵ-DNP-lysine as standard. A variety of other ingenious coupling procedures have been designed for examining the haptenic nature of small molecular weight compounds, and more especially, for conducting diagnostic procedures in radioimmunoassay and enzyme-linked immunoabsorbent assay (ELISA) (see Chapter 7). Numerous specific antibodies to compounds such as ACTH, prostaglandins, cyclic nucleotides, and steroids have been prepared to these small molecular weight compounds, which have been rendered immunogenic on appropriate carriers.

Carbodiimide Coupling. Carbodiimide reagents are of particular value in coupling amines or carboxylic acid haptens to proteins. Those compounds with the general formula $R-N=C=N-R'$, where R and R' represent aryl and alkyl groups, react with amines or carboxylic acids to form peptide bonds via a condensation reaction are shown in Figure 4-8C, with the elimination of a substituted urea, $RNHC = ONHR'$. Aqueous soluble carbodiimide solutions are readily available and have been used to couple proteins to haptens containing NH_2 or COOH residues. For example, the conjugation of bradykinin (a nonapeptide) to carrier proteins has been achieved and specific antibodies to bradykinin elicited in rabbits. Many other peptides have been coupled to protein or polypeptide carriers with carbodiimide. These include ACTH, calcitonin, gastrin, and vasopressin. The method of coupling with insolubilized and water-soluble carbodiimides appears to be easily and simply applied, is versatile, and has found wide-ranging applications, especially where the formation of peptide, ester, thioester, or phosphoester bonds is required.

Azide Coupling. Haptenic groups can be introduced into proteins, erythrocytes, viruses, and other carriers via the azide derivatives. (Figure 4-8D). The most widely used family of compounds are 3-iodo-4-hydroxy-5-nitrophenyl-acetic acid (NIP) and related derivatives. The free carboxyl group of the hapten is transformed to an acid chloride derivative with thioryl chloride ($SOCl_2$). The acid chloride is then reacted with sodium azide (NaN_3) to yield crystals of reactive haptenic azide. This compound is stable if kept frozen ($-20°C$) and stored in dimethylformamide solution. The haptenic azide can then be coupled to a protein or cell. The internal spacer of the haptenic azide minimizes carrier effects such as steric hindrance and contribution to specificity. The NIP family of haptens has been used to examine the genetics of the immune responses in mice.

Thus, coupling studies of nonimmunogenic low molecular weight compounds have contributed an understanding of the chemical basis of immunogens and, more importantly, opened doors to the advancement of clinical medicine. This is evidenced by the development of RIA procedures for assessment of polypeptide hormones in man.

Synthetic Antigens

The advent of synthetic monopolymers (a single amino acid polymer) and copolymers (two or more different amino acids) has contributed immensely to the understanding of the immunogenicity of molecules. These synthetic polymers are capable of inducing antibody synthesis in rabbits and also of reacting in vitro or in vivo by the various immunological procedures. Thus, the synthetic polymers have contributed to our understanding of the significance of charge, conformation (shape), size, optical isomerism, accessibility, and size of the antigenic determinants.

How carriers contribute to the immunogenicity of haptens is not completely understood. Carriers may contribute to the specificity of the molecule by making the hapten a complete determinant, and adding to the increase in energy of the interaction of the hapten with the B cell receptor site. On the other hand, carriers may initiate an allosteric effect in the receptor, which could be transmitted as a signal throughout the immunocyte. The hapten would be serving as the *immunodominant* point toward which antibody specificity is directed, with the carrier completing the antigenic determinent. The carrier may also contribute to the metabolizability of the hapten-carrier and thus provide appropriate hapten-carrier fragments (antigenic determinants) of enhanced immunogenic specificity.

Physicochemical Analyses for Basis of Antigenicity

Prior to the advent of synthetic immunogens, immunologists attempted to determine the basis for immunogenicity by examining the physicochemical properties of naturally occurring immunogens. Protein in particular has been examined extensively as an immunogen. Two methods have been used: (1) careful dissection of the immunogen (degradation studies) and (2) denaturation of proteins through physical and chemical means in order to change their immunogenic properties.

Degradation Studies

As has been shown, proteins consist of many antigenic determinants, which elicit high levels of antibody of varying specificities. These determinants therefore are designated *immunopotent* in contrast to *immunosilent* ones that elicit no antibody response. The primary structure of proteins, which determines their three-dimensional configuration, and molecular shape, and the accessibility and region of their immunopotent determinants makes proteins useful immunogens for studying the effects of degradation. Protein specificities reside in their antigenic determinants, and proteins may contain several different determinants (multivalent). Enzymatic degradation of proteins in vitro with proteolytic enzymes such as trypsin, chymotrypsin, pepsin, and papain has been used extensively to assess immunogenicity and to carry out structural analysis of the protein molecules. Mild enzymatic hydrolysis of proteins to large subfragments generally permits these molecules to retain their antigenicity. A case in point is the studies of IgG digested with papain, as discussed in Chapter 2. In these fragments the basic conformation of the major components (Fc and $[Fab]_2$) is essentially retained, and thus their antigenicities remain intact.

In other proteins, such as ovalbumin, exhaustive digestion of the molecules with trypsin or pepsin to smaller peptides results in complete loss of immunogenicity. Depending on the size and sequence of the small peptides they may, however, retain their antigenic determinant properties and thus behave as haptens. In fibrous proteins, "pleated-sheet" structures consisting of repeating structural units, antigenic specificity may be largely retained even after enzymatic digestion. Here the immunizing power of the fragments may or may not be comparable to the intact molecule.

Degradation studies have contributed also to recognition of the structure of proteins, especially when sequence degradation of the protein is carried out and the amino acid sequence and composition are analyzed. Thus, degradation studies have shown the antigenic significance of the primary sequence of the residues and of the conformation and size of the molecules. Unraveling of the interior residues by inversion of the original conformational structure due to degradation results in loss of antigenicity of the original molecule.

Denaturation

As in degradation studies, the treatment of proteins with a variety of physical and chemical agents can result in loss of immunogenicity. Heat, ultraviolet radiation, acid, alkali, and alcohol, for example, tend to disrupt the primary structure, especially of the globular proteins, with consequent molecular alteration. This alteration leads to modifications of the antigenic properties, in part due to unmasking of new antigenic determinants. Alterations include disruption of the three-dimensional structure with unfolding and uncoiling of the polypeptide chains. Globular structures tend to elongate to fibrous structures and occasionally dissociate to smaller nonimmunogenic molecules.

Typical findings in physical and chemical denaturation studies of proteins indicate decreased immunogenicity and changes in antigenic specificities. The changes in antigenicity are generally attributed to unmasking of new antigenic determinants on the molecular surface. In some instances there is a correlation between degree of denaturation and immunogenicity. Antibodies prepared against denatured proteins react well with the corresponding denatured antigen and in general react poorly with the native protein. On the other hand, antibodies elicited against the intact protein generally show no immunological reaction against the same denatured protein.

Table 4-9 summarizes findings on the effect of degradation and denaturation and the consequences of these effects on the immunogenicity of proteins. The immunological effects of controlled enzymatic digestion are comparable in many respects with those of denaturation on protein molecules. They both alter immunogenicity of the native molecule.

Antigenic Determinants

Throughout the discussions in this chapter much has been said about the nature of antigenic determinants. These are the smallest integral unit that contributes to the immunochemical specificity of the antigenic molecules and are dependent on accessibility, conformation, size, and position on the antigenic molecule. Antigenic determinants are also associated with the immunopotency and immunodominance of the immunogen. Table 4-10 lists some of the antigenic determinants that have been identified in natural antigens and synthetic polymers.

Summary

1. Antigens are categorized as follows: *Immunogen* is an antigen capable of evoking an immune response in a host and also of

**Table 4-9 : The Effect of Degradation and Denaturation
on the Antigenicity of Proteins**

Protein	Treatment	Immunogenicity
Ovalbumin	Pepsin	Variable, depends on degree of digestion
Monomeric flagellin	Cyanogen bromide	Fragment A—positive Fragments B, C, and D— nonimmunogenic
Nonimmunogenic amyloid	Alkali	Fragment—increase
Rabbit and human IgG	Papain	Fragments Fc and (Fab)$_2$
Rabbit serum	Heat	Immunogenic in rabbit
Ovalbumin	Alkali	Nonimmunogenic
Bovine serum albumin	Urea	Decrease
Bovine serum albumin	Heat	Increase—loss of specificity
Proteins	Heat	Increase—loss of specificity
Ribonuclease	Alkali	Decrease
Ribonuclease	Reduction or oxidation	Nonimmunogenic
Serum albumin	Reduction	Loss of antigenic specificity

reacting with its specific antibody or lymphocyte. It is synonymous with a complete antigen. *Hapten* is defined as an antigenic determinant capable of reacting with its specific antibody or lymphocyte but incapable of evoking an immune response. It is an incomplete antigen. *Tolerogen* is a monomeric form (nonaggregated) of the antigen that renders the host unresponsive (tolerant) to its immunogenic form (aggregated Ag).

2. The terms *antigen* and *immunogen* have been used interchangeably, but antigen generally has a broader connotation and includes immunogen, tolerogen, and hapten.

3. The factors that determine antigenicity include the following: foreignness of antigen to host; complexity of the molecule (bacteria or virus versus bovine serum albumin); size, charge, and conformation of the molecule; accessibility of the determinants; immunodominance and optical configuration; whether the antigen is soluble or particulate; and digestibility of the molecule.

4. Antigens can be classified as T-dependent (requiring T and B cell interaction for evoking the immune response) or T-independent. The latter require no T helper or macrophage intervention for the immune response.

5. Proteins and carbohydrates are generally considered good immunogens, whereas lipids, nucleic acids, and drugs and

Table 4-10 : Minimal Sizes of Sequentially Defined Antigenic Determinants

Antigen	Determinant	Size Extended Form A	MW	No. of Residues	Antibody in Species
Dextran	Isomaltohexose	34 X 12 X 7	990	7	Man
Poly-γ-glutamic acid (*B. anthracis*)	Hexaglutamic acid	36 X 10 X 6	792	6	Rabbit
Synthetic polymers					
Glu_{60}-Ala_{40}	Hexaglutamic acid	36 X 10 X 6	792	6	Rabbit
Glu_{60}-Ala_{30}-Tyr_{10}	"	"	"	"	"
Glu_{42}-Lys_{28}-Ala_{10}	"	"	"	"	"
Polyalanyl-BSA	Pentalanine	25 X 11 X 6.5	373	5	Rabbit
Polylysyl-BSA	Penta-(or hexa-)lysine	27 X 17 X 6.5	659	6-7	Rabbit
Polylysyl phosphoryl-BSA	Pentallysine	27 X 17 X 6.5	659	6	Rabbit
DNA	Pentathymidylate	—	1210	5	Man (SLE)
α-2, 4-dinitrophenyl-poly-L-Lysine	α-2, 4 dinitrophenyl $lysine_3$	—	632	3	Guinea pig
Myoglobulin	3-5 Amino Acids	—	~300-500	3-5	Rabbit
$(D-Ala)_n$-gly-ribonuclease	$(D-ala)_n$-Gly (n = 1-4)	—	356	4	Rabbit

chemicals are poor immunogens. The poor immunogens can be rendered antigenic by conjugation covalently to protein or synthetic polymeric carriers. Structural conformation is important in protein antigenicity. Molecular weight is of importance in carbohydrate induction of the immune response. T-independent carbohydrate antigens and PVP generally stimulate IgM antibodies.

6. Methods of chemical and physical examination of the antigenicity of molecules include use of hapten-carrier conjugates, synthetic antigens of known constituents, degradation and denaturation studies of protein antigens, and studies of the nature and size of the antigenic determinants.

Bibliography and Selected Reading

General

Goodwin, J. W. Immunogenicity and Antigenic Specificity. In H. H. Fudenberg, D. P. Stiles, J. L. Caldwell, and J. V. Wells (Eds), *Basic and Clinical Immunology* (2nd Ed.). Los Altos, Calif. Lange 1978. Pp. 39–47.

Goodwin, J. W., Fong, S., Lewis, G. K., Kamin, R., Niteck, D. E., and Balian, G. D. Antigenic structure and lymphocyte activation, *Immunol. Rev.* 39:36–59, 1978.

Landsteiner, K. *The Specificity of Serological Reactions.* Cambridge, Mass.: Harvard Univ. Press, 1945.

Nossal, G. J. V., and Ada, G. L. *Antigens, Lymphoid Cells and the Immune Response.* New York and London: Academic, 1971.

Factors Determining Antigenicity

Atassi, M. Z., and Saplin, B. J. Immunochemistry of sperm-whale myoglobulin. I. The specific interaction of some tryptic peptides and of peptides containing all the reactive regions of the antigen. *Biochemistry* 4:688, 1968.

Borek, F. Molecular Size and Shape of Antigens. In F. Borek (Ed.), *Immunogenicity.* New York: American Elsevier, 1972. Pp. 45–86.

Butler, U. P., Jr., and Beiser, S. M. Antibodies to Small Molecules: Biological and Clinical Applications. In F. J. Dixon and H. G. Kunkel (Eds.), *Advances in Immunology,* Vol. 17, New York: Academic, 1973. Pp. 255–310.

Classes, Chemicals, and Physical Basis of Antigenicity

Gill, T. J. The Chemistry of Antigens and Its Influence on Immunogenicity. In F. Borek (Ed.), *Immunogenicity.* New York: American Elsevier, 1972. Pp. 5–44.

Kabat, E. A. The nature of an antigenic determinant. *J. Immunol.* 97:1–11, 1966.

Leskowitz, S. The Immune Response to Haptens. In F. Borek (Ed.), *Immunogenicity.* New York: American Elsevier, 1972. Pp. 131–154.

Sela, M. Antigenicity: Some molecular aspects. *Science* 166:1365–1374, 1969.

Sela, M. Effect of Antigenic Structure on Antibody Biosynthesis. In S. Kochwa, and H. G. Kunkel (Eds.). *Immunoglobulins. Ann. N. Y. Acad. Sci.* 190:181, 1971.

5 : The Immune Response

The immune response associated with the T cell-mediated system was discussed in Chapter 3. The present chapter covers the elaboration of antibodies by plasma cells through the B cell (humoral) system and that system's relationship to the T cell and macrophage systems.

The factors associated with the immune response are complex and include (1) interaction and association between macrophages and T and B cells in the induction of antibody synthesis by the B cells; (2) age of the animal host; (3) quantity and type of antigen (T-independent or T-dependent); (4) route of administration; (5) health status of the host; (6) immunopotentiation by drugs and adjuvants; and (7) genetic factors (Ir genes) that regulate the ability of the host to respond to antigens. The immunogenetics of the immune response will be discussed in detail in Chapter 10.

Mode of Antigen Administration

The route of administration of an antigen can influence the nature of the immune response of the host (Table 5-1). Topical skin applications of chemicals such as dinitrochlorobenzene and its derivatives tend to induce delayed type hypersensitivity. Natural exposure to exogenous antigens via the oral or nasal cavities stimulates secretory immunoglobulins IgA and IgE and occasionally IgM. Protein antigens administered directly into the mesentery or the thymus induce tolerance or unresponsiveness in the host. Various antigens (T-independent or T-dependent) given subcutaneously, intravenously, and intraperitoneally evoke synthesis of IgG, IgM, and IgA.

General Patterns of Antigen Metabolism

Soluble Protein Antigen

Injection of a soluble antigen such as bovine serum albumin (BSA) or gamma globulin (IgG) intravenously into a normal animal sets off a metabolic process exhibiting three sharply distinguishable phases. Figure 5-1A illustrates this process following the intravenous administration of labeled (^{125}I) soluble protein. A brief equilibrium phase (Phase a) with diffusion and entrapment of the antigen in the extravascular spaces is followed by a slower phase of metabolic degradation of the antigen (phase b) which is subsequently followed by rapid immune elimination

Table 5-1 : Route of Immunization and Most Common Immune Responses of the Host to the Antigen

Route	Antigens	General Response
Topical	Chemicals	Delayed hypersensitivity
Oral or nasal	Food, pollens	Secretory immunoglobulins A or E
Mesenteric or intrathymic	Proteins	Induction of tolerance: unresponsiveness
Common routes Subcutaneous Intravenous Intramuscular Intraperitoneal	Various	IgM, IgG, IgA

resulting from the fact that the antibody synthesized has formed soluble antigen-antibody complexes (phase c).

The Ag-Ab complexes in phase c are removed by the phagocytic cells (neutrophils and macrophages). It has been demonstrated that complexes formed with the whole antibody molecule are removed from peripheral blood much more rapidly and localize in tissues in larger amounts than complexes formed with the Fab fragment. This difference in removal has been shown to be three to tenfold faster. Thus, the Fc portion of the antibody appears to play an important role in clearance of the complexes. The Fc portion of the antibody is a target for Fc receptors on phagocytic cells (neutrophils and macrophages). Antibody is detectable in the peripheral blood near the end of the clearance of the Ag-Ab complexes (phase d). The constant linear curve characteristic of phase b (see Figure 5-1) is used to determine the half-life of the antigen administered. This portion of the curve varies with the molecular size and the physicochemical nature of the soluble antigen molecules. Table 5-2 summarizes the half-life of labeled soluble proteins administered to rabbits. Phase c, the immune complex clearance, can be used to assess the immune competence and response of an animal receiving an antigen.

Particulate Antigen   Particulate antigens (such as bacteria, erythrocytes, and large viruses) injected into animals are ingested by phagocytes and thus essentially do not diffuse into extravascular compartments. The initial equilibrium phase (phase a) exhibited by soluble antigens is generally absent. An example of this is shown in Figure 5-1B for tobacco mosaic virus (TMV) labeled with [131]I. Trace fragments of particulate antigens may persist in lymphoid tissues and liver long after the antigens are no longer detectable in the blood.

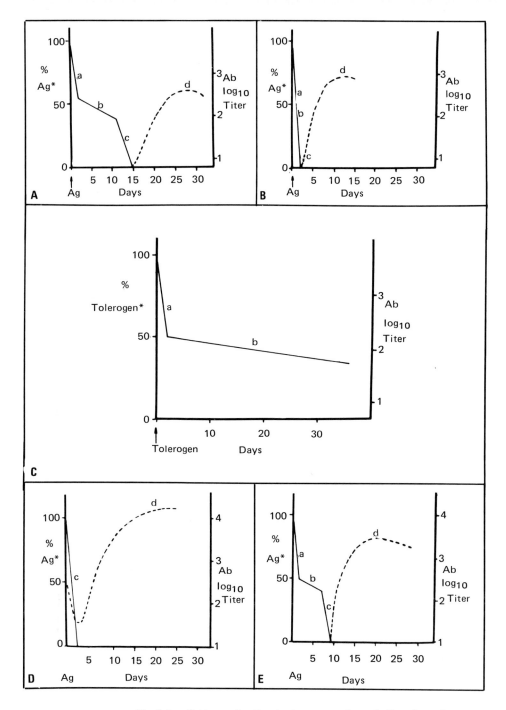

Fig. 5-1 : Patterns of antigenic clearance and metabolism shown by various kinds of antigen. A. Soluble protein Ag. B. Large colloidal TMV Ag. C. Pattern of tolerance with monomeric Ag. D. Negative phase, secondary response. E. Secondary response with soluble Ag. The antigen clearance from peripheral blood is characterized by: a = equilibrium phase; b = metabolic degradation phase; c = immune elimination phase; and d̄ = antibody synthesis phase. Solid line = antigen clearance pattern; dotted line = antibody synthesis. * = antigens labeled with radioisotopes.

104

Table 5-2 : The Half-life of Some Soluble Proteins in Peripheral Blood of Normal Rabbits

Antigen	Average Half-life (days)	Molecular Weight (daltons)
Human H-chain	4.9	50,000
Bovine serum albumin	4.3	68,000
Rabbit serum albumin	5.7	68,000
Human 7S IgG	4.7	160,000
Rabbit 7S IgG	6.0	160,000
Human IgA	2.5	160,000
Bovine thyroglobulin	2.1	670,000
Human IgM	1.6	950,000

The half-life of labeled foreign immunogens in the plasma of rabbits appear to be inversely related to their molecular weights, as shown above, the larger molecular weight molecules having a shorter half-life in plasma. The correlation coefficient was found to be −0.72. The half-life of homologous proteins appears to be dependent on their rate of metabolism. Data from Nakamura et al., 1968.

Tolerogen

Antigens that tend to persist in peripheral blood and demonstrate primarily phase a and b patterns are associated with tolerance. An example of this type of antigen (see section on tolerogen, Chapter 4) is the monomeric form of human gamma globulin (HγG), which is removed principally by metabolic means similar to those that remove autologous serum proteins. This type of pattern is demonstrated in Figure 5-1C. No immune elimination (phase c) or antibody synthesis (phase d) is exhibited. Similar patterns can be demonstrated by injection of labeled antigen into an animal rendered unresponsive by whole-body x-irradiation (500 r) or by administration of large amounts of antigen at birth (see section on tolerance, Chapter 10).

Negative Phase: Secondary Response

Animals with preexisting detectable levels of antibody, generally exhibit the pattern shown in Figure 5-1D when given the corresponding labeled antigen. Antigen-antibody complexes are formed immediately, and the clearance is that of phase c, immune elimination (negative phase). The levels of preexisting antibody decrease initially, with subsequent increase (but in some cases suppression) of antibody synthesis. High levels of preexisting antibody would tend to suppress antibody synthesis by diminishing the accessibility of the antigen to the memory cells and other aspects of the immune system. On the other hand, lower levels of preexisting antibody would enhance antibody synthesis. This concept was followed in diphtheria immunization prior to the availability of toxoid. Diphtheria toxin in an appropriate ratio to antitoxin (prepared in the horse) exhibited no toxicity. Figure 5-1E shows the labeled antigen clearance pattern in an animal with no circulating antibody but previously exposed to the antigen. A shortened phase b (metabolic degradation) and phase c (immune elimination) are demonstrated in this secondary response.

Soluble protein antigens used for metabolic and distribution studies have generally been labeled with ^{125}I or ^{131}I, although ^{3}H, ^{14}C, ^{32}P, and other radioisotopes have been used. Although the question of deiodination and catabolic formation of iodotyrosine has been raised, data using iodinated soluble proteins for metabolic and tissue distribution studies have been generally accepted.

Distribution of Antigens in Tissues

The distribution of antigens following active injection into a normal animal depends on the mode of administration, which includes the following: (1) subcutaneous, (2) intravenous, (3) intraperitoneal, and (4) intramuscular. The transport of the antigen is via blood and the lymphatics. In all cases the antigen ultimately is widely disseminated at various levels of concentration in different tissues.

Organ and Cellular Trapping and Distribution

Certain select organs and cells appear to concentrate and retain the major portion of the antigens: the reticuloendothelial cells of the liver, kidney, bone marrow, and lungs, the cells of the lymphoid systems of the gastrointestinal tract, and the lymph nodes and spleen. The major cell in the reticuloendothelial system associated with trapping of antigen is the macrophage. Its main function is to retain and digest the antigens, especially the particulate antigens. Efficient trapping of the antigen is dependent on its size and charge and on the presence of opsonic or specific antibodies. The following pattern emerges after injection of a soluble radioisotope-labeled antigen into the foot pad of a rabbit: (1) the draining small popliteal lymph node contains more radioactive antigen than other lymph nodes and even more than the spleen; but in the early phases, levels of radioactivity in lymph are equal to or slightly less than in the liver, depending on the nature of the antigen. The proportion of the antigens present in the major lymphoid system rarely exceeds a small percentage of the total administered antigen (after 48 hours), since the total lymphoid tissue of the animals (rabbit and rat) is less than 1 percent of total body weight; (2) there is no direct relationship between capacity or strength of antigenicity and degree of trapping in the lymph node; (3) however, the molecular size and physicochemical nature of the antigen show a correlation with the degree of trapping in the lymph node. For example, virus

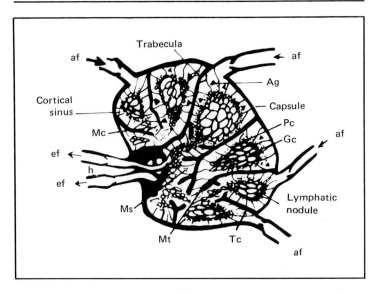

Fig. 5-2 : Localization of antigen (▲) in the popliteal lymph node of the rabbit: antigen entrapment in the region of the dendritic cells in the sinus. af = afferent lymphatics; ef = efferent lymphatics; Mc = medullary cord; Pc = paracortical; Gc = germinal center; Ms = medullary sinus; Ag = antigen; Tc = trabecula; Mt = medullary trabecula; and H = hilus.

antigens are much more readily retained in the lymph node than soluble BSA. Heat-denatured BSA is much more readily trapped than untreated BSA. Generally the larger phagocytized and denatured soluble antigens persist or are detained in the lymph nodes for longer periods by the phagocytic cells. In rabbits, foot pad injections provide an excellent route for antibody production (Figure 5-2). The trapping and drainage from the injection site, the metabolization of the antigen, and the subsequent antigen's escape through the efferent lymphatic vessels in an altered state are a dynamic process that continues until the source of antigen at the injection site is removed.

In most cases, however, antigens enter via the gastrointestinal and respiratory tracts. The lymphoid tissues are involved in the entrapment of these antigens. Induction and synthesis of antibody occurs in the lymphoid tissues lining the gastrointestinal and respiratory tracts. Entrance of antigen via these tracts stimulates production of secretory immunoglobulins such as IgA and IgE. Furthermore, it has been shown that B cells with IgA immunoglobulins are the major constituents in the lymph nodes of the gastrointestinal tract (Peyer's patches). They constitute approximately 60 to 70 percent of the B cell population in Peyer's patches.

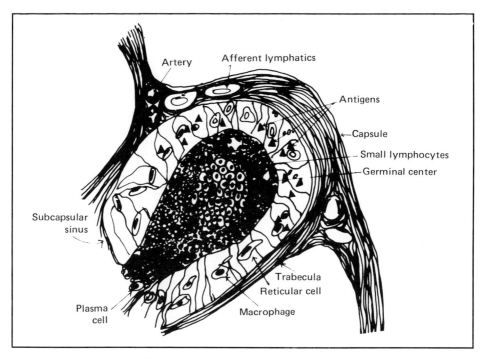

Fig. 5-3 : Enlargement in the area of the lymph node follicles showing localization of antigen (▲) in the subscapular sinus of the cortex.

Antigen Metabolism by Macrophages

The macrophages and dendritic cells constitute the important cells in the trapping of antigen. Macrophages are important also in the processing of antigen for recognition by T and B cells. They presumably present the necessary immunodeterminants for recognition by T cell and B cell receptors. The so-called *activated antigen* or *RNA immunogen* is presumably processed by macrophages. This is especially evident for particulate antigens such as bacteria and erythrocytes. These complex antigens are phagocytized and digested within the cytoplasm of macrophages in the phagosomes (vesicles). The enzymes of the macrophages found within the lysosomes (see Chapter 8) aid in the digestive process.

Antigenic Persistence in Various Cells

Judging from labeled antigen and radioautographic studies, the long-term retention of antigens in the lymph nodes happens predominantly in the medullary macrophages and the lymphoid follicles. In the macrophages the antigen is concentrated mainly in lysosomal inclusions (phagosomes) and is rapidly degraded, although significant but small amounts remain intact and stably sequestered. In the lymphoid follicles the antigen appears to be retained extracellularly between the membranes of the dendritic cells, and natural or specific antibody (passive or active) plays a significant role in this retention (Figures 5-2 and 5-3). Lack

Fig. 5-4 : Antigen
retention in the
marginal zone of
the spleen.

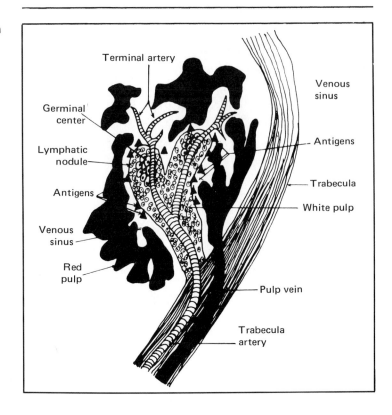

Terminal artery

Venous
sinus

Germinal
center

Antigens

Lymphatic
nodule

Antigens

Trabecula

White pulp

Venous
sinus

Red
pulp

Pulp vein

Trabecula
artery

of these dendritic cells or absence of antibody results in loss of the antigen-retentive capacity in the follicular area. However, the antibodies do not affect the retentive capacity of the medullar macrophages.

In the spleen the marginal zone appears to be the major area associated with retention of antigen, although transiently. Generally the antigens are found extracellularly in the marginal zone, and the few macrophages (in contrast to lymph nodes) may also contribute to trapping of the antigen (Figure 5-4).

It is interesting to note that the B cell—the precursor of the antibody-producing plasma cell—retains little or no antigen. Present information about antibody-synthesizing cells suggests that, although antigen can enter via the receptors and via pinocytosis into the cells, the presence of antigen is neither a necessary nor a sufficient condition for antibody synthesis.

The thymus of the young tends to retain more antigen than that of an adult. Hence tolerance is much more readily induced in young than in older animals. It is known that viruses tend to persist indefinitely in a dormant state in tissues, especially if viruses are encoded as DNA or RNA in the chromosomes or nucleic acids of cells, and to express themselves when favorable

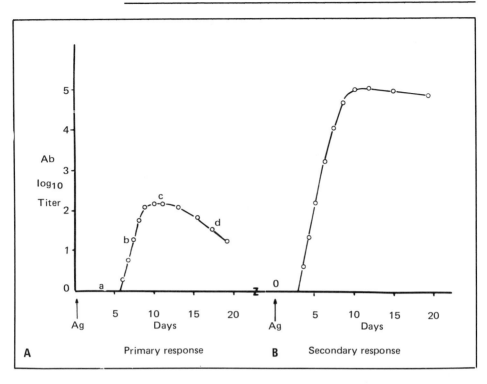

Fig. 5-5 : A. Primary and B. secondary immune responses of an animal to the same antigen. Accelerated induction and Ab synthesis phases, higher Ab level, and slower degradation are exhibited for the secondary response. Phases: a = induction phase; b = log phase; c = stationary phase; and d = degradation phase or decline.

conditions arise for their proliferation, that is, when the host's defenses are low (poor health).

Antibody Synthesis

Primary Response   An animal's initial exposure to an antigen evokes a *primary* immune response. The antibodies are first detectable 1 to 30 days after the primary antigenic stimulus. This primary response is smaller and differs somewhat from subsequent exposure to the same antigen (secondary response). A typical primary immune response is illustrated in Figure 5-5A.

This immune response can be dissected into four phases, as follows: (1) the initial lag phase (a) after antigen administration and prior to the first detectable antibody in peripheral blood; (2) the rapid log phase (b) of antibody synthesis; (3) the stationary phase (c); and (4) the subsequent degradation of the antibody (d). The lag phase is dependent on the dose, route of injection, and nature of the immunogen (soluble or particulate), and on the adjuvant used and the sensitivity of assay for the antibody.

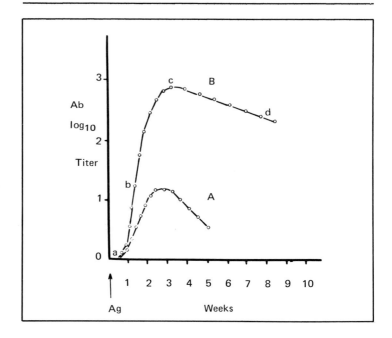

Fig. 5-6 : The enhanced effect on antibody synthesis given by adjuvant plus Ag (curve B) as compared to Ag alone (curve A). See Fig. 5-5A for designation of a, b, c, and d phases for curve B.

It is common to detect antibodies to particulate antigen by conventional agglutination or precipitation in 3 or 4 days after injection of virus or foreign erythrocytes, in 5 to 7 days for some soluble proteins, and in 12 to 15 days for bacterial suspensions. With more sensitive methods of antibody detection, such as radioimmunoassay procedures, antibodies to these immunogens can be detected much earlier. For example, the period for bacteriophage (virus 174) was demonstrated to be one day when a small dosage of antigen (0.01 μg of protein) was used and the subsequent antibody synthesis assayed by neutralization of the plaque formation of the bacteriophage against its host, *E. coli*. This study of bacteriophages demonstrated that two important features in any assessment of the lag phase are (1) the nature of the immunogen and (2) the sensitivity of the assay system for antibody detection. Virus neutralization is a much more sensitive procedure for antibody detection than agglutination or precipitation.

The exponential or lag phase of antibody synthesis (phase b), the attainment of the maximum antibody level, and the duration (peak titer—phase c) are dependent on the immunogen and the mode of administration. For example, the peak titer for erythrocytes injected into rabbits may be attained in 4 to 5 days after injection. Attainment of the peak titer varies with the immunogen and whether adjuvant is also given (Figure 5-6).

The decline (phase d, Figure 5-5A) of antibody occurs following the steady state, when the turnover (degradation) and distribution of the antibody are greater than the net synthesis by plasma cells. The steady state (phase c) exists when the synthesis of antibody equals the rate of degradation. The latter is dependent on the half-life of the antibody molecule, which varies according to Ig class (Chapter 2, Table 2-2). IgM and IgA are normally degraded much faster than IgG. Fragments of immunoglobulin, such as Fab and the light chains, are broken down ($T_{\frac{1}{2}} < 1$ day) much faster than the intact immunoglobulin. However, the $T_{\frac{1}{2}}$ of the Fc fragment is similar to that of the intact immunoglobulin. In addition, removal of the terminal neuraminic acid residues from the carbohydrate residue on the constant region of the heavy chain initiates a faster degradation of the immunoglobulin by the liver. This is similar to the effect noted for degradation of glycoproteins following removal of neuraminic acid. Degradation also is dependent on the actual serum concentration of immunoglobulin and the volume of fluid in which the Ig molecules are distributed. The total concentration of immunoglobulin in the blood is about the same as it is in extracellular fluids. The mass of immunoglobulin molecules (approximately 25 percent) that diffuse into the extravascular fluid each day is returned via lymphatic vessels intravascularly.

The decline of antibody also varies with the physical and chemical properties of the immunogen and according to whether adjuvant is used. With soluble immunogens the antibody starts to decline 2 to 3 days after the peak level. The same soluble immunogen mixed with adjuvant would decline at a much slower rate, and the antibody would persist longer in the peripheral blood.

CLASS AND PROPERTY OF IMMUNOGLOBULINS IN THE PRIMARY RESPONSE. The property and class of antibodies formed in response to a primary antigenic stimulus changes over time according to a definite sequence. The initial antibody is of the IgM class. Subsequently IgG antibody appears. This pattern is shown in Figure 5-7 for antibodies to tobacco mosaic viruses induced in rabbits. Addition of adjuvant to the antigen results in long-term synthesis of both IgM and IgG (Figure 5-7). If no adjuvant is used, the IgM is no longer detectable in peripheral blood after 1 or 2 weeks. It is highly possible that this sequence of synthesis is related to the IgM-IgG switch that has been demonstrated in B cells. It has also been shown that the IgM synthesis appears to occur during high levels of antigen in the circulation. Nevertheless, this sequence may be attributable merely to the large number of combining sites (10) on IgM molecules and to IgM's higher avidity for antigen. The IgG molecule, with two combining sites and low avidity, may be masked by the IgM reaction.

Fig. 5-7 : Sequential changes in the classes of immunoglobulins synthesized following a primary Ag stimulus such as TMV. The top curve represents the combination of IgM and IgG.

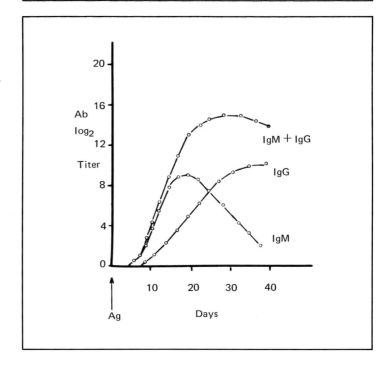

IgM synthesis can be suppressed by passively administering IgG antibody of the same specificity. This is referred to as *feedback inhibition*. The major immunoglobulin elicited by thymus-independent immunogen is IgM antibody.

In addition to the change in Ig class, the antibodies also manifest increased affinity for the immunogen. For example, the first antihapten antibodies formed after injection of the hapten-protein conjugate usually have low affinity for the hapten. Later the antibody affinity for the hapten increases. This occurs even with lower doses of hapten-protein conjugates, and the changes are especially pronounced in the IgG molecule. The increase in *affinity* is associated with an increase in *avidity* of the antibodies. *Avidity* refers to the overall tendency of antibodies to combine with antigen determinants. *Affinity* is reserved for the intrinsic association constant that characterizes the binding of a univalent antigen (see Chapter 7). This is partly attributed to the increase in antibody specificities as more and more of the immunodeterminants of the immunogens are exposed with time. That is, over time, antibodies are produced to more and more of the various determinants of the multivalent antigens. Thus, the antigen-antibody complexes formed later are less dissociable than those formed initially. Associated with the increase in avidity and affinity is the greater cross-reactivity with related ligands shown by antibodies synthesized at later periods. This is due to the increase in antibody specificities to the many determinants on the antigen molecule, some, at least, of which may be related to other antigens.

IgM-IgG SHIFT. Antibodies of IgM and IgG classes with identical affinity and specificities (combining sites) directed against oligo-D-alanine have been demonstrated in x-irradiated recipient mice given limited numbers of spleen and thymus cells from primed syngeneic donor mice. Studies with microdrop cultures using a single cell have produced antiflagellar antibodies of both the IgM and the IgG class. IgM was distinguished from IgG by the addition of mercaptoethanol. This latter compound reduces the IgM complex, thus nullifying its agglutinability, but has no effect on the IgG antiflagellar antibody. It thus was shown that a single cell can produce both IgM and IgG antibodies. About 2 percent of the spleen cells examined showed synthesis of both antibodies. Further evidence for the capability of a single plasma cell to produce more than one class of antibodies has been exhibited in cancers of the bone marrow. Plasma cells from the bone marrow of patients with multiple myeloma have demonstrated synthesis of both IgM and IgG simultaneously. Amino acid sequence analysis of the V regions of both Ig Classes revealed either complete homology or the same idiotype. Furthermore, immunofluorescence analysis with fluorescein-labeled antibodies to IgA and IgG classes has revealed synthesis of both immunoglobulins by a single plasma cell also. Thus, the evidence strongly suggests that a single precursor B cell can give rise to a clone, which can then produce similar idiotypes of IgM and IgG, although not simultaneously. This phenomenon is referred to as *IgM-IgG switch* or *shift.*

The regulatory mechanism for the IgM-IgG switch has not been defined. Recent evidence suggests, however, that the switch may be modulated by prostaglandins elaborated by adherent cells. Synthesis of IgG increased in spleen cells primed with SRBC when prostaglandin F_{2a} ($PGF_{2\alpha}$) was given after sensitization (Figure 5–8). This effect is reflected in a greater number of IgG plaque-forming cells (PFC) expressed in both the primary and the secondary responses $PGF_{2\alpha}$ may act on the B cell directly, or it may act on the T cell regulating the shift from IgM to IgG. The prostaglandins may have their effect on the cyclic nucleotides. c-AMP and c-GMP, acting as second messengers, have been shown to affect DNA-mRNA transcription and RNA-protein translation. Therefore the repressor μ-gene and the depressor γ-gene may be affected, as depicted in Figure 5–9. Whatever the mechanism, $PGF_{2\alpha}$ appears to have a pronounced effect on the increase of IgG.

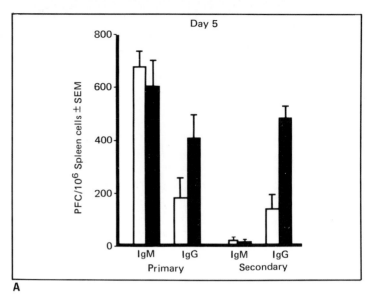

A

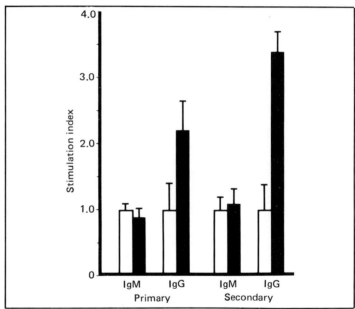

B

Fig 5-8 : Analysis of IgM and IgG synthesis by plaque-forming cell
(PFC) assay. Figure 5-8A shows the number of IgM and IgG PFCs, from
mice spleen cells formed by control (open bars) and prostaglandin $F_{2\alpha}$
treated (solid bars) during primary and secondary responses. Figure 5-8B
shows the stimulation index (SI = mean PFC/10^6 spleen cells of experimental mice divided by mean PFC/10^6 spleen cells of control mice) of
the data in Fig. 5-8A. In these studies, the experimental mice (BDF$_1$) received 100 μg prostaglandin $F_{2\alpha}$ 24 hours after 1 x 10^8 SRBC administration. In the primary response studies, mice were sacrificed 5 days after
injection of SRBC (4 days after 100 μg PG$F_{2\alpha}$). Mice in the secondary
response study were treated as in the primary response, but were rechallenged with SRBC only 27 days after the initial injection and then sacrificed 5 days after the second administration of SRBC.

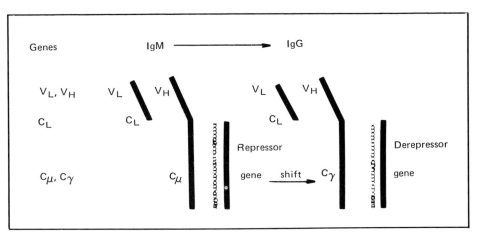

Fig. 5-9 : Schema of polypeptide chains modulated by genes specifying a shift from IgM to IgG within one B cell. The IgM and IgG V regions of the L- and H-chains have the same genes and, therefore, similar idiotypes. The change is in the isotype, from μ to γ, in the C region of the H-chain and requires a total of five genes. The shift can be expressed by gene action repressor for μ and depressor for γ of the C_H chains.

A total of five genes is sufficient to explain the shift from μ to γ heavy chain according to the two-gene polypeptide concept. Since the idiotypes are similar, the V region of the H-chain and the complete L-chain will be similar, only the shift from C_μ to C_γ is required (Figure 5–9).

ANTIGENIC COMPETITION AND PROMOTION. When two or more unrelated antigens are administered to an animal simultaneously, antibody synthesis to one is suppressed. For example, poly-L-alanyl-protein given at the same time as poly-D-alanyl-protein will cause synthesis of antibody to poly-D-alanyl-protein, and little or no antibodies will be detected against poly-L-alanyl-protein. This is referred to as *antigenic competition,* and more specifically as *intermolecular competition. Intramolecular competition* can also occur. In this instance two molecular determinants in the same molecule compete for receptors on the B cell. A D-amino acid and an L-amino acid polypeptide conjugated to the same molecule will, when administered to a host, evoke antibody in greater amounts to the D-amino acid polypeptide determinant than to the L-amino acid polypeptide determinant. This is due in part to the immunodominant characteristics and greater affinity of the poly-D-amino acid peptide for the B cell receptors.

Intermolecular competition cannot be explained by the mechanism given for intramolecular competition. It may be due to the suppressive effect of T cell on B cells, or the *allotypic suppression* discussed later in this chapter (p. 125–126).

Increased antigenic response to immunogen (W) is exhibited when it is given at the same time as another antigen (Z). This is especially pronounced when the host has been exposed previously to antigen Z. This antigenic promotion to immunogen (W) has been attributed to the activation by immunogen (Z) of T cells previously exposed to immunogen (Z) and the subsequent release of lymphokines that stimulate neighboring B cells bound via their receptors to immunogen W.

The Secondary Response

The secondary response is evoked in a host that has been primed previously with the same immunogen. Antibodies may or may not be detectable in the animal from the initial priming or exposure. The secondary response is sometimes called the *anamnestic* (memory) or *recall response* (see Nonspecific stimulation later in this section). In contrast to the primary response, it is characterized by (1) a lower required concentration of immunogen; (2) a shorter lag phase; (3) a high rate and longer duration of antibody synthesis; (4) high levels of antibody concentration; and (5) a slower rate of decline (see Figure 5-5B). In addition, IgG antibodies with high affinity are synthesized in greater proportion than are antibodies of the IgM class. The capacity for the secondary response can persist for many years, depending on the nature of the immunogen. This accounts for the long-lasting immunity seen against viral infection. Even long after antibodies are no longer detectable, reexposure to small amounts of antigen can usually evoke prompt synthesis of relatively large amounts of highly efficient antibody. In the primary response, antibody synthesis occurs at a slower rate and antibodies are generally initially of lower binding quality. Overall the secondary response is associated with a shorter lag period, faster clearance of antigen from the circulation (see Figure 5-1E), more rapid synthesis of antibody, and peak levels of antibody of possibly one hundred-fold or greater than the primary response. The expansion of immunocytes at the cellular level following primary and secondary exposure to antigen can be seen schematically in Figure 5-10.

IMMUNOLOGICAL MEMORY. The concept of immunological memory is based on the observed characteristics of the secondary response. Initial exposure to an immunogen triggers the appropriate clones, which have specific Ig receptors for the immunogen and which are subsequently transformed into B blast cells. The latter cells either become plasma cells and synthesize and secrete the antibodies or become memory cells (small lymphocytes) retained within the lymphoid system. A second challenge will activate both the primary B precursor cells and the committed memory T and B cells, resulting in a greater number of cells producing antibody in the secondary response.

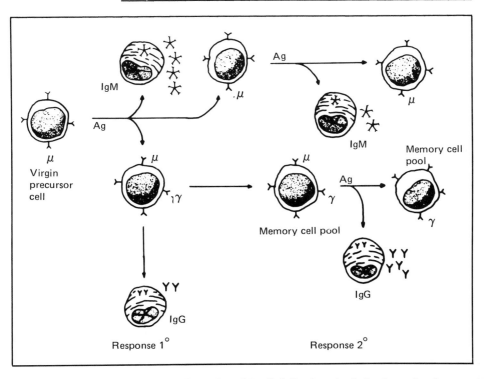

Fig. 5-10 : Expansion of B cells following stimulation by antigen in primary and in secondary exposure to a given immunogen.

This proliferation of plasma cell and memory cell is illustrated in Figure 5-10 for both the primary and the secondary response. The nature of the regulatory mechanism(s) for the proliferation of these cells is still uncertain; that is, what regulates the number of memory cells and/or plasma cells? Recent observations suggest that prostaglandins produced by adherent cells (macrophages and monocytes) may play a significant role in specifying the expression of memory and/or plasma cells. Administration of $PGF_{2\alpha}$ (100 μg) to BDF_1 mice 24 hours after they had been primed with sheep red blood cells caused a significant increase ($p < 0.01$) in IgG plaque-forming cells in mice challenged with SRBC 24 days (secondary response) after the initial injection (Figure 5-8). The data suggest that the increase in IgG in the secondary response is a reflection of an increase in IgG memory cells, induced by the $PGF_{2\alpha}$ administered 24 hours after the initial injection of SRBC. The basis for the prostaglandins' effect on the IgM-IgG shift is presently unknown (see previous section on IgM-IgG shift). They may act directly on the primed blast cells (memory cells containing IgM and IgG receptors [see Figure 5-10]) or act on the T cell, which has been suggested as a possible regulator of the IgM-IgG switch. Both T and B cells have been demonstrated to have receptors for prostaglandins of the E series and for histamine and catecholamines. Via their action on the membrane receptors, these compounds appear to increase cyclic nucleotides. This receptor, however, is not β-adenyl cyclase.

In the secondary response, memory is exhibited by both B and T cells. The antihaptenic secondary effect can generally be demonstrated in rabbits using the same hapten on another carrier. The nature of the carrier is of importance; it must be able to stimulate the T helper cell (carrier effect). For example, one year after rabbits are primed with DNP–BIgG a vigorous secondary response to DNP can be elicited with DNP-hemocyanin conjugate. Memory is present in the B cells, which promptly stimulate high-affinity anti-DNP antibodies. Memory in the T cells is exhibited by T-dependent antigens.

SECONDARY RESPONSE STIMULATED BY RELATED ANTIGENS. A secondary response can be stimulated by a closely related hapten on the same carrier. The antibodies formed in this secondary response are primarily reactive to the initial haptenic determinant administered in the primary response. This phenomenon of cross-stimulation is referred to as *original antigenic sin* and has been seen in epidemiological studies of antigenically related strains of influenza viruses. It has also been demonstrated in closely related viral strains of herpes and many others. An example of cross-reacting stimulation was demonstrated in rabbits given DNP-BIgG in the initial stimulation and challenged 8 months later with TNP-BIgG. The rabbits exhibited a marked increase in anti-DNP-BIgG rather than anti-TNP-BIgG antibodies.

This phenomenon has been employed to study past histories of viral infections. Various strains of the virus have been used to examine the antibody levels of the current infections. In many cases antibody titers to the current infecting strains are found to be lower than titers to related viral strains that presumably infected the individuals in the past. This is especially demonstrable in older individuals. Furthermore older individuals are better protected against past strains they have been exposed to than younger individuals not previously exposed to the viruses. This has been observed in the periodic waves of influenza viral infections due to different strains.

NONSPECIFIC STIMULATION. Anamnestic responses can be elicited by nonspecific stimulation in animals. In these cases the stimuli have no immunogenic relationship to the initial priming antigen. In numerous disease processes (liver, collagen diseases, etc.) increases in immunoglobulins occur. These have been referred to

**Table 5-3 : Monocytic Factors ("Monokines")
in Modulation of the Immune Response**

Factors	Effect
Lymphocyte-activating factor (LAF)	Stimulatory
Genetically restricted factor (GRF)	"
Stem cell–differentiating factor	"
Lymphocyte-trapping factor	"
B cell-activating factor (BAF)	"
Normal macrophage (MAF)	"
Prostaglandins	"
DNA synthesis	Inhibitory
Cytotoxins	"
Prostaglandins	"

**Table 5-4 : Serum Factors ("Cytokines") That
May Modulate Immune Response**

Factors	Effect
Complement components	Stimulatory
Fetuin	"
Transferrin	"
C-reactive protein (CRP)	"
Normal immunosuppressive protein (NIP)	Inhibitory
α-Fetoprotein, fetuin (AFP)	"
Immunoregulatory α-globulin (IRA)	"
C-reactive protein	"

as *polyclonal gammopathy.* They are generally associated with acute inflammatory reactions, and the release of immunoregulatory factors (Tables 5-3 and 5-4) may stimulate the memory cells to become plasma cells that secrete immunoglobulins. For example, serum taken from rabbits after x-irradiation has been shown to elaborate an endotoxin-like glycoprotein when given to rabbits earlier primed with TMV-induced stimulation of a secondary antibody response to the TMV antigen (Figure 5-11). Sera from adjuvant-treated animals have also shown similar nonspecific effects. Agents capable of inducing the mitogenic effect, such as PHA and PWM, can also induce anamnestic responses in animals primed previously with immunogens. This is represented in Figure 5-12 and expresses the polyclonal expansion of B cells. Clinically this phenomenon has been utilized in the diagnosis of rickettsial infections (typhus fever). Evidently

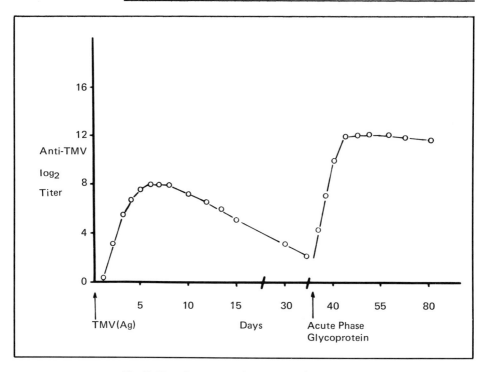

Fig. 5-11 : An anamnestic response of rabbits to TMV antigen, induced by a nonspecific acute phase glycoprotein isolated from post-x-irradiation serum.

individuals with this infection and with fever produce high levels of an antibody that reacts with *Proteus* OX-19 antigen (nonmobile strain).

The term *anamnestic (recollection)* is best used to refer to non-specific stimulation of the secondary antibody response, whereas the specific response stimulated by antigen is best referred to as the *secondary response.*

Lymphocyte Interactions in the Immune Response

T and B Cell Interrelationship: T-Dependent Antigen

Evidence presented in the literature suggests that, for some immunogens (thymus-dependent), antibody synthesis by the B cell requires the intervention of the T helper cell: that is, an interaction of the T and B cells, either directly or through soluble mediators released by T cell acting on B cell receptors. An example of a T-dependent immunogen is aggregated human γ-globulin (AHGG), a naturally occurring protein that requires the action of T helper cell for the blastogenic transformation of the B cell and the subsequent elaboration of antibody by the

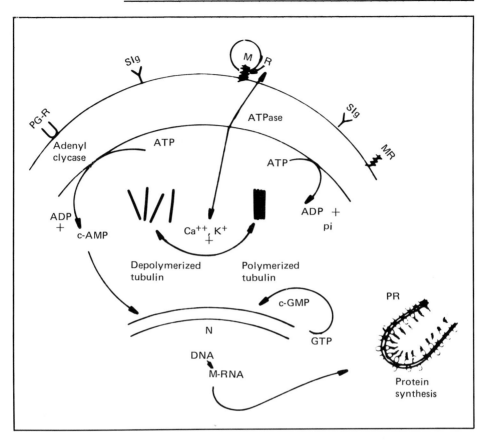

Fig. 5-12 : The nonspecific mitogenic effect (at the molecular level) on memory B cells, with subsequent antibody (protein) production. SIg, MR, and PG-R = surface immunoglobulin, mitogen receptor, and prostaglandin receptor, respectively.

plasma cell (Figure 5-13). The immunodominant determinant of the immunogenic AHGG binds to its specific receptor on the committed, but unprimed, B cell clone, while through the carrier effect the AHGG immunogen relates to receptors on the T helper cell. The receptors on the T cells have as yet not been defined, although Ig-like receptors or HLA have been suggested as possible candidates. The T helper cell either aggregates the immunogen on the B cell or transmits a signal via a soluble messenger for the B cell to undergo blast transformation. The next step involves the formation of memory cells and plasma cells. The memory cell is a small lymphocyte specifically committed to, or encoded for, the production of antibody to the immunogenic determinant exposed to initially. When reexposed to the same or cross-reacting determinants (secondary response), the memory cell is transformed to plasma cell. The plasma cells elaborate either IgM or

Fig. 5-13 : T and
B cell interrela-
tionships following
antigenic stimula-
tion by aggregated
human gamma
globulin (AHGG).
Th = T helper cell;
B = B cell.

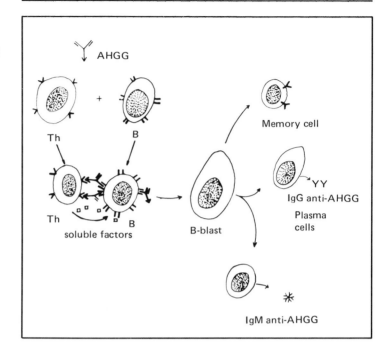

IgG antibodies with similar idiotypes if the determinants are homogeneous in structure.

B Cell Response: T-Independent Antigen

T-independent antigens presumably stimulate B cells directly without the intervention of T helper cells, although antibody synthesis may be regulated by T suppressor cells. It has been suggested that the repeated polymeric units of immunodeterminants common to T-independent immunogens are the major contributing factor in the triggering of B cells to blastogenic transformation and to antibody synthesis. The T-independent antigens include bacterial LPS (gram-negative microorganism), pneumococcal polysaccharide (gram-positive microorganism), levan, Ficoll (copolymer of sucrose and epichlorohydrin), dextran, polymerized flagellin, and various synthetic polypeptides (see Chapter 4). An alternative explanation of how T-independent antigens activate B cells to synthesize antibodies is based on the mitogenic property of the antigens and their ability to activate polyclonal B cells. It has been suggested that the mitogenic property of the T-independent immunogens is associated with the transmission of a signal that is required for B cell transformation to blast cell and subsequent antibody synthesis. Recent experiments utilizing lipopolysaccharide isolated from *Salmonella* lacking the repeated oligosaccharide units when coupled to SRBC after coupling with TNP (TNP-LPS) stimulated similar plaque-forming cells in animals as that induced by intact LPS

Fig. 5-14 : T-independent antigen stimulation of B cell.

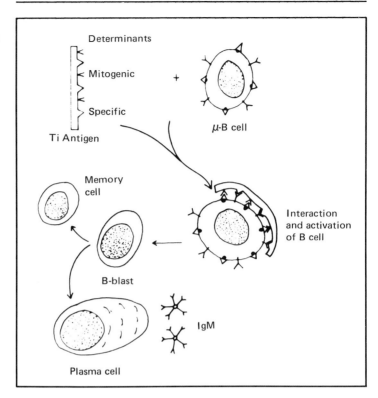

with repeating oligosaccharides. This TNP-LPS nevertheless retained the mitogenic property. Thus, it has been suggested that B cell triggering by T-independent antigens is dependent on their mitogenic property rather than on their repeating array of immunodeterminants. Triggering by T-independent antigen is depicted in Figure 5–14.

The nonspecific polyclonal expansion of immunoglobulins by B cells also appears to be dependent on the nonspecific mitogenic signal expressed by the T-independent antigens such as LPS. The theory supposes that T-independent macromolecules having repeated *epitopes* (determinants) trigger B cells directly, because they are capable of cross-linking the specific immunoglobulin receptors. The triggering would be done by the aggregated or concentrated Ig receptors on the membrane surface of B cells. For T-dependent antigens lacking repeated epitopes, macrophage surface or T helper cells presumably aid in the concentration of the immunoglobulin receptors and thus transmit the necessary signal for blast transformation of the B cells and antibody synthesis. The question as to whether two signals or one signal activates the B cell to blastogenesis is merely one of designation. If the specific immunoglobulin receptor binding to the B cell is considered to be signal 1, then the mitogenic effect of the T-independent antigen and/or of the T helper cell or macrophage for the T-dependent antigen is considered to be a second signal. It has been shown, however, that the initial specific binding of the antigen to the immunoglobulin receptor of a B cell does not in itself trigger blastogenesis or synthesis of antibody. This would imply that the mitogenic signal of T-independent antigens and/or the T helper or macrophage signal for T-dependent antigens is the single signal, required for blastogenesis and antibody synthesis.

Role of Macrophages in T and B Cell Interaction

An interplay of T cells, B cells, and macrophages is a prerequisite for antibody synthesis with particulate antigens. The macrophages appear to play a major role in processing the antigen—giving it appropriate antigenic determinants so that it becomes *activated antigen*—before T and B cells begin antibody synthesis.

The macrophages can also release immunoregulatory factors (Table 5-4), which may control the quantity or the class of antibody synthesized. Evidence has been presented in vitro and in vivo that removal or blockade of macrophage function abrogates antibody synthesis to SRBC in the presence of T and B cells. Macrophages, in addition to carrying out phagocytosis, preparation, and concentration of antigen, release immune response regulatory factors collectively referred to as *monokines* (Table 5-4). The other major functions of macrophages are presented in Chapter 8. The active immunogen prepared by the macrophage is acted upon by the T and B cells, as was demonstrated for soluble AHGG immunogen. This sequence of events is presented in Figure 5-15.

Current evidence generally supports the concept that immunoglobulin receptors on B cells are specific for a given antigenic determinant (clonal selection) and that the subsequent binding itself does not trigger blast transformation of B cells and resultant antibody synthesis; but, rather, that a signal (first if Ig receptor Ag-binding is not considered as signal one or second if the IgR-Ag binding is considered as first) is transmitted from the mitogenic moiety of a T-independent antigen (Figure 5-14) or from the T helper cell (Figures 5-14 and 5-15) in T-dependent antigen. That all three cells are required seems evident from studies in which it was found that deletion of any one of the three cells, either in tissue culture or when transplanted to x-irradiated animals, abrogated antibody synthesis to SRBC. In these studies antibody synthesis was determined by analysis of the number of plaque-forming cells in the spleen in the presence of SRBC with guinea pig complement. Hemolysis of the SRBC around a single spleen cell constitutes the plaque-forming cell (PFC).

Fig. 5-15 : Inter-
relationship of
macrophages (Mθ)
and T and B cells
in the synthesis of
antibody to SRBC
antigen. Th = T
helper cell.

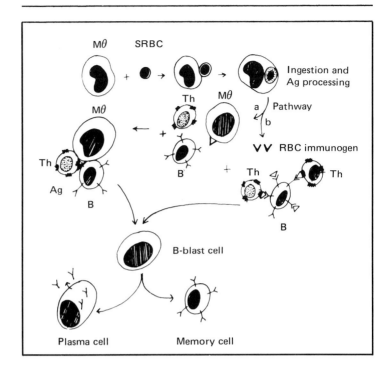

*Role of Antibody
in Modulation of
the Immune Response*

Measurable passively administered or active antibodies in the peripheral blood of animals tend to suppress further antibody synthesis by keeping the administered immunogen from binding to the specific receptors on B cells. This is one of the rational bases for administration of human anti-D (RhoGAM) to an Rh-negative mother after the birth of her Rh+ infant: to prevent the infant's RBC from reacting with the immunocompetent cells of the mother (see Chapter 11). Additionally, via feedback mechanisms, antibodies also suppress further antibody synthesis. Whether this suppression is directed to the B cells or to enhancement of T suppressor cell activity has not been clearly defined. Apparently the antibody binds to the reactive immunodominant determinant and renders it inaccessible to the Ig receptors of B cells.

*Isotype
Suppression*

The isotypic antibody anti-μ, when given to an animal prior to sensitization with immunogen, will inhibit synthesis of IgM, IgG, and IgA antibodies. Anti-Igγ or anti-Igα similarly administered will inhibit the synthesis of only their own isotypes; however, that is IgG and IgA, respectively. These antiisotypic antibodies, however, have no effect on animals previously primed with antigen.

*Allotype
Suppression*

Allotypic suppression is characterized by the inability of an individual to synthesis allotype immunoglobulin [for example,

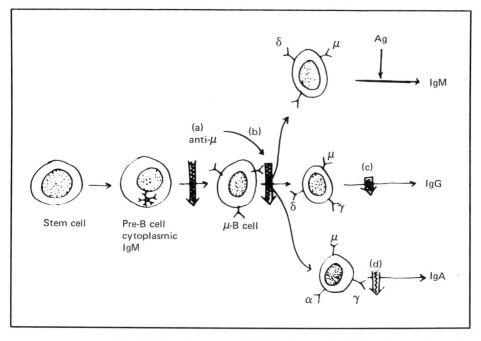

Fig. 5-16 : Ontogeny of the B cell as deduced from the use of specific antibodies to the heavy chains. Anti-μ given at point (a) would result in no IgM, IgG, or IgA syntheses; anti-μ given at point (b) would result in no IgG and IgA syntheses: anti-γ given at point (c) would show no IgG synthesis; and anti-α given at point (d) would show no IgA synthesis.

IgG, Gm(1)] after receiving by passive administration the antibody to the allotype [in this case IgG, Gm(1)]. The mechanism of this inhibition appears similar to that discussed for the RhoGAM therapy in the preceding paragraphs.

Idiotype Suppression

Idiotypic suppression is characterized by the inability of an individual to produce antibody of a particular idiotype (specific antibody to an antigen), if the individual has been previously immunized (actively with the idiotype or passively with the anti-idiotype antibody) against the idiotype. The anti-idiotype antibody acts by suppressing the anti-idiotype clones, either by eliminating them or by blocking the reaction between the idiotype and the anti-idiotype clones.

The mechanisms for the Isotypic, allotypic and idiotypic suppressions all appear to be similar.

These antiisotypes have been used to assess the sequential development (ontogeny) of the B cell system in developing chicks (Figure 5-16). Presumably the sequence is as follows; μ-B cells,

Table 5-5 : Normal Values of Immunoglobulins IgG, IgM, and IgA in Serum of Children and Adults

Age	Mean Value and (Range) (mg/dl)			
	IgG	IgM		IgA
Month of birth	1250 (800-1800)	Male 10 (0-25)	Female 12 (0-25)	3 (0--6)
1	713 (450-1188)	40 (19-75)	51 (24-96)	6 (3-17)
3	438 (263-688)	60 (29-119)	77 (37-152)	25 (11-57)
4	413 (244-663)	66 (31-131)	84 (40-168)	27 (12-67)
6	475 (281-763)	72 (36-144)	92 (46-184)	32 (14-76)
8	550 (325-875)	78 (39-156)	100 (50-200)	36 (15-88)
10	650 (388-1025)	84 (41-169)	108 (53-216)	40 (17-101)
12	719 (450-1188)	88 (44-175)	112 (56-224)	44 (21-126)
Year				
2	875 (538-1400)	103 (54-206)	131 (69-264)	59 (26-147)
4	1025 (625-1650)	110 (59-225)	141 (75-288)	92 (37-231)
8	1188 (725-1938)	115 (60-226)	146 (77-288)	137 (61-336)
12	1213 (750-2000)	119 (60-238)	151 (77-299)	179 (78-420)
15	1225 (750-2000)	125 (63-250)	157 (80-320)	210 (84-483)
Adult	1250 (800-1800)	125 (60-250)	160 (70-280)	210 (90-450)

γ-B cells, and finally α-B cells. Administration of anti-μ in the early phase of the development of the bursa of Fabricius results in the suppression of IgM, IgG, and IgA synthesis in the chicken. Administration of anti-μ at a later period results in the formation of IgM, but no IgG or IgA.

This evidence is further supported by studies of cord serum and serum in the developing infant. The sequence of synthesis as reflected in the newborn infant is IgM, IgG, and IgA. The initial high levels of IgG reflected in the sera of the newborn are attributable to the mother. The concentrations of the serum immunoglobulins of man from birth to age 15 are tabulated in Table 5-5.

Role of T Suppressor Cell

It has been clearly demonstrated that an important subset of T cells (see Chapter 3) play a significant role in regulating both the cellular and the humoral immune responses. This is evident when, for example, there is a loss of T suppressor function either through deficiency of these T suppressor cells or through a temporary loss of suppressor activity that leads to serious pathological conditions. Such conditions are reflected in the autoimmune diseases (see Chapter 14), in hypersensitivities (see Chapter 13), in severe infections (see Chapter 17), and in malignancies (see Chapter 16) involving malfunctions of both the humoral and the cell-mediated systems.

The mechanism of suppressor cell activity has not been clearly defined, but the following mode of T suppressor action has been suggested (Figure 5-17): (1) T suppressor cells have a direct effect on B or T effector cells; (2) T suppressor cells produce lymphokines, such as interferon-like substance or chalone, which can act on the target cells (B or T cell); (3) T suppressor cells compete with B cells or T effector cells for immunogenic determinants; (4) T suppressor cells interfere with T helper function directly by competing for the T helper antigenic receptor and thus suppressing the triggering signal; and (5) T suppressor cells interfere with the mitogenic signal transmitted by the T-independent antigen. T suppressor cells themselves may be regulated by stimuli such as histamines, catecholamines, and prostaglandins. It has been demonstrated that T suppressor cells have receptors for these active physiological agents and that these agents can induce synthesis of c-AMP independently of the β-adenylcyclase pathway. The macrophages that synthesize prostaglandins may also play a significant role in immunoregulation and suppression in both the CMI and the humoral system.

Nonspecific Humoral Regulators

Many factors in normal and pathological serum and fluids have been shown to affect the immune response. Some investigators have categorized these factors on the basis of cellular origin. Factors arising from monocytes have been referred to as *monokines*; those from other cells, as *cytokines;* and those from lymphocytes (see Chapter 3), as *lymphokines.* Examples from each category are shown in Tables 5-3, 5-4, and 5-6, and their negative or positive effects on antibody synthesis presented.

Summary

1. Antigens can be administered by several routes to induce an immune response in an animal: orally, nasally, intraperitoneally, intravenously, intramuscularly, subcutaneously, and topically. The major natural routes for entrance of antigen are through the respiratory (nasal) and gastrointestinal tracts (oral).
2. Administration of antigens through these various routes leads to various types of immune response (see Table 5-1).
3. The various antigens administered to animals intravenously give various blood clearance and metabolic patterns. These are examined by use of radiolabeled antigens. Blood clearance patterns of antigens vary according to the physical and chemical properties of the antigens. Clearance of soluble protein antigens is characterized by three phases: (1) a rapid equilibrium of the antigen with the fluid phase of the tissue compartments; (2) a constant metabolic clearance phase from which the half-life in blood of the antigen may be deduced; and (3) an immune elimination phase. Blood clearance patterns of particulate or large complex antigens differ from those

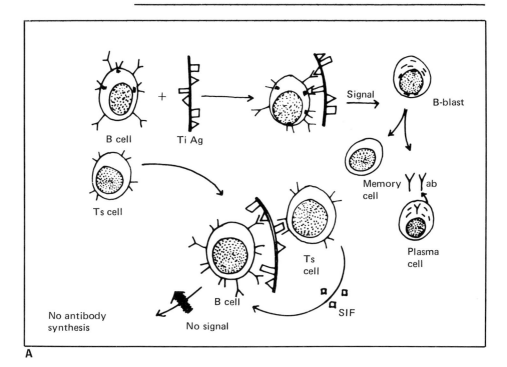

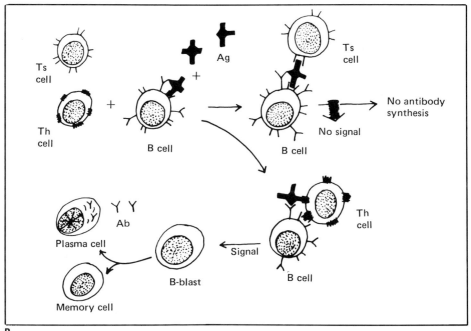

Fig. 5-17 : Hypothetical model of T suppressor cell action. A. Intervention between B cell and T-independent antigen. B. Intervention between T helper and B cell. Ts = T suppressor cell; Ti Ag = T-independent antigen; Th = T helper cell.

**Table 5-6 : Lymphocytic Factors That
May Modulate the Immune Response**

Factors	Effect
T cell–replacing factor (TRF)	Stimulatory
Allogeneic effect factor (AEF)	"
Helper factor for IgE	"
Thymus hormone	"
IgE suppressor factor	Inhibitory
Allotypic suppression	"
Inhibitor of DNA synthesis (IDS)	"
Chalones	"
Feedback inhibition factor (FIF)	"
Lymphoblastogenesis inhibition factor (LIF)	"
T-cell-suppressive factor (TSF)	"

of soluble protein antigens. Clearance of antigens also differs according to whether the antigenic stimulation is primary or secondary. Preexisting antibodies will induce a negative phase. Tolerogens show no immune elimination phase.

4. Antigens administered to animals are found in various tissues. Examination of the lymph node and spleen, the major tissues involved in antibody synthesis, shows the following: in the lymph node, antigens localize in the subcapsular region (see Figure 5-3), in association with the dendritic cells; in the spleen, they localize in the marginal region (see Figure 5-4).

5. It is interesting to note that antigens are rarely found in the proximity of the B cells that ultimately synthesize the antibodies following maturation to plasma cells.

6. Macrophages process particulate and T-dependent antigen and probably regulate the immune process via the monokines.

7. Antigen given to an animal for the first time elicits a *primary immune response* in the animal. Antibody synthesis has the following phases: (a) an induction or lag period (antigen processing, T and B cell and macrophage activation), whose duration varies with the nature of the antigen; (b) a log phase of rapid antibody synthesis; (c) a peak level or stationary phase, during which rate of antibody synthesis equals rate of antibody degradation; and (d) a phase of antibody decline, when rate of degradation is greater than rate of antibody synthesis. In the primary response, IgM antibodies are synthesized initially, then IgG. A single plasma cell can produce IgM initially, then switch to synthesis of IgG. When two or more antigens are given simultaneously, either competition or enhancement of antibody synthesis occurs.

8. The *secondary response* is engendered in a previously primed animal given the same antigen or related antigens again, after an interval of rest since the first exposure. The phases of antibody syntheses are shorter in the secondary than in the primary response and greater amounts of antibody are synthesized. The rational basis for booster treatment in vaccination processes is based on the phenomenon of the secondary response.

9. Secondary or anamnestic responses can also be induced by nonspecific factors such as unrelated antigen, mitogens, adjuvant, lipopolysaccharides, and almost any inflammation-inducing agents.

10. Tremendous advances have been made in the analysis of the relationship of T and B cells and macrophages in the immune response. T-independent antigen reacts with B cells directly and stimulates antibody synthesis. These antigens appear to possess properties of immunogenicity and mitogenicity that trigger antibody synthesis. T-dependent antigens appear to lack this mitogenic property. Macrophage is required for antigen processing and possibly for modulation via monokines. The interaction of T and B cells and macrophages may require direct contact or, as evidence seems to indicate, modulation via the lymphokines of T and B cells and the monokines of macrophages.

11. Antibody can modulate the immune response via a feedback mechanism (unknown) or by sequestration of antigen and thus prevent antigenic access to immunocytes (RhoGAM treatment) (allotypic suppression).

12. Evidence for the modulation of antibody synthesis has been found for T suppressor cells.

13. Nonspecific immunoregulators include monokines, cytokines, and lymphokines.

Bibliography and Selected Reading

General

Edelman, G. M. (Ed.). *Cellular Selection and Regulation in the Immune Responses,* Vol. 29. Soc. Gen. Physiol. Series. New York: Raven, 1974.

Golub, E. S. (Ed.). *The Cellular Basis of the Immune Response, An Approach to Immunobiology.* Sunderland, Mass.: Sinauer, 1977.

Parker, C. W. Control of lymphocyte function. New Engl. J. Med. 295: 1180, 1976.

Uhr, J. W., and Moller, G. Regulator Effect of Antibody on the Immune Response. In F. J. Dixon, Jr., and H. G. Kunkel (Eds.), *Advances in Immunology,* Vol. 8. New York: Academic, 1968. P. 81.

Unanue, E. R., and Calderon, J. Evaluation of the role of macrophage in immune induction. *Fed. Proc.* 34:1717, 1975.

Weinstein, Y., and Melman, K. Z. Control of Immune Response by Cyclic AMP and Lymphocytes that Adhere to Histamine Columns. In B. Cinader (Ed.), *Immunology of Receptors.* New York: Dekker, 1977. Pp. 115-130.

Antigen Metabolism and Tissue Distribution

Hokama, Y., Coleman, M. K., and Riley, R. F. Cx-reactive protein response in rabbits during immunization with foreign proteins. *J. Immunol.* 85:72, 1960.

Nakamura, R. M., Spiegelberg, H. L., Lee, S., and Weigle, W. O. Relationship between molecular size and intra- and extravascular distribution of protein antigens. *J. Immunol.* 100:176, 1968.

Nossal, G. J. V., and Ada, G. L. (Eds.). *Antigens, Lymphoid Cells, and the Immune Response.* New York: Academic, 1971.

Antibody Synthesis

Hokama Y., Matsuo, M., Lam, M. P., Joyo, B. S., Siu, C. E., Morita, A. H., Teraoka, J., Oishi, N., and Kimura, L. H. Regulatory Role of Prostaglandins in the Primary and Secondary Immune Response to SRBC in Mice. The In Vivo and In Vitro Effect on Plaque-Forming Cell Response of Primed Spleen Cells. In B. Samuelson, P. W. Ramwell, and R. Paoletti (Eds.), *Advances in Prostaglandin and Thromboxane Research.* New York: Raven, 1980. Pp. 1669–1673, Vol. 8.

Janeway, C. A., Jr. Cellular cooperation during in vivo antihapten antibody responses. I. The effect of cell number on the response. *J. Immunol.* 114:1394, 1975.

Kishimoto, T., and Ishizaka, K. Regulation of the antibody response in vitro. VI. Carrier-specific helper cells for IgG and IgE antibody response. *J. Immunol.* 111:720, 1973.

Kolb, A., and Bosma, M. J. Clones producing antibodies of more than one class. *Immunology* 33:461, 1977.

Matthias, R., Wabl, M. R., Forni, L., and Loor, F. Switch in immunoglobulin class production observed in single clones of committed lymphocytes. *Science* 199:1078, 1978.

Mitchison, N. A. The carrier effect in the secondary response to hapten-protein conjugates. II. Cellular cooperation. *Eur. J. Immunol.* 1:18, 1971.

Origins of Lymphocyte Diversity. Cold Spring Harbor Symposia on Quantitative Biology, XLI (Parts 1 and 2). Cold Spring Harbor Laboratory of Quantitative Biology, Cold Spring Harbor, L. I., New York, 1977.

Riley, R. F., and Hokama, Y. Appearance of a substance in acute phase serum which elicits Cx-protein responses. *Science* 132:1894, 1960.

Lymphocyte Interactions in the Immune Response

Baker, P. J., Reed, N. O., Stashak, P. W., Amsbaugh, D. F., and Prescott, B. Regulation of the antibody response to type III pneumococcal polysaccharide. I. Nature of regulatory cells. *J. Exp. Med.* 137:1431, 1973.

Janossy, G., and Greaves, M. F. Lymphocyte activation. I. Response of T and B lymphocytes to phytomitogens. *Clin. Exp. Immunol.* 9:483, 1971.

Katz, D. H. Adaptive differentiation of murine lymphocytes: Implications for mechanisms of cell-cell recognition and the regulation of immune responses. *Fed. Proc.* 38:2065, 1979.

Moller, G. 19S antibody production against soluble lipopolysaccharide antigens by individual lymphoid cells in vitro. *Nature* 207:1166, 1965.

Mosier, D. E., Johnson, M. B., Paul, W. E., and McMaster, P. R. B. Cellular requirements for the primary in vitro antibody response to DNP-Ficoll. *J. Exp. Med.* 139:1354, 1974.

Rosenthal, A. S., Lipsky, P. E., and Shevach, E. M. Macrophage-lymphocyte interaction and antigen recognition. *Fed. Proc.* 34:1743, 1975.

Rosenthal, A. S., Blake, J. T., Ellner, J. J., Greineder, D. K., and Lipsky, P. E. The Role of Macrophage in T Lymphocyte Antigen Recognition. In A. S. Rosenthal (Ed.), *Immune Recognition.* New York: Academic, 1975. Pp. 539–554.

Skelly, R. R., Munkenbeck, P., and Morrison, D. C. Stimulation of T-independent antibody responses by hapten-lipopolysaccharides without repeating polymeric structure. *Infect. Immun.* 23:287, 1979.

Woodland, R. T., and Cantor, H. Idiotype specific T helper cells are required to induce idiotype positive B memory cells to secrete antibody. *Eur. J. Immunol.* 8:600, 1978.

6 : Modulation of the Immune Response

The delineation of the immune response has been achieved to a certain extent by use of a variety of agents, physical and chemical, nonspecific and specific, in the modulation of the immune processes. These included x-irradiation, immunopotentiators, immunosuppressive drugs, and surgical ablation of specific organs and tissues. This chapter will discuss in brief those factors which have contributed to our understanding of immunological processes.

Tests for Evaluation of Immunocompetency In order to evaluate and assess the effects of the immunopotentiators and the immunosuppressive agents, it was necessary to decide what are considered normal values for immunocompetence in animals. Both in vitro and in vivo test procedures have been established for the assessment of immunocompetency of the cellular (T cell) and humoral (B cell) systems. These methods are summarized in Table 6-1.

Immunopotentiation Immunopotentiation is the augmentation or enhancement of the immune process by use of a variety of substances, especially drugs and immunoadjuvants, which have a positive effect on the responses of both the cellular- and humoral-mediated systems. The development of agents for immune augmentation was spurred by a need to combat cancer, to reverse iatrogenic immunosuppression, and to treat immunodeficiency diseases and chronic infections. *Immunopotentiators* circumscribes a large number of therapeutic agents. The term, however, does not describe the action of the drugs adequately, since they have other nonpotentiating effects, that is their actions are not restricted to potentiation. The paragraphs to follow include brief discussions of the recently discovered immunopotentiating drugs and the role of adjuvant. The latter has been used traditionally for boosting immunological responses. Delineation of the mechanism of adjuvant and immunopotentiator actions, may be the key to an understanding of the immune response.

Adjuvants MYCOBACTERIUM. Immunogens persisting for a long time in tissues enhance antibody and prolong synthesis in the peripheral circulation. Thus, a series of multiple injections at low doses

Table 6-1 : Tests for Evaluation and Assessment of Immunocompetency in Man

Assessment	Antigens, Target Cells, or Reagents
I. In vivo	
A. Humoral responses	
1. Primary antibody responses	Bacteriophage T4, hemocyanin, influenza virus vaccine, xenogeneic red blood cells
2. Secondary antibody responses	Toxoid; tetanus, diphtheroids; polio and other viral vaccines (rubella, influenza); *Salmonella typi*, 4 antigens
B. Cell-mediated responses	
1. Primary	Skin reactions DNCB, hemocyanin, PPD
2. Secondary	Skin reactions to mumps, candidin, trichophytin, streptokinase, streptodornase, PPD
C. Nonspecific responses	
1. Inflammatory response	Skin window, use of various antigens or mitogens
II. In vitro	
A. T cell analysis	
1. Mixed lymphocyte reaction (MLR or MLC)	Allogeneic lymphocytes
2. Blastogenesis	
a. Specific	Specific antigens
b. Nonspecific	Mitogens: PHA, Con A, lentinan, PWM
3. Mitogen-induced leukocytotoxicity (Con A or PHA)	Allogeneic lymphocytes or tumor cells
4. Enumeration	
a. E-rosette	SRBC
b. Immunofluorescence	Anti-Thy, anti-T1 (labeled with fluorescein agents)
c. EA-rosette (Fc receptor	EA-SRBC (antibody-coated SRBC)
d. Cytotoxicity	Specific antibodies to T subsets plus complement

5. Lymphokines
   a. MIF — Macrophage migration
   b. Interferon production — Viral inhibition

B. B cell analysis
   1. Blastogenesis
      a. Specific — Anti-Ig
      b. Nonspecific — Mitogen, PWM, LPS
   2. Mitogen induction — Polyclonal Ig synthesis
   3. Enumeration
      a. EAC-rosette — Antibody + SRBC + complement
      b. Immunofluorescence — Specific anti-Ig-labeled with fluorescent agents
      c. Ea-rosette (Fc receptor) — EA-SRBC
      d. Immuno-beads — Immunobeads, anti-Ig-sepharose-beads
   4. Cytotoxic antibodies — + Complement: lymphocytes (as in HLA typing)

C. Macrophage analysis
   1. Leukocyte cytotoxicity—direct — Various target cells
   2. Leukocyte cytotoxicity—(Fc receptor) — Antibody-coated
   3. Phagocytosis — Various target cells or inert practices, bacteria

D. Analysis for other cells
   1. Natural killer cell (no complement or Ig requirement) — Various target cells (tumors)
   2. Leukocyte cytotoxicity
      a. ADCC killer cells — Antibody-coated
      b. Neutrophils — Target cells
   3. Null cells (Ig⁻ and C⁻) no receptors — E-SRBC and EAC-SRBC (negative reactions to these tests)

137

Table 6-2 : Immunoadjuvants Used in Immunopotentiation of the Immune Response

Substances	Composition or Chemical Nature
Freund's complete adjuvant (CFA)	Water-oil emulsion and killed *Mycobacterium tuberculosis* mixture
BCG	Bacillus of Calmette-Guérin (attenuated *Mycobacterium*)
Water-soluble adjuvant (WSA)	Muramic acid–containing polymer linked to arabino-galactan
Synthetic S-MDp	Muramic dipeptide (*N*-acetyl-muramyl-L-alanyl-D-isoglutamine)
Polymeric anions	Poly A:U, double-stranded RNA (dsRNA); poly I:C, dextran sulfate
Bacteria	*Corynebacterium parvum; Bordetella pertussis*
Toxins and polysaccharides	Lipopolysaccharides (endotoxins); lentinan, glucan

is more effective than a single moderate or large dose. Addition of adjuvant to the immunogen whether in single or multiple low doses, however, will enhance synthesis and prolong antibody in the peripheral blood. Adjuvants in the form of alum gels, aluminum hydroxide or phosphate have been used effectively in immunization with diphtheria toxoid. Broadly speaking, adjuvant is a substance that enhances or increases the immune response to the immunogen with which it is mixed or added. The various adjuvants used in animals for the increased production of antibody are listed in Table 6-2. The most effective adjuvants appear to be the water-oil emulsions containing killed *Microbacterium tuberculosis.* The water-oil adjuvants following subcutaneous administration tend to disseminate as small oil droplets. Antibody synthesis occurs earlier and persists longer as depicted in Figure 6-1 (curve B), than in the response to soluble protein antigen alone (curve A). Freund's complete adjuvant (FCA) is not used for immunization in man due to its irritating effect and tendency to induce delayed type hypersensitivity and formation of granulomatous lesions at the site of injection. It may also stimulate lymph node enlargement and possibly induce lymphomas (cancer of the lymphoid cells). The mechanism of adjuvant action has been examined by many investigators. Two major conclusions can be drawn: adjuvant mixed with immunogen (1) promotes the maintenance of low effective antigen levels in tissue; that is, encourages a slow absorption rate of the antigen entrapped in the lipid micelles; and (2) provokes a chronic inflammatory response. As a result of inflammation, macrophages are activated, and enhanced phagocytosis and preparation or presentation of the antigen to the T and B cells occurs. Activation of macrophages would also lead to the induction and release of monokines,

Fig. 6-1 : The effect of adjuvant (curve B) on the primary immune response in an animal given soluble protein antigen. The control response is shown in curve A.

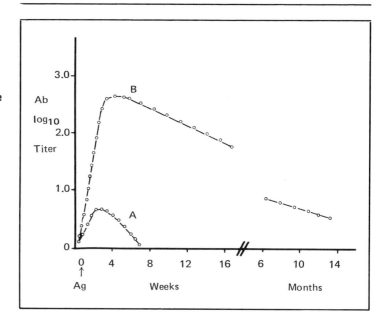

which can affect T and B cell stimulation and proliferation. The mycobacteria in FCA tend to enhance only the T cells by acting as immunogens themselves for the T cells or as carriers for the soluble protein antigen. Mycobacteria induce T cell proliferation, as evidenced by the hyperplasia in the paracortical region of the lymph node. Activation of the T cells would engender the release of B cell–stimulating factors (lymphokines) and thus enhance antibody synthesis. The major effect of the acid-fast microorganism may be on the T helper cells also. Furthermore, T cell lymphokines would stimulate macrophages in a variety of ways, and the activated macrophages in turn would contribute to enhancement of the immune response directly or via its monokines.

LOW MOLECULAR WEIGHT COMPOUNDS RELATED TO *MYCO-BACTERIUM*. Chemical fractions obtained from *Mycobacterium* have also proved to be useful adjuvants, especially the water-soluble fractions, since they induce none of the granulomatous lesions exhibited by the intact organism. Synthetic low molecular weight, water-soluble adjuvants have been prepared that simulate the immunoadjuvanticity of the fractions obtained from *Myco-bacterium.* They are presently being examined for human use in vaccination against various microorganisms and in cancer immunotherapy. Some of these low molecular weight synthetic adjuvants and their selective immunopotentiating effects on different immune responses are shown in Table 6-3. The structure of a synthetic low molecular weight adjuvant is shown in Figure 6-2.

Table 6-3 : Synthetic Adjuvants with Selective Immunopotentiation

Compound	MW	Activity (Effect on Immune Response)			
		DTH[a]	CML[b]	Humoral (PFC)[c]	Pyogenic Activity[d]
6-o-Mycoloyl-N-acetylmuramyl-L-serine-D-iso-glutamine	1,666.91	++	++	–	–
6-o-Mycoloyl-N-acetylmuramyl-glycyl-D-iso-glutamine	1,666.91	–	++	–	–
6-o-Mycoloyl-N-Acetylmuramyl-L-alanyl-D-iso-glutamine	1,686.95	++	++	–	++

[a]Ag = M-(4-(4'-arseno-phenylazo)-phenyl)-N-acetyl-L-tyrosine administered to guinea pigs and allogeneic mice; DTH, delayed type hypersensitivity.

[b]Enhanced cell-mediated lympholysis (CML) shown in allogeneic mice.

[c]PFC = plaque-forming cell for humoral system evaluation.

[d]Pyogenicity demonstrated in rabbits.

Fig. 6-2 : The chemical structure of a low molecular weight synthetic adjuvant, 6-o-stearoyl-N-acetyl-muramyl-dipeptide.

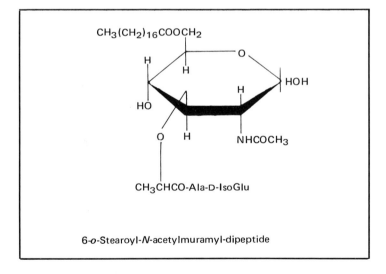

6-o-Stearoyl-N-acetylmuramyl-dipeptide

CORYNEBACTERIUM. Mice (C57B/6J) given heat-killed *Coryne-bacterium parvum* showed maximum levels of increase in prosta-glandin E (PGE) in spleen cultures 5 to 10 days after injection of the adjuvant. The increased synthesis of PGE appeared as early as 30 minutes after initiation of the culture, with the maximum level attained after 48 hours of incubation. Treatment of the culture with indomethacin abolished the synthesis of PGE, and removal of the adherent cells or macrophages significantly decreased the synthesis of PGE. Treatment with another strain of *Corynebacterium,* one that does not affect the lymphoreticular system, had no effect on PGE synthesis by spleen cells. These findings suggest that adjuvant must have an effect on the lymphoreticular system, perhaps more specifically on the macrophages. Zymosan added to spleen cell cultures previously treated with *C. parvum* also enhanced PGE synthesis. PGE appears to have a significant effect on immune or mitogenic responses via stimulation of c-AMP. Thus, the immunostimulating and immunosuppressive properties of *C. parvum* may be due to this increase elaboration of PGE, an important mediating molecule in inflammation. It is likely that all adjuvants that have a similar effect to *C. parvum* on macrophages and PGE synthesis may modulate the immune and mitogenic responses in a similar way, although the time of increase and the maximum level of PGE may vary with each adjuvant. It remains to be established whether the major pathway of adjuvant action is as found with *C. parvum* activation of macrophages, PGE synthesis, increase in intracellular cyclic nucleotides, and enhanced immune response. This sequence, however, would be compatible with the chronic inflammatory properties of adjuvant action.

OTHER ADJUVANTS. Poly A:U appears to act on the cell-mediated system (increases T helper cells, probably via c-AMP) and also, but in doses toxic for animals, induces production of interferon.

BCG has been used for immunotherapy in the treatment of melanoma (a malignant form of skin cancer that spreads rapidly and systematically and produces a melanin pigment [dark]) and for augmentation of the immune system. Its major effect appears to be on the T cell system, although it is not a good immunoadjuvant per se.

Lipopolysaccharides (LPS) have been used in cancer therapy, but their use is limited by their toxicity. LPS appear to stimulate the humoral immune response system. They are also involved in the activation of complement in the alternative pathway (see Chapter 9). The polysaccharide lentinan, derived from *Lentinus edodes* (mushroom), appears to stimulate the antibody-dependent cytotoxic cells but has no effect on the immune responses. On the other hand glucan, a polysaccharide obtained from zymosan (*Saccharomyces cerevisiae*), induces macrophage activation and T cell enhancement. It is also involved in the activation of complement via the alternative pathway.

Immunopotentiating Drugs

LEVAMISOLE. Levamisole (LMS) is a phenylimidazothiazole used therapeutically as an antihelmintic agent. The structures of

Fig. 6-3 : The chemical structures of two immuno- potentiators, levamisole and inosiplex.

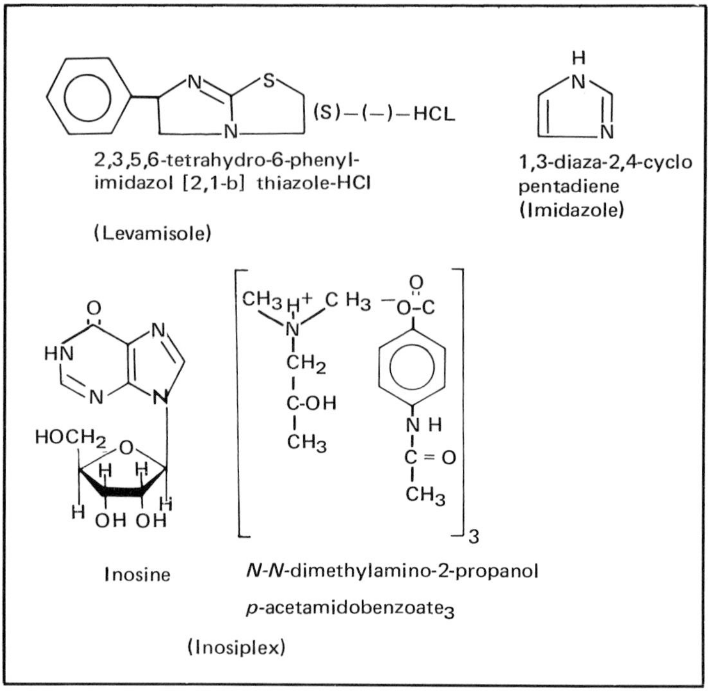

2,3,5,6-tetrahydro-6-phenyl-
imidazol [2,1-b] thiazole-HCl

(Levamisole)

1,3-diaza-2,4-cyclo
pentadiene
(Imidazole)

Inosine

N-N-dimethylamino-2-propanol

p-acetamidobenzoate$_3$

(Inosiplex)

LMS and its parent compound imidazole are presented in Figure 6-3. An enormous amount of experimental and clinical investi- gation into the immunopotentiating capabilities of this com- pound has yielded the following reports: (1) in man, LMS was reported to restore and augment the delayed hypersen- sitivity reactions to DNCB and PPD and to increase DNA synthesis of lymphocytes to mitogens and antigens in vitro. Some studies showed, however, that the effect of mitogen re- sponses in vitro was dependent on the time of addition and dose of LMS. Thus, variable results have been obtained in the reported literature. (2) Lymphokine production was shown to be in- creased by LMS, and augmentation of E-rosette and T suppressor cell activity has also been attributed to LMS. The accumulated evidence appears to indicate that the cell-mediated system is preferentially responsive to LMS. (3) A thymosin-like activity has been attributed to levamisole, also. The reticuloendothelial system has been shown to be responsive to the action of LMS, as manifested by an increase in carbon clearance, enhanced phagocytosis, and bactericidal effects on peritoneal macrophages in animal studies. (4) LMS also augments the chemotaxic re- sponses of neutrophils and macrophages. (5) Furthermore, ad- ministration of LMS to 10-day-old suckling rats induced a sig- nificant protection against herpes virus and a virulent strain of Staphylococcus. It was thought that the mobilization and increased maturation of the neutrophils and macrophages augmented the protective effect against these microorganisms in the newborn rats.

The mechanism of levamisole's action is presently unclear. It has been suggested that, like its parent compound imidazole, LMS acts on the cyclic nucleotide diphosphoesterases and promotes an increase in breakdown of c-AMP. Theophylline, which suppresses the action of c-AMP diphosphoesterase, would be expected to reverse the LMS effect. This indeed appears to be the case. LMS has also been shown to suppress and stimulate enzymes of the citric acid cycle in *Tetrahymena pyriformis* and the glucose metabolism of leukemic cells (myeloblastic). In addition, LMS has exhibited inhibition of human platelet aggregation stimulated by the prostaglandin precursor arachidonate, an analog of endoperoxide, as well as by epinephrine and hydrogen peroxide. This inhibition of platelets has also been demonstrated by imidazole.

Present investigations have suggested that levamisole is not generally effective against primary bacterial or viral infections in immunocompetent adult animals but may be of benefit in the treatment of chronic or recurrent infections in immunodeficient individuals or newborn animals. Since LMS has no intrinsic antimicrobial effect, its action appears to lie in the potentiation of the defects of the various arms (refers to CMI, humoral and nonspecific systems) of the immune response.

INOSIPLEX. Inosiplex, a complex of inosine with *p*-acetamidobenzoic acid-*N*, *N*-dimethylaminoisopropanol, has been shown to have immunopotentiating properties. The structure of this complex is shown in Figure 6-3. Its antiviral efficacy appear to be at a maximum when it is given to patients therapeutically during the course of a viral infection. When given prophylactically, its antiviral protection seems to be of no value. The action of the drug appears to be on the efferent arm, that is, probably on the lymphocytes interacting with the virus or those primed by the virus. Inosiplex appears to stimulate these lymphocytes to proliferate. This is reflected by increases in antiviral titers in patients given the drug. Increase in lymphokine production has been noted with inosiplex. Immunopotentiation has been ascribed to this drug, and it may prove to be a useful antiviral agent.

Immune System Products in Potentiation

Certain products of the immune system are associated with immunopotentiation. These are discussed throughout this text: the lymphokines, especially transfer factor and interferons (see Chapter 3), and the thymic hormone thymosin. These biological compounds all play a significant role in the immuno-regulation of the host defense system.

The few agents just discussed, as well as others too numerous to present in this text, offer a wide spectrum of degree, mode, and mechanism of action. Differences in action of these agents provide for some degree of specificity, and when their mode of action is delineated, they may be used for selective actions and ultimately for combination therapy designed to achieve a multiciplicity of action for correcting the defect in the immune response.

Immunosuppression   The acute and chronic suppression of the immune process can be achieved by a variety of physical and chemical agents, by specific surgical removal of immunocompetent and immunoregulating tissues, and by the use of specific antibodies to various cells or products of the immune processes. Immunosuppression is practiced in attempts to control and ameliorate hypersensitivities (humoral and CMI), autoimmune diseases, allogeneic transplantation of organs and tissues, and in the treatment of lympho-proliferative disorders (lymphoma, myeloma, and leukemia). In general, it is used to suppress only the active immune processes associated with the pathogenesis of the disease.

Agents used for immunosuppressive therapy and for the under-standing of the immune processes in experimental animals have also been used in cancer chemotherapy. Many of these drugs act during the proliferation phase of the cell cycle, which appears to be the part of the cycle most susceptible to drug action. The sequence of events following antigenic or mitogenic stimulation of the immune system and the subsequent burst of mitotic division (in synchrony) make for better understanding of the drug action in the immune processes. Thus, selective toxicity for the immune proliferation of immunocytes can be achieved in the suppression of the immune process in organ transplantation. In contrast, tumor cells proliferate randomly and thus make it more difficult to achieve selective toxicity of proliferating tumor cells. Furthermore, immunosuppression drugs are given at lower doses and for longer periods, while in cancer chemotherapy drugs are given at higher levels and at longer intervals of rest due to the adverse side effect of these drugs.

Drugs can affect various phases of the cell cycle and can be broadly categorized as cell cycle-specific (CCS) and cell cycle-unspecific (CCNS). The CCS drugs appear to affect cells only during the active cell-cycling phase, therefore presumably not during the G_0 phase, whereas CCNS drugs are capable of inhibition and killing at all phases. CCNS drug actions are generally

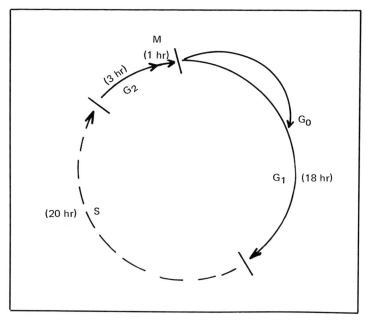

Fig. 6-4 : The cell cycle: G_1 is the phase between mitosis and the DNA synthesis phase (S); G_2 is the period between the end of S and the beginning of M (the mitotic phase); and G_0 is a quiescent phase. If the cell remains in the G_0 phase, further proliferation does not occur until the cell is back in the cyclic G_1 phase.

manifested by slowing of the S phase and an irreversible effect on the G_2 phase rendering the cells incapable of division.

Figure 6-4 of the cell cycle indicates the parts that are affected by the immunosuppressive agents discussed here. The G_1 phase (18 hours) precedes the S phase, and during this period various enzymes, including those necessary for DNA synthesis (DNA polymerase), are synthesized. The long S phase (20 hours) constitutes the period of DNA replication for the various chromosomes (commitment to DNA synthesis in this phase). The G_2 phase is the period of specialized protein and RNA synthesis and manufacture of the mitotic spindle apparatus prior to the short (1 hour) phase of mitosis. The G_0 phase constitutes the long period of resting state in which cells are not cycling (pre-G_1 phase).

Figure 6-5 represents immunocyte expansion following antigenic stimulation. Examination at the level of replication affords insight into the mechanism of action of immunosuppressive drugs. These immunosuppressive drugs and their mode of action on the immune processes and immunological injury are listed in Table 6-4.

Fig. 6-5 : Immunocyte expansion following antigenic stimulation in the primary response. Numbers in circles indicate region of drug action listed in Table 6-4.

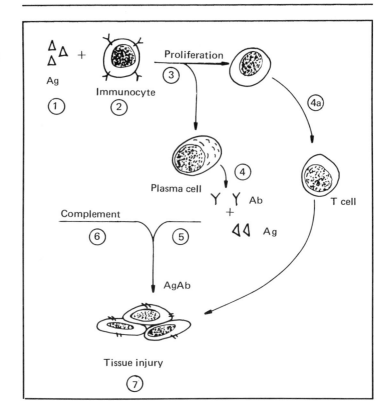

X-irradiation

Classic studies conducted on rabbits in the mid-1950s showed that animals given sublethal whole-body x-irradiation 24 to 48 hours before administration of an immunogen such as SRBC will have a loss or suppression of antibody synthesis to the immunogen as demonstrated by a lack of anti-SRBC (hemolysin) titers. Suppression of antibody synthesis is noted even when x-irradiation is given 2 to 4 hours prior to antigen injection. Antibody synthesis is less affected when x-irradiation is given 24 to 48 hours *after* antigen stimulation, however, although the induction and rate of antibody synthesis are somewhat prolonged. The major effect of x-irradiation is on the bone marrow cells and, therefore, on both T and B cells precursors and on the lymphoid system. A temporary immune suppressed state is engendered until the cells recover some weeks later. Whole-body x-irradiation and selective radiation have been used for suppression of the immune system, especially of the bone marrow, prior to organ transplantation, and in diseases such as aplastic anemia and leukemia. X-irradiation has little or no effect on the secondary immune system. Low levels of x-irradiation given with the booster immunogen that stimulates the secondary response have had an adjuvant effect in animal studies but have not been used clinically.

Table 6-4 : Drugs and Their Mode of Action
(Refer to Figure 6-5 for the Numbers in Parentheses)

Drug or Agent	Mode of Action
X-irradiation	(2) Effect on immunocyte, prior to antigen administration
Prednisone	(2), (3), (7) Effect on immunocyte and on proliferation, anti-inflammatory effect (injury site)
Azathioprine	(3) Effect on proliferation (expansion)
Methotrexate	(3) '' ''
Cyclophosphamide	(2), (3) Effect on immunocyte and on proliferation
Dactinomycin	(3), (4) Effect on proliferation and synthesis of antibody and protein synthesis in T cells
Antibody (anti-Rho, anti-D)	(1), (2) Sequestration of antigen and negative feedback in immunocyte
Antilymphocyte	(2), (3), (4), (4a) Cytotoxicity to T or B cells
Dicromoglycate	(5) Effect on Ag-Ab complexes
PGE$_1$	(5) '' '' '' ''
Anticomplement	(6) Effect on C system
Tirolone	(4a), (7) Suppressed or delayed hypersensitivity

Immunosuppressive Drugs

CORTICOSTEROIDS. Animal responses to corticosteroid administration are not uniform. It has been demonstrated that man, guinea pigs, and primates are resistant to steroids, while rodents—mice, rats, and rabbits,—are highly sensitive. The side effects attributed to corticosteroids in general are sodium retention, edema, hypokalemia, hypoglycemia, hirsutism, hypertension, and occasionally psychic disturbances.

Early experimenters with corticosteroid administration to animals observed a significant decrease in the peripheral lymphocytes, engendered by a lymphopenia. This finding was attributed to lympholysis, especially with high dosages. It is also reflected by a reduction in size of various lymphoid tissues (spleen, lymph node), after administration of prednisone and dexamethasone. Other alterations induced by corticosteroids include: (1) redistribution of lymphocytes; (2) an effect on protein synthesis; and (3) stabilization of membrane, especially the lysosomal membrane, thus preventing the release of inflammatory factors from the granules of PMN and macrophages. Adrenocorticotropic hormone (ACTH) secreted by the pituitary has been used in suspected autoimmune diseases such as myasthenia gravis. ACTH acts by stimulation of endogenous corticosteroids, which in turn cause immunosuppression. Presumably the antiacetylcholine receptor antibodies are suppressed and thus alleviate the clinical manifestations associated with myasthenia gravis.

Table 6-5 : Drugs Used in Immunosuppressive Therapy

Disease	Agents Used
Autoimmune	
1. Acute glomerulonephritis	Prednisone, 6-mercaptopurine, cyclophosphamide
2. Autoimmune hemolytic anemia	Prednisone, cyclophosphamide, azathioprine, chlorambucil, 6-mercaptopurine
3. Idiopathic thrombocytopenia purpura	Prednisone, vincristine, mercaptopurine, azathioprine
Organ transplant	
1. Renal and heart	Azathioprine, prednisone, antilymphocytic globulin, dactinomycin, cyclophosphamide
2. Bone marrow	Cyclophosphamide, prednisone, methotrexate, antilymphocyte globulin, total body x-irradiation

Corticosteroids affect both the T and the B cells and hence the cell-mediated and humoral-mediated immune processes. The most greatly affected appear to be the thymocytes and the subsets of T cells, including the Ts and Th cells. At least in the spleen of mice, B cells appear to decrease more rapidly than T cells following administration of hydrocortisone acetate. In mouse spleen the B cells appear to be affected to a greater extent than the T cells, although both are affected by hydrocortisone acetate. In general, the plasma cells are less sensitive to corticosteroid. Therefore corticosteroids have less effect in secondary responses than in the primary response. Prolonged administration of prednisone, however, will diminish antibody synthesis with depletion of precursors of Th and B cells.

The major advantage of corticosteroids is their lack of effect on the myeloid and erythroid precursors of the bone marrow. Thus prednisone, a synthetic corticosteroid, is widely used as an immunosuppressive drug (Table 6-5). The effect of chronic administration of prednisone and other corticosteroids should be considered, especially of adrenal suppression and the feedback effect on the pituitary (diminished ACTH output). The structures of hydrocortisone and predisone are shown in Figure 6-6.

ANTIMETABOLITES. Azathioprine (Imuran) is an imidazolyl derivative of 6-mercaptopurine (6-MP) and acts as a structural analogue or antimetabolite. Azathioprine is metabolized to 6-mercaptopurine, which is the active factor in the immunosuppression exhibited by this agent. It acts on the proliferative stage of the cell cycle following antigenic stimulation (see Figure 6-5).

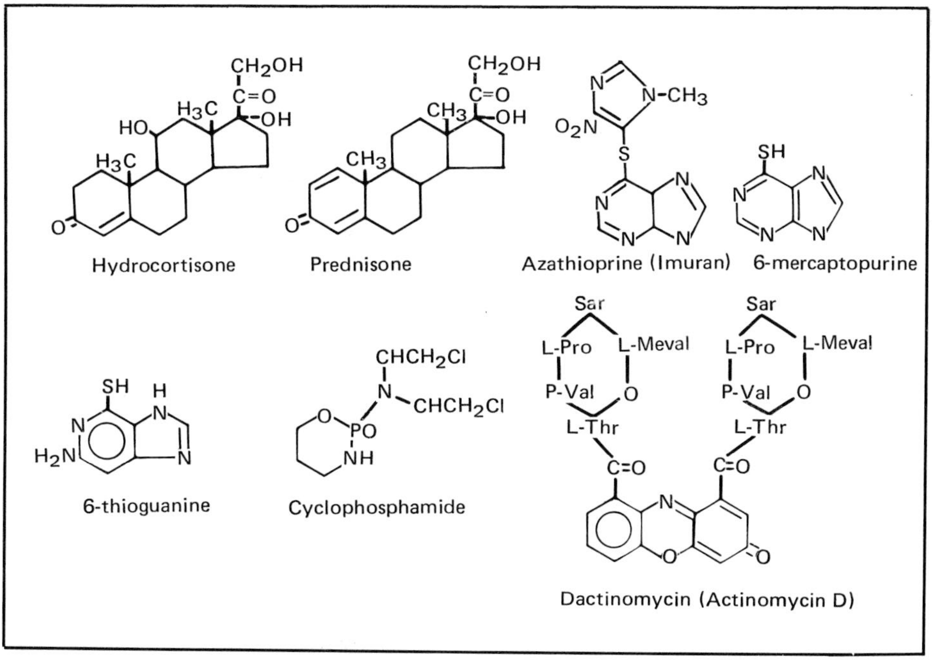

Fig. 6-6 : Chemical structures of some immunosuppressive agents.

Azathioprine is absorbed readily from the gastrointestinal tract and is metabolized to 6-mercaptopurine, the active compound in vivo. 6-MP is further metabolized to 6-thiouric acid by xanthine oxidase prior to excretion through the urine. Low levels of intact azathioprine and 6-MP are excreted through the urine, thus increasing the toxicity two-fold in patients with anephric or anuric kidney problems. Use of azathioprine in such patients should be regulated. For patients receiving allopurinol, a xanthine oxidase inhibitor, the levels of administered azathioprine should also be regulated: doses generally should be reduced to one-fourth or one-third of the usual. Allopurinol is used for control of hyperuricemia. Unlike the corticosteroids, azathioprine and 6-MP are toxic to the bone marrow. This is manifested primarily by leukopenia with occasional anemia, thrombocytopenia, and bleeding, sometimes accompanied by skin rashes, drug fever, nausea, and vomiting and occasionally vomiting with gastrointestinal symptoms. This last is generally manifested with high doses of the drug. Hepatic dysfunction, with very high serum alkaline phosphatase levels and mild jaundice, occurs occasionally.

As indicated earlier, azathioprine, like 6-MP acts on nucleic acid synthesis (antimetabolite), the proliferative stage following antigenic stimulation. The agents are essentially cytotoxic and irreversibly destroy the cells in proliferation (CCS drugs). They affect cell-mediated and humoral responses in both primary and secondary phases. The major clinical uses of azathioprine are listed in Table 6-5. 6-Mercaptopurine is an antimetabolite (purine analogue) and affects the immune responses during the proliferative phase when DNA synthesis is at its peak (phase S of the cell cycle). Administration of 6-MP results in the formation of the 5'-phosphate ribonucleotide of 6-MP (thioinosinate [T-IMP]). This metabolite may inhibit a number of vital metabolic pathways in purine metabolism. T-IMP can block the conversion of inosinate (IMP) to adenylsuccinate (AMPS), a key reaction in the formation of adenylate. Also, T-IMP inhibits or reacts with inosinic dehydrogenase, the enzyme that catalyzes the conversion of IMP to xanthylate (XMP), a key step in the formation of guanylate (GMP) from IMP. Thus, T-IMP inhibits or blocks the synthesis of AMP and GMP from the key metabolite IMP. T-IMP may have its key effect on the first committed de novo pathway of purine synthesis—the reaction of glutamine and 5'-phospho-α-D-ribosyl-pyrophosphate (PRPP) to form ribosylamine-5'-phosphate, catalyzed by 5'-PRPP-amidotransferase. This enzyme (ribosyl amidotransferase) controls a major part of purine biosynthesis and is highly responsive to intracellular concentrations of 5'-monophosphate ribonucleotides via feedback inhibition. *Analogues* as well as normal nucleotides can inhibit this key enzyme. Thus, T-IMP can have a major effect on it and thereby on purine biosynthesis (Figure 6-7). The half-life of 6-MP in blood is 90 minutes. It is rapidly metabolized by xanthine oxidase and excreted via the urine.

6-Thioguanine (6-TG) is metabolized via the nucleotide corresponding to guanine. Its major effect appears to be the displacement of guanine and the resultant formation of functionally altered polynucleotides. It also inhibits purine metabolism but less effectively than 6-MP. It is absorbed rapidly, with a half-life of 1 to 1½ hours and is excreted in urine as β-thiourate and methylated 6-TG.

A major obstacle to the use of purine analogues is acquired resistance to the drugs. This appears to be due to the deficiency of the enzyme inosinic-guanylic pyrophosphorylase, which is required for the "lethal" synthesis of fraudulent ribonucleotides of guanine or hypoxanthine analogues.

CYTOTOXIC AGENTS. The alkylating agent cyclophosphamide (see Figure 6-6) is one of the useful immunosuppressive drugs employed as an antineoplastic agent for the treatment of lymphoproliferative malignancies. These include lymphoma and certain leukemias. Cyclophosphamide acts on the proliferating lymphoid

Fig. 6-7 : Thio-inosinate (T-IMP), a derivative of 6-mercaptopurine and 5'-monophosphate ribose, in the inhibition of purine metabolism.

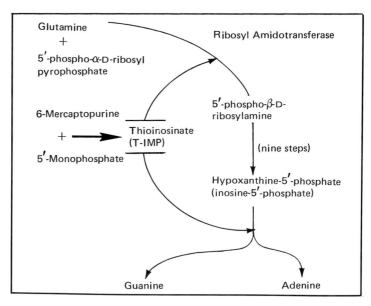

cells (step 3 in Figure 6-5) and alkylates some resting cells. Cyclophosphamide, like other alkylating agents, affects DNA synthesis by alkylation of the purines and thus tends to be mutagenic as well. Inhibition of glycolysis, cellular respiration, the activity of various enzymes, and protein synthesis has been attributed to the alkylating agents. The major effects are on proliferating cells and include cytotoxicity and mutagenicity. The side effects of cyclophosphamide are less severe on the CNS than those of the typical nitrogen mustards and include nausea, alopecia, hepatic dysfunction, and frequently leukopenia. Cyclophosphamide in larger doses may induce an apparent specific tolerance to a new antigen if administered with or shortly after the antigen. Large doses may carry a considerable risk of pancytopenia and hemorrhagic cystitis. Nevertheless, large doses are used in addition to x-irradiation to prepare patients for bone marrow transplants. This, however, makes the recipient vulnerable to GVH reaction, if the HLA comptability is improperly typed. In smaller doses cyclophosphamide has been effective in autoimmune disorders (Table 6-5).

Other cytotoxic agents used in immunosuppression include vincristine, methotrexate, and dactinomycin.

OTHER DRUGS. The enzyme L-asparaginase (L-asparagine amidohydrolase EC 3.5.1.1) isolated from *E. coli* may be of value in selective immunosuppression of precursors of the lymphoid series. It has been shown that lymphoblasts in acute lymphoblastic leukemia require the amino acid L-asparagine for growth.

Most normal differentiated tissue can synthesize its own L-asparagine. The enzyme L-asparaginase hydrolyzes catalytic L-asparagine to aspartic acid and ammonia, thus depriving the lymphoblast of L-asparagine and causing its demise. The enzyme has had limited use because of its antigenicity, which can induce hypersensitivity. Nevertheless, significant numbers of remissions of lymphoblastic leukemias in children have been observed. The side effects of the drug include chills, fever, allergic reactions, fatty degeneration of liver, defects in blood coagulation, and occasional CNS toxicity.

Tilorone can show antitumor and antiviral activities in animal models. In rodents the activities of tilorone have been associated with its interferon-inducing capacity. Tilorone seems to have a paradoxical effect on the immune response, exhibiting an adjuvant-like effect in humoral immunity and an ability to suppress cellular immunity. The effect on CMI is associated with temporary lymphopenia restricted to the T cells. The chronic administration of Tilorone with antigen appears to alter the expression of delayed type hypersensitivity at step 7 in Figure 6-5.

Specific Suppression of the Immune System

Xenogeneic antibodies can be used to specifically suppress various target cells within the immune processes. Antimacrophage, antilymphocyte, antiplasma, and anti-Ig heavy chain sera have all been used for neutralization of both humoral and cell-mediated immune responsiveness. Antilymphocyte globulin (ALG) has been used clinically in abrogation of the recipient's immune system in organ transplantation. Each of these antisera for specific cells has been used in numerous experiments to delineate the sequence of events in the immune processes.

Allotypic Suppression

An interesting phenomenon observed endogenously in rabbits is the *allotypic suppression* associated with anti-IgG, antibodies. The maternal rabbit produces specific antiallotype IgG antibodies against a fetus with paternal allotype IgG markers, thus suppressing the expression of the paternal allotype immunoglobulin G in the newborn rabbit. This suppression of paternal allotype IgG in the rabbit offspring persists for months, even after the disappearance of the maternal antiallotype in the peripheral blood of the offspring. This can be explained as follows: A female rabbit with a homozygous allotype b_4 is mated with a male with a (homozygous) allotype b_5; therefore the offspring would have the allotype $b_4 b_5$. This mating results in the production of anti-b_5 by the female rabbit. This antibody passes the placental barrier and hence induces suppression of allotype b_5 expression in the fetus and subsequently in the newborn. This is referred to as *allotypic suppression.* The administration of xenogeneic anti-allotype antibody to the newborn animal does not cause the same phenomenon. The mechanism of allotypic suppression is presently unclear, though an autoimmune concept has been postulated. That is, low levels of antiallotype antibodies (example, anti-b_5) may be produced by the unsuppressed lymphocytes against the suppressed in the newborn. Evidence for this idea, however, is lacking, as no anti-allotype antibodies have been detected after the disappearance of the initial maternal anti-allotype antibody (anti-b_5), nor have antibodies been detected in in vitro studies.

Antibodies

Anti-immunoglobulin heavy chain antibodies can induce suppression of heavy chain isotypes. Thus anti-μ antibody panspecifically suppresses IgM, IgG, and IgA humoral responses of B cells uncommitted to antigen. This same antibody has no effect on IgG production by B cells previously primed by antigen. In mice, anti-γ and anti-α antibodies suppress class-specifically; that is, IgA and IgG, respectively, are suppressed by anti-γ and anti-α. In chickens, however, anti-α antibody suppresses both IgA and IgM synthesis. Heavy chain isotype suppression is restricted to humoral responses only. Thus cell-mediated immune responses are not affected by anti-heavy–chain antibodies. The mode of effect of these antibodies on the B cells is not clear, but it appears to be direct, since no T suppressor cells are involved. These anti-heavy–chain antibodies appear to have no deleterious effect on the host except for the isotypic suppression. On the basis of these observations and through the use of anti-heavy chain antibodies in neonate mice, the ontogeny of B cells as shown in Figure 6-8 has been suggested. The model (Figure 6-8) stresses the separation (two precursor cells instead of one) rather than sequential development postulated by others from data in chicken studies. The chicken model suggests that the IgA and IgM synthesizing cells come from a common precursor, whereas the mouse model suggests two separate precursors, 1 for IgG and 1 for IgA (Figure 6-8).

Surgery

Surgical methods of immunosuppression have been utilized to assess functions of various tissues in the immune response. Studies of the consequences of thymectomy (T cell deletion) and bursectomy (B cell deletion) have been discussed in Chapter 1. These surgical removals in experimental animals, associated with studies of congenital defects in the development of the thymus and deletion of specific B cells in humans, have contributed to the understanding of various immunological deficiency diseases (see Chapter 15). Chronic thoracic duct drainage contributes to immunosuppression and is attributable primarily to T cell deficiency, since T cells are the major constituent of the lymphatic system.

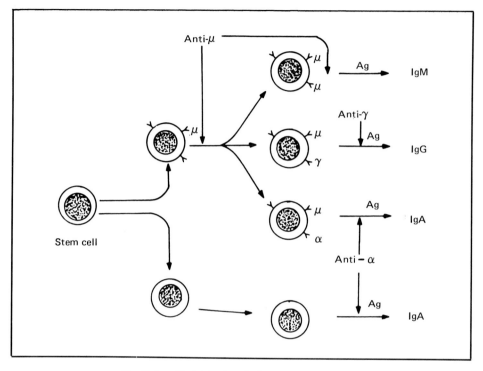

Fig. 6-8 : Model for B cell clonal development, showing probable sites of anti-Ig heavy chain and antigen actions.

Nonspecific blockage of macrophages of the reticuloendothelial system by carbon particles, Thorotrast (the α-emitting compound, thorium dioxide), and other nondigestible particulate substances can suppress the immune system. Animals incapacitated in this manner are highly vulnerable to infections and especially to the endotoxins (lipopolysaccharides).

Summary

1. Delineation of the immune response has been aided by the use of immunopotentiators and immunosuppressors.
2. Immunopotentiators include natural and synthetic adjuvants and various chemicals.
3. Adjuvants are substances that enhance or increase the immune response in the host to the antigen administered with the adjuvant. They promote slow absorption of the antigen (enhance its persistence) and provoke the activation of the amplification and ancillary systems of the host (macrophages, complement, neutrophils, etc.).
4. Natural adjuvants include the mycobacteria in Freund's complete adjuvant, BCG, bacteria, and bacterial products such as the lipopolysaccharides (see Table 6-2).

5. Synthetic adjuvants have been prepared that stimulate the major structural entity in *Mycobacterium tuberculosis* that is associated with immunoadjuvanticity properties. These include muramic dipeptide and the 6-*O*-mycolyl-N-acetylmuramyl peptides (see Tables 6-2 and 6-3). Other adjuvants include poly A:U and poly I:C, which appear to act on the cell-mediated system.

6. Drug immunopotentiators of interest include levamisole (a derivative of imidazole) and inosiplex. LMS has shown enhancement of the CMI in deficient individuals with essentially no significant effect on the immune system of normal individuals. Inosiplex appears to potentiate the primed immune cells after initiation of the viral infection.

7. Physical and chemical agents have been used for suppression of the immune response. These agents have been used principally in transplantation and cancer chemotherapy.

8. X-irradiation has been widely used for suppression of the immune response of the recipient in organ transplants, especially in bone marrow transplants. X-irradiation essentially destroys the lymphoid cells, the T and B cells, and the stem cells in the bone marrow. It is essentially a nonspecific and nonselective destruction of the immune system.

9. Immunosuppressive drugs include corticosteroids, the antimetabolites, cytotoxic compounds, and many others. The corticosteroids include the naturally occurring hydrocortisone and the synthetic analogues such as prednisone and dexamethasone. The antimetabolites azathioprine, 6-thioguanine, and 6-mercaptopurine affect the purine metabolic pathway at the cellular proliferative stage of the cell cycle. The cytotoxic drug cyclophosphamide appears to affect the resting and proliferative phase of the immunocyte. L-Asparaginase acts by hydrolysis of asparagine to aspartic acid and ammonia, thus depriving lymphoblast cells that appear to require L-asparagine.

10. Specific suppression of the immune response can be achieved by use of xenogeneic specific antibodies to immune cells such as horse antilymphocyte antiserum. Endogenous specific immune suppression by the mother against the fetal immune system has been demonstrated in rabbits. This is referred to as *allotypic suppression.* Surgical removal of a specific organ such as the thymus in neonates can induce immunodeficiency—for example, in the T cell system of a thymectomized animal.

11. The use of specific immunopotentiators and immunosuppressive drugs will undoubtedly contribute to the understanding of the various complex phases of the immune processes.

156

Bibliography and Selected Reading

General

Bloom, B. R., and David, J. R. (Eds.). *In Vitro Methods in Cell-Mediated and Tumor Immunity.* New York: Academic, 1976.

Chirigos, M. A. (Ed.). *Immune Modulation Control of Neoplasia by Adjuvant Therapy, Progress in Cancer Research and Therapy,* Vol. I. New York: Raven, 1978.

Gabrielsen, A. E., and Good, R. A. Chemical Suppression of Adaptive Immunity. In F. J. Dixon, Jr., and J. H. Humphrey (Eds.), *Advances in Immunology,* Vol. 6. New York: Academic, 1967. Pp. 92-230.

Gilman, A. G., Goodman, L. S., and Gilman, A. (Eds.). *The Pharmacological Basis of Therapeutics* (6th ed.) New York: Macmillan, 1980.

Nakamura, R. M. (Ed.). *Immunopathology, Clinical Laboratory Concepts and Methods.* Boston: Little, Brown, 1974.

Pardee, A. B., Dubrow, R., Hamlin, J. L., and Kletzien, R. F. Animal cell cycle. *Annu. Rev. Biochem.* 47:715, 1978.

Rose, N. R. and Friedman, H. (Eds.). *Manual of Clinical Immunology.* Washington, D. C.: Am. Soc. Microbiol., 1976.

Immunopotentiation

Allison, A. C. Effects of Adjuvants on Different Cell Types and Their Interactions in Immune Responses. In Ciba Found. Symp., *Immunopotentiation.* New York: Elsevier, 1973. P. 73.

Chirigos, M. A. (Ed.). *Immune Modulation Control of Neoplasia by Adjuvant Therapy, Progress in Cancer Research and Therapy,* Vol. I. New York: Raven, 1978.

Fischer, G. W., O'Brien, J., Hokama, Y., Maybee, D., and Chou, S. C. Effect of levamisole on metabolism of phagocytic cells. *Cancer Treat. Rep.* 62:1637, 1978.

Frost, P., and Lance, E.M. The Relation of Lymphocyte Trapping to the Mode of Action of Adjuvants. In Ciba Found. Symp., *Immunopotentiation,* New York: Elsevier, 1973. P. 29.

Grimm, W., Seitz, M., Kirchner, H., and Gemsa, D. Prostaglandin synthesis in spleen cell cultures of mice injected with *Corynebacterium parvum. Cell. Immunol.* 40:419, 1978.

Hokama, Y., Morita, A. H., Abad, M. A., Joyo, B. S., Uchida, D. A. and Fischer, G. W. Effect of levamisole on aggregation of platelets stimulated with compounds associated with the prostaglandin synthetic pathway. *Res. Commun. Chem. Pathol. Pharmacol.* 19:141, 1978.

Janossy, G., and Greaves, M. F. Lymphocyte activation. II. Discriminating stimulation of lymphocyte sub-populations by phytomitogens and heterologous anti-lymphocyte sera. *Clin. Exp. Immunol.* 10:525, 1972.

Kettman, J. R. Modulation of the acquisition and expression of immunity by Tilorone: I. Delayed-type hypersensitivity responses. *Immunopharmacol.* 1:21, 1978.

Symoens, J., and Rosenthal, M. A review: Levamisole in the modulation of the immune response: The current experimental and clinical state. *J. Reticuloendothel. Soc.* 21:175, 1977.

Uemiya, M., Sugimura, K., Kusama, T., Saiki, I., Yamawaki, M., Azumi, I. and Yamamura, Y. Adjuvant activity of 6-*O*-mycolyl derivatives of N-acetylmuramyl-L-seryl-D-Isoglutamine and related compounds in mice and guinea pigs. *Infect. Immun.* 24:83, 1979.

Immunosuppression

Bach, J. F. *The Mode of Action of Immunosuppressive Agents.* Amsterdam, North Holland, 1975.

Claman, H. N. Corticosteroids and lymphoid cells. *N. Engl. J. Med.* 287:388, 1972.

Dumont, F., and Bischoff, P. Differential effect of hydrocortisone on lymphocyte populations in the mouse spleen. *Biomedicine* 29:28, 1979.

Fauci, A. S. Mechanism of corticosteroid action on lymphocyte subpopulations. II. Differential effects of in vivo hydrocortisone, prednisone, and dexamethasone on in vitro expression of lymphocyte function. *Clin. Exp. Immunol.* 24:54, 1976.

Spreafico, F., and Anaclerio, A. Immunosuppressive agents. In J. W. Halden, R. G. Coffey, and F. Spreafico (Eds.), *Immunopharmacology.* New York: Plenum, 1977. P. 245.

Taliaferro, W. H. Modification of the Immune Response by Radiation and Cortisone. In O. V. St. Whitelock (Ed.) *Immunology of Cancer,* New York: Ann. N. Y. Acad. Sci., 1956. Pp. 745–764, Vol. 69.

Webb, D. R., Jr., and Winkelstein, A. Immunosuppression and Immunopotentiation. In H. H. Fudenberg, D. P. Stites, J. L. Caldwell, and J. V. Wells (Eds.), *Basic and Clinical Immunology* (2nd ed.). Los Altos, Calif.: Lange, 1978. P. 308.

Specific
Immunosuppression

Lance, E. M., Medawar, P. B., and Taub, R. N. Anti-lymphocyte Serum. In F. S. Dixon, Jr., and H. G. Kunkel (Eds.), *Advances in Immunology,* Vol. 17. New York: Academic, 1973. P. 2.

Manning, D. D. Heavy chain isotype suppression: A review of the immunosuppressive effects of heterologous anti-Ig heavy chain antisera. *J. Reticuloendothelial Soc.* 18:63, 1975.

Najarian, J. S., and Simmons, R. L. The clinical use of anti-lymphocyte globulin. *N. Engl. J. Med.* 285:158, 1971.

Primi, D., Smith, C. I. E., and Hammarstrom, L. Role of suppressor T cells in autoimmune responses induced by polyclonal B cell activators. *Scand. J. Immunol.* 7:121, 1978.

7 : Antigen–Antibody Reactions

W. Stephen Nichols, Jr.
Robert M. Nakamura

The antigen-antibody (Ag-Ab) reaction was first recognized by the early bacteriologists. The idea of specificity in antibody recognition of antigen arose from the finding that sera from patients infected with certain bacteria showed a tendency to bind to the infecting organism, while sera of unexposed individuals did not react with the bacteria. This observation led to the formulation of the existence of antibodies. Subsequently, establishment of the Ag-Ab reaction as a principle in host defense against invasion by foreign elements rapidly led to knowledge regarding the nature of the humoral immune system. This was accompanied by the development of numerous ingenious immunological techniques applicable to a wide array of topics in clinical medicine and research as well as by the discovery of the nature of several diseases mediated by the immune system, such as common allergies and autoimmune disease.

Antigen Binding Specificity is the capacity of antibodies to discern different antigenic determinants. Initial curiosity concerning specificity and the nature of the Ag-Ab bond led to a study of low molecular weight (incomplete) antigens known as *haptens*. Haptens are small, single-valency molecules that, alone, do not raise an antibody response. When haptenic molecules are attached to protein carrier molecules, however, antibodies are formed to the carrier as well as to the haptenic determinant. Landsteiner first used haptens such as 2,4-dinitrofluorobenzene (DNP) to investigate the specificity of immunoglobulins generated in response to single haptens by reacting the haptenic antibody with other, but similar, haptens. It became apparent that occasionally slight cross-reactivity exists among antibodies to somewhat different haptens. Moreover, it was soon recognized that a wide variation in the strength of antigen-antibody bonding exists among host antibodies raised to a single antigenic stimulus. Altogether, these findings demonstrated that, upon immunization with a single antigenic determinant, a variety of antibody combining characteristics arise among the responding antibody molecules. This is the *heterogeneity* of the immune response. The *diversity* of the immune response refers to the large array of separate antibody specificities that may be generated by an organism in response to the large number of different antigenic stimuli existing in nature.

The heterogeneity and diversity of the antibody response at first argued both for and against the so-called *instructional theory* of antibody formation suggested by Pauling. According to the instructional theory, the diversity of antibodies arises from direct instruction of protein synthesis of antibody to conform to different antigen templates. The large number of antibody responses to many different antigens in nature can be explained in this way; however, the heterogeneity of the antibody response to a single antigen is difficult to explain by this theory. The discovery of specific amino acid sequences of the antigen-binding regions of antibodies—in portions of the heavy and light chains of antibodies—led to the hypothesis that genes are involved in the instruction of variable regions (V regions) of antibodies and function as a mechanism for generating heterogeneity as well as diversity of antibody responses. The instructional theory thus gave way some time ago to theories concerned with genetic mechanisms for generating antibody diversity. It is now accepted that hypervariable regions spaced throughout the V regions determine specificity through the folding of these intramolecular domains into unique three-dimensional structures. A cluster of amino acids in apposition to antigen produces specificity of antigen binding. Slight genetically controlled variations of the amino acid sequences of different antibody combining sites that participate in the immune response to a single antigen result in the heterogeneity of the immune response and provide the possibility for cross-reactivity of antibodies with other similar antigens.

The number of genes encoding specific antibody recognition sites for the large number of antigens encountered in nature is impressive. There are possibly 10^8 or more antigens in nature. Depending somewhat upon the responding organism, the immune system is capable of responding to the majority of them. The strength of the diversity of this system, acting as a host defense mechanism, is enhanced by the heterogeneity of the response. Heterogeneity ensures the presence of a best fit between antigen and antibody and, ultimately, promotes an effective protective response to foreign material. Following the initial immunization period, and following the switch from IgM to IgG production, the antibody response appears to narrow in heterogeneity, increasing in specificity. Anamnestic recall of an antigen also results in relatively specific antibody production.

Primary Ag-Ab Reactions

The combination of antibody and antigen constitutes the primary reaction, the result of which is formation of a simple Ag-Ab complex. The strength of binding depends upon the complementary geometry of molecules—the closeness of fit of the corresponding parts of the antigen determinant and the recognition site on the antibody. *Specificity* almost exclusively depends upon the character of geometric fit. It also depends upon a closely related factor, the *affinity* of the Ag-Ab reaction. Affinity is the thermodynamic attraction between antigen and antibody molecules. Affinity depends upon the combined sum of short-range, noncovalent, intermolecular, attractive and repulsive forces. A successful primary reaction is a statement of the affinity of an Ag-Ab interaction. Affinity differs from specificity in that specificity denotes the likelihood of cross-reactivity between antibody and different antigens. Specificity is qualitative, and considers the character of an antibody in relation to multiple antigens, while affinity is more or less a quantitative characteristic of single Ag-Ab systems.

Since Ag-Ab bonding is weakly electrostatic (noncovalent) involving ionic interaction, hydrogen bonding, and van der Waals forces, it is important to remember that the primary reaction is reversible and that the Ag-Ab complex dissociates to a degree following the combination of individual molecules of antigen and antibody. To investigate relative differences among antibody affinities, equilibrium dialysis may be used to study the reversible Ag-Ab reaction and to establish the affinity constant. An antigen—for example, a hapten—and the antibody under study may be separated from one another by a semipermeable membrane. As the hapten or other small molecule diffuses across the membrane, the reaction proceeds toward the right of equation (1):

$$Ag + Ab \; \underset{K_2}{\overset{K_1}{\rightleftharpoons}} \; Ag\text{-}Ab \qquad (1)$$

Eventually equilibrium is reached, and the reaction may be thought to consist of a constant small number of antibodies reacting to form complexes with antigen, while equal numbers of molecules of Ag-Ab complex dissociate to form free antigen and antibody. K_1 and K_2 are constants expressing the tendency of the equilibrium reaction to move in one direction or the other. This is a statement of the *Law of mass action*, and the events in equation (1) may be rewritten as (2):

$$\frac{[Ag\text{-}Ab]}{[Ag]\,[Ab]} = \frac{K_1}{K_2} = K_{1,2} \text{ (equilibrium constant)} \qquad (2)$$

where the left-hand expression denotes the concentration of complex in the numerator, with the product of free antigen and antibody concentrations in the denominator. $K_{1,2}$ denotes the equilibrium constant and is an expression of the tendency for equation (1) to flow to the right. K_1 approximates the affinity of the reaction under consideration and is most accurate when monovalent hapten and antibody are used.

Table 7-1 : Sensitivity of Immunological Tests

Test	Minimum of Antibody Nitrogen (μgN/ml) Needed
Precipitation	
Tube	0.1
Immunodiffusion	0.1-0.3
Agglutination	
Qualitative	0.05
Hemagglutination	
Passive	0.001
Inhibition	0.001
Coombs reaction	0.01
Complement fixation	0.05
Fluorescent-antibody assay	
Qualitative	1.0
Radioimmunoassay	$<$0.001
Enzyme immunoassay	$<$0.001
Anaphylaxis, cutaneous (local)	.003

Source: Modified from Kwapinski, *Methodology of Immunochemical and Immunological Research.* New York: Wiley, 1972.

The affinity of an Ag-Ab reaction is estimated using colored or radioactive hapten in equilibrium experiments, measuring the amount of bound or free hapten on the antibody side of the dialysis membrane and then later measuring unbound antigen on the opposite side of the membrane. *Avidity* defines the degree of stability of Ag-Ab complex. It is partially dependent upon affinity; i.e., factors concerned with binding. But avidity is also associated with presence of multivalent binding and other factors that do not necessarily contribute to primary binding. The rate of disassociation of Ag-Ab complexes is used to approximate complex factors governing avidity. A two-dimensional graphic representation of equilibrium measurements, expressed using the law of mass action for primary Ag-Ab reactions, yields information concerning the heterogeneity of the antibody tested as well as the strength of affinity and avidity. These determinations characterize primary Ag-Ab reactions.

Detection and Application of Primary Reactions

Techniques for detection of primary Ag-Ab reactions offer some of the most sensitive means for detecting antibody or antigen (Table 7-1). These tests are not dependent upon a series of reactions or biochemical processes that are necessary for procession of the antigen-antibody reaction to the secondary or tertiary phases of humoral mediated immunity (Figure 7-1). Requirements for detecting the primary reaction include (1) a purified antigen or antibody preparation; (2) a technique for labeling or

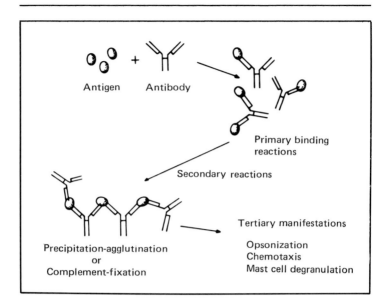

Antigen   Antibody

Primary binding
reactions

Secondary reactions

Tertiary manifestations

Precipitation-agglutination
or
Complement-fixation

Opsonization
Chemotaxis
Mast cell degranulation

Fig. 7-1 : Antigen-antibody reactions. Initial binding of antigen and antibody is the primary reaction. Secondary manifestations of the primary reaction arise from cross-linkage of separate antigen molecules (precipitation or agglutination) or complement fixation. Tertiary events arise as physiological manifestations of the primary reaction.

possibly quantitating bound antibody or antigen, and (3) separation of the antigen-antibody complex from free antigen or antibody. The primary tests include fluorescent antibody techniques, radioimmunoassay, and enzyme immunoassay. Such tests are commonplace in the laboratory today.

IMMUNOFLUORESCENCE (IF) ASSAY. Fluorescent-labeled antibody (FA) was first used by Coombs and his coworkers in 1941. In the immunofluorescence (IF) test, the primary reaction between antigen and antibody is detected by using a fluorescent molecule (fluorescein or rhodamine) attached to antibody. The endpoint is measured by detection of fluorescent Ag-Ab, either with fluorescence microscopy or with spectrophotometry.

The principles of IF tests are simple. One of the most frequently used tests is tissue immunofluorescence assay, with antigen in tissue or cells labeled with a FA specific for the antigen. The excess FA is washed off, and then the material is examined for the presence of fluorescence with an ultraviolet microscope (Figure 7-2). Positive (fluorescence) staining denotes an Ag-Ab reaction and demonstrates the presence of antigen in the tissue.

The direct IF assay uses direct labeling of various antigens with FA (Figure 7-3). The indirect IF assay is used to detect either

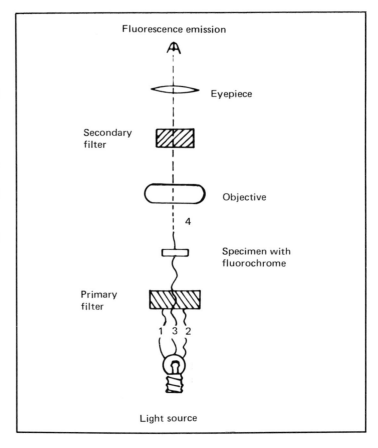

Fig. 7-2 : Fluorescence microscopy. An ultraviolet light source excites fluorescence in a specimen containing fluorochrome label. The primary filter selects a suitable wavelength (3). Excitation results in release of visible light (4), filtered for optimal visibility (secondary filter) and presented at the eyepiece for detection of fluorescence emission.

unknown antigen or antibody in a test medium. In the indirect assay, the FA reagent serves as a second antibody in a kind of sandwich of reactions between known antigen substrate, unknown antibody, and reagent FA. The reaction of antigen plus unknown antibody plus FA to immunoglobulin reveals the presence of an immunoglobulin in the test medium specific for the substrate.

The FA inhibition technique relies on interference of a positive (direct) FA reaction with a substrate by an unknown antibody with specificity for the antigen substrate. Most fluorescence techniques are easily characterized and are specific, sensitive, and easily run.

Direct IF testing may be used for detection of previously formed immune complexes. Since immune complexes in the circulatory system often localize in tissue, sections from organs of patients suspected of having circulating immune complexes are examined with FA directed toward the immunoglobulin of the Ag-Ab complex. The tissue is again washed free of excess unattached

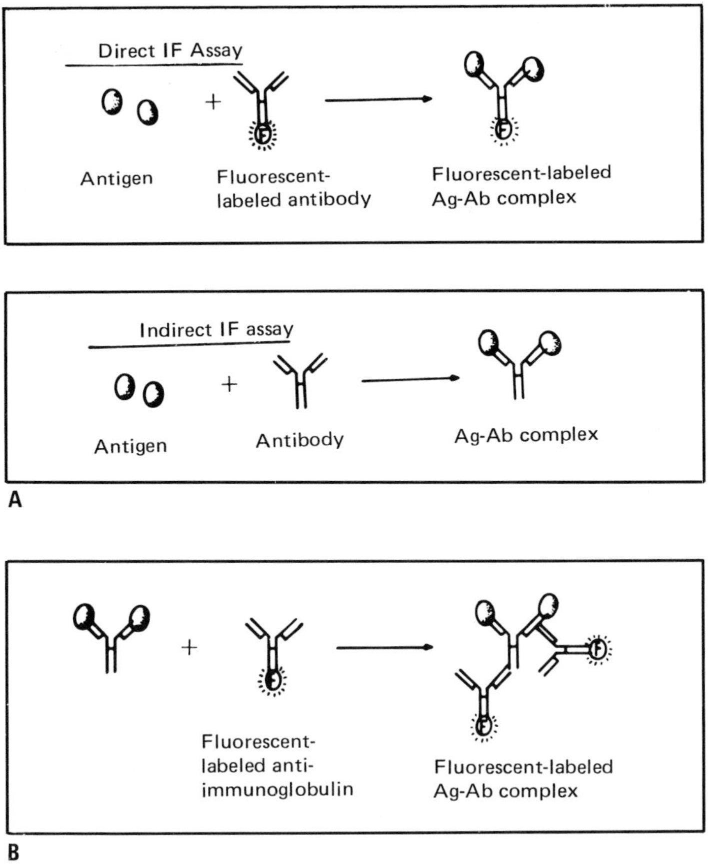

Fig. 7-3 : Immunofluorescence assays. The direct assay involves direct labeling of an antigen with a fluorescent antibody. In the indirect assay, (A) antigen is first reacted with a nonlabeled antibody (test medium); and (B) the resultant Ag-Ab complex is identified by using a second antibody, which is specific for immunoglobulin and is labeled with a fluorescent tag.

FA, and a microscopic search is made for fluorescence. The presence of fluorescence suggests the presence of an immune complex. This kind of finding suggests the pathogenesis of what is known as immune complex disease. Direct IF tests are useful for identifying antigens on the surface, or in the cytoplasm, of cells.

One of the most valuable of the indirect IF procedures is that used to detect autoantibodies. Autoantibodies are those that attach to various host antigens, soluble or insoluble. Antibodies to insoluble antigens are best detected by using tissue-bound antigen, or by attaching the antigen to a carrier adsorbent in a solid phase. Presently, some of the most frequently used tests for autoantibodies are IF tests for antibodies to various nuclear antigens in the collagen vascular diseases. In these tests, patient serum is screened for antibodies to nuclear antigens in tissue sections. Mouse tissue is often used, and indirect IF is employed to identify antibodies in test serum that attach to nuclei in tissue substrate. This constitutes a test for a primary reaction of specific antibody with nuclear antigen and suggests the possibility of antinuclear autoantibody in the patient's serum. The spectrum of autoimmune diseases is covered in Chapter 14.

Another IF procedure is commonly employed to identify antigens in solution. After addition of the FA, fluorescent immune complexes may be separated from solution physically or chemically. Fluorescence is detected in the separation phase by photometric methods.

Using diverse adaptations of the IF methods, direct identification of Ag-Ab reactions is carried out. Moreover, localization of injected antigens or infectious organisms, or measurement of various enzymes or hormones in sera or other fluids, may all be carried out.

RADIOIMMUNOASSAY (RIA). Radioimmunoassay (RIA) was developed by Yalow and Berson in 1960. It is of the utmost sensitivity and is easily adapted to various Ag-Ab systems. A variety of substances presently measured by RIA techniques are listed in Table 7-2. Radioimmunoassay uses the principle of competitive inhibition of binding of a marker molecule and often employs a radionuclide as a marker for an antigen that is reacted with antibody in the first phase of the test (Figure 7-4). [125]I is a convenient marker for many of these tests. In the second phase of the test unlabeled antigen is added in excess, and the reaction between labeled and unlabeled antigen and antibody is equilibrated. The resultant immune complex is precipitated. This separates immune complex-bound radioactive antigen and soluble free radioactive antigen. By varying the amount of unlabeled antigen added to the test reaction in the second phase, a graphic relationship may be established between the original concentration of unlabeled antigen and the ratio of radioactive antigen bound up in immune complexes to radioactive antigen free in solution. The concentration of an unknown quantity of antigen may be determined through use of this standard curve. The concentrations of known antibody and labeled antigen are held constant in this procedure.

Radiolabeled antibody may also be used in RIA reactions. In this procedure, radiolabeled antibody is generally added to soluble antigen. Unbound labeled antibody is removed, and then the number of counts in the solution of precipitate of labeled immune complex is measured and compared to standard curves with the amount of unknown antigen determined. This test may be manipulated to measure amounts of unknown antibody.

One of the most useful RIA techniques, solid phase immunoadsorbance—which employs a solid adsorptive surface such as

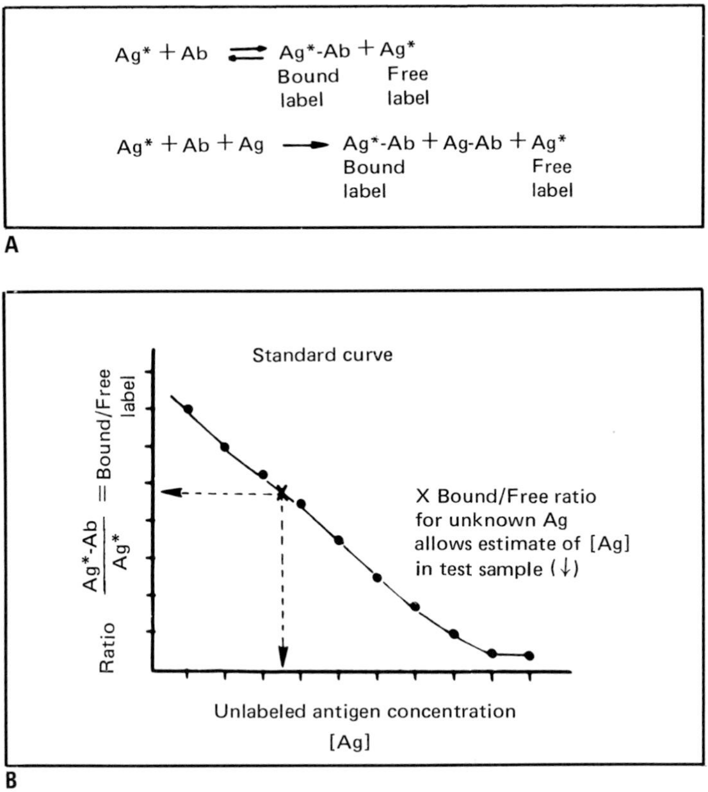

A

B

Fig. 7-4 : Radioimmunoassay. A. Radiolabeled antigen (Ag*) is reacted with Ab to form bound (Ag*-Ab) and free (Ag*) labeled antigen. **B.** If unlabeled Ag is present, competitive inhibition of binding between Ag* and Ab allows determination of an unknown antigen concentration. The ratio of bound to free label is plotted on a standard curve, using standard Ag concentrations. Subsequently, the bound/free ratio is determined for a test solution of unknown Ag; and, from the curve, unknown Ag concentration is calculated.

the surface of a plastic tube to bind antigen or antibody—is growing in popularity. The reaction between known antigen that is bound to the plastic surface and free-unknown antibody is carried out on the solid surface, which is then washed free of unreacted reagents in the aqueous phase (Figure 7-5). Determination of the presence of unknown antibody (antibody bound to antigen on solid surface) is done by causing a labeled antibody to the unknown antibody to react with the Ab bound to Ag, then washing and measuring the amount of radiolabeled marker present. The amount of radioactivity present is proportional to that of the bound unknown antibody. By reversing the situation cited, that is, specific known antibody abount to the solid surface, unknown Ag can be determined. This RIA procedure is referred to as "solid phase" RIA.

Fig. 7-5 : Radio-
immunoadsorption.
A. Antigen is
attached to a solid-
phase adsorbent.
B. The adsorbed
antigen reacts with
an unknown anti-
body. C. The
unknown antibody
in the Ag-Ab
complex is quanti-
tated with a radio-
labeled antibody
to immunoglobulin.

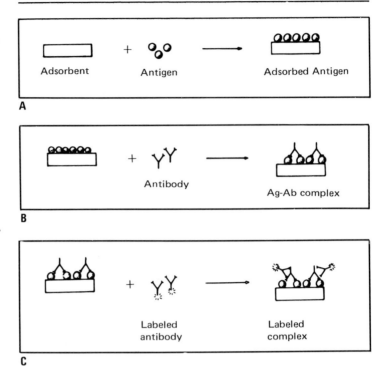

ENZYME IMMUNOASSAY (EIA). Enzyme immunoassay (EIA)
uses techniques similar to those of IF assay and RIA, with many
of the same modifications and uses. These tests are replacing the
spectrophotometric IF and the RIA tests.

In principle, a purified enzyme is linked to antibody (or antigen)
and serves as the marker. The activity of the enzyme marker is
detected by cytochemical or photometric assays (Figure 7-6).
Horseradish peroxidase and alkaline phosphatase are enzymes
commonly used in these procedures.

When peroxidase is used, the most common method, the marker
enzyme is detected by reacting hydrogen peroxide with diamino-
benzidine. A black color indicates the presence of the enzyme.
The enzyme can be detected in tissue, so that the test can be used
much as the direct tissue IF tests, except that light microscopy is
used in the enzyme test.

The activity of enzyme systems (horseradish peroxidase or alkaline phosphatase) is usually diminished when enzyme is conjugated to antibody. This may be due to stain hindrance between
enzyme and substrate caused by the antibody. However, the techniques of EIA are tremendously valuable because numerous modifications exist for light and electron microscope based EIA. Solid
phase enzyme-linked immunosorbent assay (ELISA) is extremely

Fig. 7-6 : Enzyme immunoassay. Enzyme-labeled antibody serves as a marker for the presence of an Ag-Ab complex. Enzyme substrate is supplied to develop a precipitate or color change in the presence of enzyme-labeled antibody.

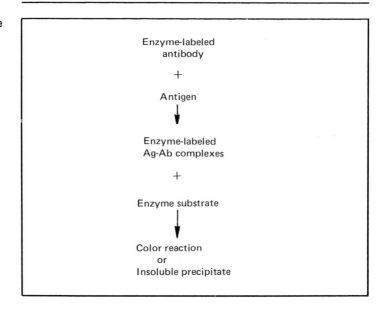

Enzyme-labeled
antibody

+

Antigen

↓

Enzyme-labeled
Ag-Ab complexes

+

Enzyme substrate

↓

Color reaction
or
Insoluble precipitate

popular and is based on the same principle as the solid phase RIA test (pp. 166-167). The enzyme techniques are easily automated to perform large numbers of tests rapidly, and the potential hazards of radioisotopes do not plague EIA.

These tests are extremely sensitive and therefore offer a means of measuring hormone, enzyme, serum protein, and drug levels. EIA is supplanting even RIA in several of these areas, including drug level monitoring. It is also useful in detection of antibody to various infectious organisms, such as human hepatitis B virus.

Secondary Manifestations of Ag-Ab Reactions

The primary reaction consists of simple antigen-antibody recognition. Following the combination of antigen and antibody, secondary reactions may take place, if there is cross-linkage of Ag-Ab complexes (see Figure 7-1). Manifestations of secondary reactions depend upon the conditions under which combining antigen and antibodies associate. The kind of antibody involved, IgG or IgM, is often important in bringing about secondary manifestations, as is the kind of antigen. The size and solubility of the antigen help determine the likelihood that primary reactions will develop into secondary reactions. The reaction of some Ag–Ab complexes with complement components in the serum leads to secondary manifestations such as cell lysis.

Primary reactions are measured simply by identification of the antigen-binding event. Detection of secondary manifestations consists of observation of the effects of secondary binding shown in Figure 7-1. These include precipitation and agglutination.

An antibody bringing about one of these reactions is named, accordingly, a *precipitin* or an *agglutinin.* Corresponding antigens arousing specific secondary events are named with the suffix -ogen; hence, *precipitinogen* and *agglutinogen.*

Detection of secondary reactions was performed during the very first in vitro observation of Ag-Ab reactions (see Wilson and Miles, 1965). These were the precipitin and agglutinin reactions.

Detection and Application of Precipitin Reactions

The precipitin reaction was discovered by Kraus in 1897 (see Wilson and Miles, 1965) when he observed that a precipitate formed when serum taken from typhoid patients was mixed with the cell-free filtrate of cultured organisms. The technique was later modified several times and led to useful information concerning the nature of Ag-Ab reactions and infectious disease immunity. Individuals contributing to knowledge in this area include such investigators as Ehrlich, Heidelberger, Pauling, and Landsteiner. Importantly, Heidelberger extended the precipitation technique to quantitatively measure total antibody protein nitrogen, and immunology took its place among the exact sciences. Today, precipitin techniques remain sensitive and accurate methods for quantitating immune responses. Applications of immunoprecipitin reactions are numerous and include procedures for quantitation of major serum proteins and detection of antibodies in the diagnosis of infectious diseases.

The lower range of sensitivity of the precipitin assays is about 0.1 to 0.3 mg N/dl. This compares favorably with other immunological procedures, although detection of trace molecules and certain endocrine factors requires more sensitive means, such as RIA (Table 7-2).

EQUIVALENCE REACTIONS. The precipitation reaction takes place when antibody attaches to soluble antigen. Usually, naturally occurring antigens contain multiple antibody attachment sites. In the precipitation reaction, antibodies bind to the several attachment sites on each molecule of antigen, thus effectively bridging soluble antigen. A lattice structure of antigen and antibody is formed which varies in size depending on the amount of bridging that takes place. Since the solubility of Ag-Ab complexes is partly dependent on the size of the complex, the reaction may form insoluble complexes that fall out of solution as precipitate. *Flocculation* is a word sometimes used to characterize the formation of a rather loose precipitate as the result of a secondary reaction.

Naturally occurring antibodies all have two or more combining sites. IgG has two identical antibody combining sites (divalent),

Table 7-2 : RIA in Laboratory Medicine

Pharmacological	Peptide hormones
Digoxin	ACTH
Digitoxin	Agiotensin
Cyclic nucleotides	Bradykinin
Prostaglandins	Glucagon
Folic acid	Growth hormone
Vitamin B_{12}	B-subunit (hCG)
Steroid hormones	Insulin
Aldosterone	Oxytocin
Cortisol	Parathyroid
Estriol	Renin
Progesterone	Thyroglobulin
Testosterone	Thyroxine
	Triiodothyronine

the Fab portions of the molecule. IgM has five identical combining sites, and IgA two or three. It follows that natural antibodies all have the potential for cross-linkage of antigenic sites on different antigens. Different antibodies precipitate the same antigen to varying degrees according to various antibody characteristics such as affinity and specificity, the charge of the molecules involved, and the shape of the complex.

In general, the likelihood of precipitation of antigen with antibody also depends upon the relative concentration of antigen and antibody. The reaction between antigen and antibody is described in terms of three zones of precipitin reactivity (Figure 7-7). In the first, or *prozone,* the zone of relative antibody excess, antibody molecules combine primarily with individual antigens, sometimes to the extent that all antigenic sites are covered by antibody. The concentration of antibody is such that individual antigen sites are covered so extensively that no cross-linkage of antigens takes place. The Ag-Ab reaction results in soluble complexes in this case.

In the second zone of reactivity, the relative concentration of antigen is increased, and forms with the antibody a maximal degree of cross-linkage of separate antigen molecules. There is insoluble lattice formation, and precipitation takes place. This is the *zone of equivalence* of antigen and antibody. At the point of equivalence, the antigen and antibody concentrations are about equal. If a divalent antibody is used, virtually every antibody is attached to two different antigen molecules. All of the antigen and antibody in the reaction precipitates. The third zone is

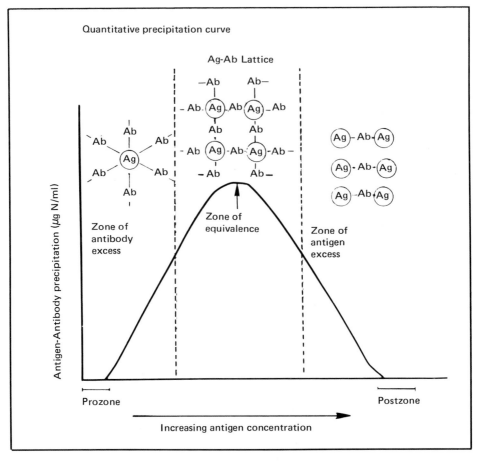

Fig. 7-7 : The quantitative precipitation curve. Lattice formation due to Ag-Ab cross-linkage causes a precipitate that varies according to the relative excess of antigen or antibody. Maximal precipitate forms at the point of equivalence (↑).

the *postzone,* the zone of relative antigen excess. The antigen binds all the antibody, but there is little lattice formation, owing to the paucity of available antibody combining sites for cross-linkage of antigen.

The three phases of the precipitin reaction are part of a spectrum of Ag-Ab reactivity that varies with different ratios of antigen to antibody concentration. The three zones may be identified by reacting serial dilutions of antibody with antigen and observing, initially, the zone of negative precipitation, then the development of precipitate (zone of equivalence), and finally the point of disappearance of precipitation with diluted serum. The identification of the point of equivalence, with maximal precipitation, is useful for quantitation of antibody, assuming use of a standard

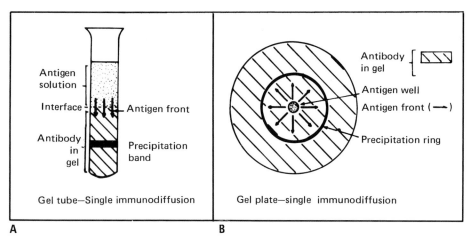

Fig. 7-8 : Single gel immunodiffusion. A. Antigen moving from a solution into a tube of a gel containing antibody causes a precipitation band at the zone of equivalence. B. Antigen moving from a solution onto a plate of antibody gel causes a ring of precipitation at equivalence.

antigen reagent. The total protein N is determined at the point of equivalence, and the known antigen N subtracted. The remaining protein N is that of the antibody present at equivalence.

Natural antibodies of considerable concentration may arise, with test sera occasionally precipitating antigen at very high dilutions, or titers. The *titer* of an antibody is the reciprocal number of the highest serial dilution of the antibody still yielding an observable Ag-Ab reaction with a constant amount of antigen. Testing for the presence of antibody to natural antigens, such as those encountered in infectious disease, may result in negative precipitin reactions among the first dilutions of a very high titer antibody due to the prozone phenomenon.

GEL IMMUNODIFFUSION. Immunoprecipitation methods have proved extremely valuable to research and clinical diagnosis. Several simple techniques have evolved from the classic precipitation reaction. Primarily, these involve precipitation in a gel such as agar. The classic gel technique of Oudin is the simple gel diffusion method (Figure 7-8). Antigen is first incorporated into a gel, either in a tube or in a flat plate. Antibody is then layered over the gel in the tube or placed in a hole, or well, cut in the gel in the plate. A precipitate forms as antibody diffuses into a gel and meets the antigen. The principle of the equivalence zone is important in understanding precipitation of Ag-Ab complexes in gel. Concentrated antibody diffusing into the gel is gradually diluted by the volume of gel. The front of diffusing antibody briefly forms complexes with antigen, only to have the wave of antibody excess behind the front rapidly resolubilize the complexes according to the law of mass action. A visible precipitate is not formed in such a prozone. With time, the moving front of antibody is diluted and reaches an optimal concentration for formation of a precipitate at the zone of Ag-Ab equivalence in the gel. The thickness of the precipitin line is a function of the concentration of complexes formed.

The line of precipitation is linear in a gel tube overlayered with antibody and circular in a gel plate with antibody diffusing radially from a well in the agar. Immunoprecipitation carried out in a flat of gel in this fashion is known as *radial immunodiffusion (RID) precipitation.* The distance that the antibody front travels through gel prior to establishment of an equivalence zone is proportional to the concentration of antibody. Given constant conditions of volume, of serum applied to agar, temperature, pH, antigen concentration, and agar concentration, the distance of migration of an unknown antibody may be compared to the distance of migration of various concentrations of known standard serum antibody plotted on a graph from which the unknown antibody concentration can be extrapolated. The conditions of the precipitation reaction in gel can be reversed, using antibody in gel and antigen as the mobile front, to determine concentrations of common substances such as serum proteins.

Interestingly, when antigen and antibody are both applied to wells in a plate of agar, a line of precipitation forms between the two wells (Figure 7-9). The line may be situated closer to one well than the other, depending on the concentrations of antigen and antibody and the point of equivalence. If antibody is present in high concentration, the antibody front is concentrated relative to antigen, and the antibody pushes the line of precipitation toward the well containing the less concentrated antigen. This kind of procedure is called *double immunodiffusion precipitation.* If multiple antigens are applied to a gel and run against a common antiserum or antibody, separate precipitin lines form between the antibody well and the antigen-containing wells, since separate conditions of equivalence develop depending on the nature and concentration of the antigen and antibody in each precipitin system. This finding is of great practical use and was extended by Ouchterlony.

In the Ouchterlony technique, two or more wells adjacent to one another are situated around a central antibody well. These are filled with antigens under study for properties of possible identity of antigenic structure. When two identical antigens in adjacent wells are diffused against a precipitating antibody, precipitation lines formed at separate adjacent zones of equivalence fuse continuously at a point central to the antigen wells. A line of common

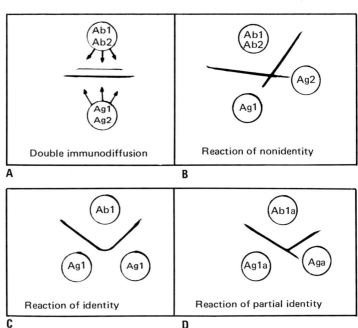

Fig. 7-9 : Double gel immunodiffusion. A. Multiple lines of precipitation result from simultaneous immunodiffusion of multiple antigens and antibodies on a gel plate. B. Different Ag-Ab systems precipitate as intersecting lines in the reaction of nonidentity of antigens. C. The reaction of identity of antigens results in a smooth continuous line between wells. D. The reaction of partial identity of antigens results in a spur between wells with extra antigen (Ag1a).

precipitation exists for the two antigens. Although the antigen concentrations may differ, central fusion of precipitin lines is maintained because a smooth continous gradient of equivalence conditions exists between the adjacent antigen fronts. Where the average concentration of the two colliding antigen fronts meet requirements of equivalence, a common line of precipitate forms. This is the *reaction of identity* between antigens. Nonidentical antigens do not form common points of equivalence, in the area of collision between diffusing antigen fronts, so that no common line of precipitation forms. Two separate lines of equivalence form in this case. This is the *reaction of nonidentity* of antigens. When antigens containing several antigenic determinants are used in this test, with one of the antigens containing at least one but not all of the determinants of the other, a *reaction of partial identity* may take place. The line of precipitation forms between the antibody and the antigen with multiple specificities, while a second line of precipitation forms between the antibody and the antigen of limited determinants. This line forms a point of continuity with the first precipitin line but does not extend beyond the first. A spur effect is formed by the complete and incomplete precipitin lines.

Immunodiffusion methods offer some of the most convenient methods for measuring serum proteins. Single radial immuno-diffusion, for example, is frequently used to quantitate serum complement components, individual immunoglobulins, hapto-globin, ceruloplasmin, etc.

IMMUNOELECTROPHORESIS. Another extremely useful immuno-diffusion technique is that of immunoelectrophoresis (Figure 7-10). Protein, lipoproteins, or other charged constituents of serum and other fluids are placed in a well in a gel flat or in a similar material and then subjected to an electrical potential placed across the gel. Negatively charged proteins such as albumin migrate by a process of electrodiffusion, or *electrophoresis,* moving rapidly toward the anodal pole of the gel. Relatively positive or weakly negative molecules such as immunoglobulins migrate only slowly or remain within the fluid. Separation of multiple proteins in solution may be done by electrophoresis. Staining electrophoretically separated proteins allows study and quantitation of the individual proteins.

Following gel electrophoresis, the current may be removed and a trough in the gel paralleling the migration of proteins through the electric field may be formed by removing a strip of the gel. An antiserum is then placed in this trough, and the separated proteins passively migrate through the gel toward the antiserum, which in turn migrates toward the multiple advancing fronts of the proteins. This last process is similar to double immuno-diffusion. Where diffusing proteins encounter an antibody front, a precipitin arc forms. These combined processes, electrophoresis and passive immunodiffusion, are termed *immunoelectrophoresis* (IEP). IEP effectively separates numerous molecules and allows identification and study of them. Rabbit or goat antiserum to human serum allows development of over twenty separate pre-cipitin arcs through IEP of human serum. This process has im-mense applicability in the clinical laboratory, as it can be used to identify certain abnormal serum proteins on the basis of the aberrant precipitin arcs that they manifest. Monoclonal anti-bodies in such diseases as multiple myeloma are identified by IEP.

Monoclonal immunoglobulins, or *paraproteins,* occur in serum or urine. Monoclonal proteins arise in multiple disorders. Pri-marily they appear in malignant lymphoproliferative diseases such as multiple myeloma, Waldenström's macroglobulinemia, lymph-oma, and chronic lymphocytic leukemia. *Monoclonal* simply refers to the progeny of a single cell.

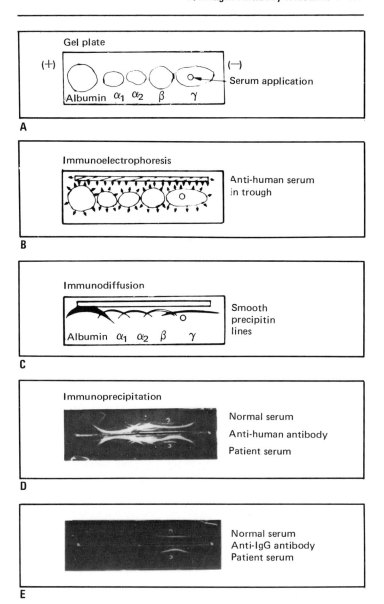

Fig. 7-10 : Immunoelectrophoresis. A. Serum proteins are separated by migration through an electrical field. B. The electrical field is removed, and separated proteins are immunodiffused toward a trough containing antibody to serum proteins. C. Precipitin arcs form between serum protein antigens and antibody. D. A patient's monoclonal immunoglobulin is identified as a restricted aberrant zone over one precipitin arc (compared to normal serum precipitin arcs). E. By using anti-IgG antibody, the abnormal precipitin arc is identified as an IgG immunoglobulin (compared to normal serum IgG precipitin).

Monoclonal immunoglobulins are homogeneous in size, charge, and amino acid sequence, since they derive from a single clone of lymphocytes or plasma cells. The homogeneous protein migrates in a narrow restricted area electrophoretically. Serum protein studies by IEP are of use in documenting the presence of monoclonal proteins, and they identify the heavy and light chain structure of the abnormal protein, aiding in distinguishing between polyclonal and monoclonal protein abnormalities. Due to the homogeneous charge and size of paraproteins, a localized abnormal precipitin line develops on IEP in the monoclonal disorders.

Occasionally, light chains of a plasma paraprotein spill into the urine (Bence-Jones protein), and IEP or urine is useful for detection of such monoclonal light chains. Very rarely, paraproteins consist of a heavy chain alone or of isolated light chains. The distribution of the immunoglobulin classes of paraproteins is similar to the distribution of antibody classes normally present among antibodies; i.e., $IgG(\kappa) > IgG(\lambda) > IgA(\kappa)$, etc.

Electrophoresis and IEP of serum are also used for documenting immunodeficiency of humoral immunity. Immunoglobulins are decreased in the congenital or acquired antibody deficiency disorders.

COUNTERCURRENT ELECTROPHORESIS (CEP) uses electrophoresis of antigen and antibody from separate wells, in opposite directions, speeding the rate of precipitation (Figure 7-11). Precipitation with double immunodiffusion takes place over a period of time, up to 24 to 48 hours. CEP produces a precipitin line in as short a time as 30 to 60 minutes and increases sensitivity severalfold. The diagnosis of infectious disease may now be speeded by use of this technique. Serum or CSF containing antigen from microorganisms is counterelectrophoresed with reagent antibody. Formation of a precipitin line suggests the identity of the infection. Among others, cryptococcal, *Hemophilus,* and meningococcal antigens in CSF may be identified with this test, suggesting an etiology of bacterial meningitis. Viral diseases may also be diagnosed in this fashion.

NEPHELOMETRY. Nephelometry is the measurement of the turbidity of suspensions. Dilute solutions of antigen and antibody may react to produce slight turbidity. This precipitin reaction scatters incident light, and the degree of scatter is proportional to the amount of precipitation and, therefore, to the amount of unknown antigen or antibody present. Optical density measurements of antigens are performed most accurately

Fig. 7-11 : Countercurrent immunoelectrophoresis. Ag and Ab gel diffusion and precipitation of Ag-Ab complex are accelerated, using an electrical field.

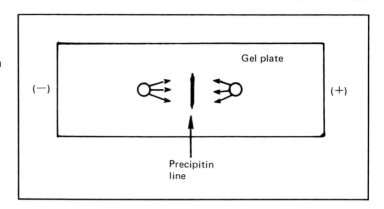

along the ascending limb of the region of antigen excess. High concentrations of antigen may be diluted in order to facilitate these kinds of measurements.

Automated immunoprecipitin techniques are particularly well applied to nephelometry. Presently, laser nephelometers are quite popular, with light sources from helium-neon laser beams. The disadvantage of nephelometry is that optically active material present in solutions may interfere with the measurement of precipitation.

Automated immunoprecipitin techniques are particularly well applied to nephelometry. Presently, laser nephelometers are quite popular, with light sources from helium-neon laser beams. The disadvantage of nephelometry is that optically active material present in solutions may interfere with the measurement of precipitation.

Agglutination Reactions

Agglutination reactions consist of the clumping of visible particulate material such as cells or synthetic matter by antibody. The Ag-Ab reaction takes place at the surface of particles, with antigen located in such a manner as to be available to specific binding by antibodies. The first agglutinin reactions were carried out with bacteria and specific agglutinins. Agglutination reactions with red blood cells led to the discovery of the ABO blood groups. Several ingenious modifications of agglutination techniques find ubiquitous use in contemporary medicine and research today.

Agglutination takes place in fluids in two phases: (1) combination of particulate antigen and antibody (the primary reaction) and (2) aggregation of antigen through cross-linkage, with formation of a lattice of particles. The first phase depends upon a specific reaction between antigen and antibody, while several factors such as particle surface charge and antibody type, may influence aggregation. Particles such as red cells or bacteria bear a slight negative charge (the zeta potential) in suspension and therefore tend to repel each other. The surface potential of such particles is such that, due to electrical repulsion between adjacent particles, cross-linkage of antigen-coated particles by a molecular bridge of antibody is at times prevented. Since the IgM molecule is larger than the IgG molecule, IgM is about 750 times more effective than IgG in bridging particles in solution. The failure of bridging and aggregation of particles following successful primary Ag-Ab reaction is called "incomplete agglutination."

INCOMPLETE AGGLUTINATION REACTIONS. Manipulation of the relative ionic strength of the test medium in agglutination reactions may reduce the strength of the zeta potential, thus decreasing the distance between particles and increasing cross-linkage and aggregation of particles. Addition to the test medium of charged low weight molecules such as albumin increases the likelihood of complete reactions. Factors such as viscosity of test medium are also important in aggregation, and addition of polymerized molecules such as dextran augments viscosity and increases agglutination in some systems.

The chief disadvantage of agglutination testing is that it is semi-quantitative. Although agglutination may be carried out with standardized reagents repeated results are accurate only to a fourfold difference in titers. The sensitivity of the reaction is good, and the test may be modified for use in a microsystem, with tests carried out in small wells and the results read with a microscope or magnifying mirror.

CLASSIFICATION OF AGGLUTINATION REACTIONS. The various types of agglutination reactions are outlined in Table 7–3.

Direct Agglutination Tests. The simple reaction is brought about by specific antibody linkage of suspended particulate antigen. Modifications of the test medium may be necessary to bring about aggregation in incomplete reactions. Amplification of the sensitivity of hemagglutination reactions, by modifications of charge and viscosity with 5–30% bovine albumin additive, is frequently employed in the blood bank for identification of incomplete IgG antibodies to blood group antigens. Enzyme treatment of bacteria and red cells also augments agglutination, with enzyme removal of structures blocking antigen expression and accessibility, or through enzyme-mediated hydration or charge alteration of surface membranes. These procedures are now commonplace in the blood bank in the workup of atypical antibodies.

Table 7-3 : Classification of Agglutination Reactions

Direct agglutination tests
  Simple
  High viscosity
  Enzyme-augmented

Indirect (passive) agglutination
  Red cell
  Inert particles (latex, bentonite)
  Chemically linked antigen

Agglutination inhibition

Antiglobulin tests
  Direct Coombs
  Indirect Coombs

Direct agglutination reactions are also of immense use in detecting serum antibodies to numerous antigens. Some of the most useful tests are those for antibodies developing in salmonellosis, brucellosis, rickettsiosis, and several other infectious diseases.

Widal Test. The Widal test, useful in the diagnosis of common infectious diseases, tests for serum antibody agglutination of whole inactivated microorganisms. Antibody screening is carried out against selected species of *Salmonella.* Sera are studied for the presence of antibody to one or more of several different somatic, flagellar, or capsular antigens. A serum titer of 1/80 or greater against somatic or flagellar antigens indicates the possibility of active infection. Lower titers may indicate early infection or the fact that the test organisms do not play a role in the disease under investigation. Antibody titers are followed over a number of days or weeks to determine if antibody levels are increasing or falling. Significant changes (fourfold) in the titer of an antibody often have a correlation with recent development of the disease and an ongoing immune response to the stimulus of the organism. *Brucella, Franciscella, Shigella, Bordetella* and other bacteria are also easily adapted for direct agglutination testing for diagnosis of the corresponding infectious diseases.

Weil-Felix Test. The Weil-Felix test employs strains of *Proteus vulgaris* to detect cross-reacting antibodies to Rickettsiae, such as those responsible for the spotted fevers. Rocky Mountain spotted fever is the most important example of rickettsial disease in the United States. High titers of agglutinins occurring in other rickettsial diseases such as typhus and Q fever are also detected by this test.

Indirect (Passive) Agglutination. Development of the technique of passive agglutination has had numerous ramifications in the laboratory. This technique utilizes particles or cells passively coated with soluble antigen (Figure 7-12). Agglutination is then brought about by exposing particles with adsorbed antigen to

Fig. 7-12 : Indirect (passive) agglutination. Antigen is passively adsorbed onto a carrier particle. Subsequently, antibody agglutinates the insoluble (particulate) antigen.

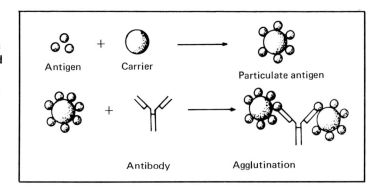

specific antibody. The reverse process can also be used: antibody is passively adsorbed to carrier particles (reverse passive agglutination).

Although many substances adsorb spontaneously to red cell surfaces, several proteins adsorb relatively poorly to cells. Mild treatment of red cells with tannic acid or other similar reagents increases adsorption of many proteins. For nonadsorbable substances, chemical bonding of antigens to carrier cells is extremely useful. Several chemicals such as bisdiazobenzidine (BDB) allow covalent bonding of proteins to the cell membrane.

Agglutination systems using inert particles (immunoadsorbents) such as latex (polystyrene polymer) and bentonite (potters' clay) are also very useful. Small particles of latex or bentonite readily adsorb protein and act as colloidal antigen in passive agglutination tests.

Indirect hemagglutination assays exist for testing and identification of agglutinins to several infectious organisms. Numerous noninfectious antigens have proved useful in hemagglutination assays for antibodies in autoimmune diseases. In these tests, various extracts of nuclei are used to coat carrier particles such as red cells. Hemagglutination performed with patient sera identifies the presence of autoantibodies. These tests are somewhat limited in sensitivity as compared to RIA or EIA.

Agglutination Inhibition Reactions. In agglutination inhibition reactions, quantitation of antigen is carried out by assessment of competitive inhibition of agglutination of a particulate antigen by a soluble unknown antigen (Figure 7-13). In this test, antibody reacted with particulate antigen causes agglutination. If antibody is first reacted with identical soluble antigen, then, after addition of the insoluble antigen coated on carrier particles, there is failure of agglutination to take place due to insufficient amounts of available antibody. Soluble antigen may be quantitated on the basis of the degree of inhibition of agglutination of

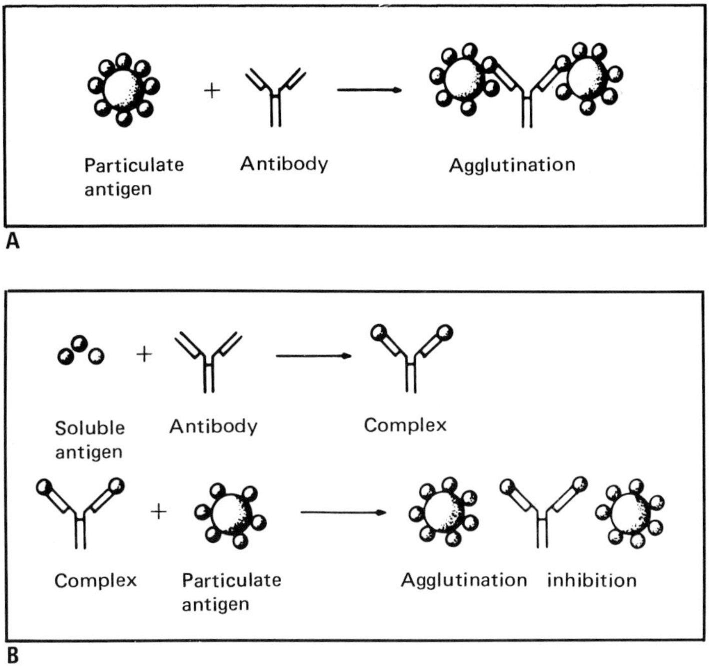

Fig. 7-13 : Ag-
glutination inhibi-
tion. A. Particulate
antigen is agglutin-
ated by antibody.
B. Unknown soluble
antigen, when
reacted with anti-
body, inhibits
agglutination of
the particulate
antigen.

Particulate   Antibody   Agglutination
antigen

A

Soluble   Antibody   Complex
antigen

Complex   Particulate   Agglutination   inhibition
           antigen

B

the particle system. A commonly used variation of the agglutination inhibition test employs antibody and closely related soluble
antigens to identify the specificity or cross-reactivity of antibody
to families of antigens as judged by the relative degrees of inhibition of agglutination.

Agglutination inhibition tests are of use in detecting human
chorionic gonadotropin (hCG) present in serum and urine in
pregnancy. Detection of hCG is useful in the confirmation of
pregnancy. Basically, pregnancy tests use hCG-coated latex or
red cells and antibody to hCG to generate agglutination of these
particles. Urine examined for the presence of hCG is mixed
with antibody to hCG. Following this, particulate hCG indicator
particles are added to the urine. Agglutination of the particles
by antibody is inhibited if hCG is present in the urine. This
test result is consistent with pregnancy.

Virus Hemagglutination Assays. A useful variation of the agglutination inhibition test uses the property of certain viruses, such as
influenza virus, which adheres to and agglutinates red cells. Serum
antibody mixed with the virus forms an immune complex inhibiting the agglutination of red cells by the virus. This result
indicates presence of serum antibody to the virus. This assay is
presently utilized to test patient's serum for antibody to rubella
virus and is useful in recognizing women at risk for the tera-
togenic effects of in utero rubella infection. A titer equal to or

Fig. 7-14 : Coombs
testing. In the
direct test, incom-
plete hemagglutinins
attached to red cells
are identified by
using antibody to
immunoglobulin
to bring about
agglutination.
A. In the indirect
test, red cells are
first reacted with
unknown serum to
test for the presence
of free incomplete
agglutinins. B. The
second antibody
(anti-immunoglobu-
lin) is then applied
to bring about
hemagglutination.

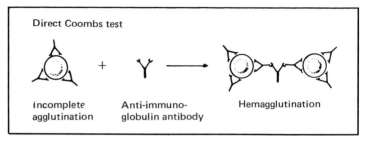

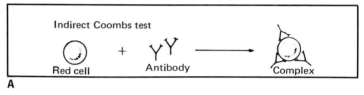

A

B

greater than 1:8 to 1:10 of rubella antibody is ordinarily protective against the disease. Women without significant titers of
rubella antibody benefit from immunization against rubella.

Antiglobulin-Mediated Assays. A useful mode of detecting incomplete agglutinins was developed by Coombs et al., 1945, who
used an anti-immunoglobulin antibody to bridge incomplete
agglutinins hooked to red cells (Figure 7-14). The result was that
red cells with attached incomplete agglutinins were rapidly aggregated. This is the direct antiglobulin test, or *direct Coombs
test,* which is used frequently by blood banks in the study of
antigen-antibody systems. The direct Coombs test is commonly
employed using reagent antibody to detect antibody-sensitized
red cells in vivo. There are numerous modifications of the Coombs
technique. The most important is the indirect Coombs test.

The indirect Coombs test allows a search for free (unattached)
incomplete antibodies to red cells in serum. Incomplete antibodies are identified in this context by mixing cells of known
antigenicity with the unknown serum. The cells are then washed,
and the second antibody (antiglobulin) is added. Free serum
antibody is detected by agglutination of the reagent cells with
the second antibody.

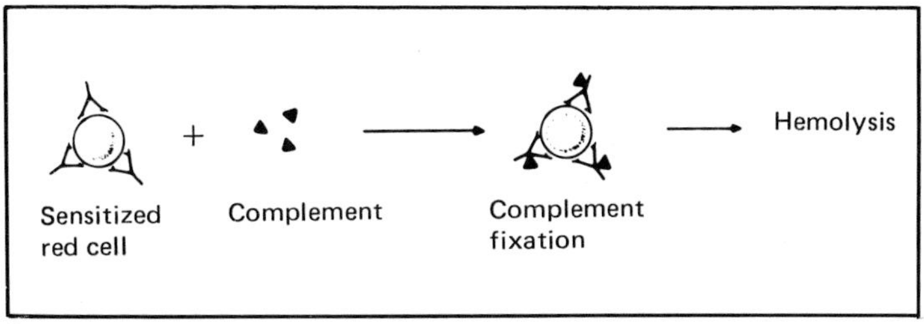

A

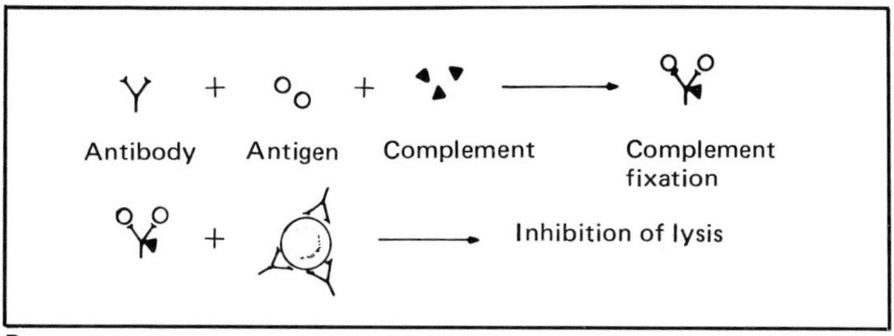

B

Fig. 7-15 : Complement-fixation. A. Cells sensitized with specific anti-erythrocyte antibody undergo lysis in the presence of complement. B. Unknown antibody in the presence of specific antigen forms Ag-Ab complexes that fix complement. This reaction exhausts complement, inhibiting complement-mediated hemolysis of sensitized red cells.

COMPLEMENT FIXATION. One of the most useful secondary manifestations of Ag-Ab reactions depends upon complement-mediated lysis of erythrocytes following red cell sensitization with specific antibody for either naturally occurring membrane or antigens adsorbed to membrane. (Figure 7-15). The combination of Ag-Ab reaction and complement fixation produces small cell membrane defects, loss of cytoplasmic contents, hypotonic swelling of the cell, and lysis (see Chapter 9). The reaction may be quantitated by holding antigen, red cell number, and complement concentration constant. The degree of complement-mediated lysis of cells, the indicator for the Ag-Ab reaction, is then a function of antibody titer and specificity for antigen on red cells.

The most useful complement-related test employs inhibition of complement fixation. This test serves to identify complement-fixing antibody to numerous antigens. Red cells are sensitized with antierythrocyte antibody. Subsequently a solution of antigen and complement is mixed with unknown serum, then with the red cells. If complement activity is removed by an initial Ag-Ab reaction, then complement-mediated lysis of sensitized red cells, the indicator systems, is abrogated. An antibody with specificity for the soluble antigen in the system is identified.

This test is quantitated on the basis of the degree of inhibition of the indicator system (complement-mediated lysis of reagent red cells) and is adaptable to many antigen-antibody systems. Requirement for use of this test is simply that the Ag-Ab reaction under study fix complement. Antibody-sensitized erythrocytes in this test are prepared with nonlysing antibody to a red cell membrane component. Most often sheep erythrocytes prepared with rabbit antisheep erythrocyte antibody (hemolysin) erythrocytes are employed.

The complement fixation test is particularly useful in detecting antibodies to various infectious organisms. It is an important technique for diagnosis of certain parasitic diseases. The complement-mediated lysis test can be modified to take place in agar, so that lymphocytes producing hemolysing antibody may be detected by the presence of lytic areas in agar containing erythrocytes, complement, and hemolysin-producing lymphocytes.

Antibody-mediated hemolysis is also a useful screening test for complement levels in serum. Hemolysis is measured spectrophotometrically, with the results generally expressed as the quantity of serum complement necessary to cause lysis of 50 percent of the red cells present (CH_{50} test). The test is useful in studying or diagnosing diseases in which there are decreased serum complement levels. In such cases, red cells sensitized with specific antierythrocyte antibody are first standardized. Unknown serum is tested as a source of complement, and the CH_{50} test result is measured by titering the patient's serum for lysis of the red cells. Diseases associated with decreased serum complement are usually immunological in nature and generally reflect the immunological consumption of complement in vivo. There are also hereditary diseases with a decrease or absence of individual complement components. Since activation of the several complement components (C1–C9) must take place to cause lysis of red cells, a deficiency of one single component will decrease apparent complement levels in the CH_{50} test.

Several other nonimmunological diseases are associated with somewhat increased complement levels, although the reason for this is not completely clear.

Tertiary Manifestations of Ag-Ab Reactions

Tertiary manifestations of the Ag-Ab reaction include those reactions due to the physiological effects of the antigen-antibody reaction. In vitro tests are used to detect Ag-Ab reactions through observation of the tertiary effects of the primary reaction.

Detection and Application of Tertiary Reactions

Tertiary reactions may also be observed in vivo as manifestations of antigen-antibody reactions. They are usually adaptive (protective). When tertiary reactions are exaggerated in severity in vivo, they are occasionally pathological. Several techniques are

Fig. 7-16 : Opsonization. Particulate antigen coated with opsonizing antibody promotes activation of macrophages and phagocytosis of antigen.

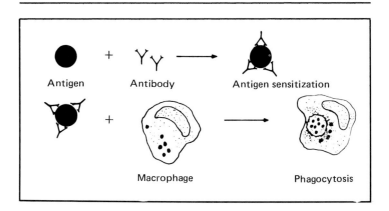

Antigen   Antibody   Antigen sensitization

Macrophage   Phagocytosis

useful in testing for the presence of antibodies stimulating tertiary reactions as well as for the ability of patients' peripheral white cells to act in certain of these reactions.

OPSONIZATION. Opsonization is a tertiary reaction following attachment of antibody and in some cases complement to particulate antigen or microorganisms (Figure 7-16). The primary Ag-Ab reaction subsequently augments phagocytosis of antigen by macrophages. The stimulus for phagocytosis during opsonization occurs through changes in a portion of the attached antibody or through complement fixation. Recognition of attached opsonin activates the phagocyte, possibly by increasing hydrolytic enzymes in the cell. The reaction is quantitated through comparison of test serum with normal serum to indicate the level of opsonizing antibodies. Usually the reaction is run with standard numbers of particles or organisms, macrophages, and complement, if necessary. The index of opsonization between test and normal serum is related to the relative titer and specificity of opsonin. This reaction is similar to events that take place in vivo where opsonization plays an important role in eradicating infection.

Opsonizing antibodies are often measured for their degree of presumptive protection against specific bacteria. Opsonizing antibodies against *Staphylococcus, Streptococcus, E. Coli,* etc., are often measured. By using normal serum as well as normal and patient-derived neutrophils and monocytes, a patient's capacity for a phagocytic response to opsonizing antibody and bacteria may also be indexed.

IMMOBILIZATION TESTS. Certain antibodies immobilize organisms to which they attach. A once-popular procedure was the *Treponema pallidum* immobilization (TPI) test for syphilis. The organism is normally quite mobile until exposed to antibody under special conditions. The measure of its immobilization against antibody titer provides knowledge concerning previous exposure to the disease. The test is specific but difficult to perform. It is used only when primary or secondary tests for syphilis such as the IF and agglutination tests, respectively, are equivocal.

NEUTRALIZATION REACTIONS. Neutralizing antibodies bind to infectious agents such as viruses. Antibody attached to virus-coated protein prevents adsorption to and penetration of cell membranes as well as uncoating of the virus in the cell cytoplasm. The effect of neutralizing antibody is to block infection of host cells at several levels. The virus is neutralized in vivo in the blood stream, in other fluids, or, often, at musocal and cell surfaces. Neutralizing antibody is occasionally enhanced by complement fixation.

The in vitro test for neutralizing antibodies uses standard virus and tissue culture methods. Dilutions of serum are mixed with infectious antigen and subsequently placed in tissue culture. A measure of neutralizing antibodies is carried out by later searching for signs of specific virus-associated tissue culture infection. The titer of protective antibody is measured by observing the degree of lysis or disruption of normal tissue culture cells (cytopathic effect). Testing for neutralizing antibodies to such viruses as influenza, measles, mumps, polio, and others is commonly carried out in this fashion.

CHEMOTAXIS. Chemotaxis is the directional movement of cells across a chemical gradient. Chemotaxis of monocytes and polymorphonuclear leukocytes may follow Ag-Ab reactions that fix complement. C5a, a fragment created from the C5 complement component during complement-fixation, provides a powerful chemotactic stimulus. The effect is to actively mobilize and localize phagocytes in the vicinity of an Ag-Ab reaction. The effects of opsonizing antibody are magnified by chemotaxis. Individuals with defective chemotaxis, in diabetes and possibly in sickle cell anemia, show an increased prevalence of certain infections.

In vitro, chemotaxis is tested by placing patient's phagocytes on the other side of a barrier (such as a Millipore filter) from a potent chemotactic stimulus, the chemotaxin. The number of phagocytes traversing the barrier in the direction of the chemotaxin is an index of chemotactic response. In vivo, a so-called skin window may be created, placing a coverslip and chemotactic stimulus or immunogen over interrupted skin. The number of phagocytes reaching the local skin reaction and adhering to the coverslip is partially indicative of the chemotactic response.

MAST CELL DEGRANULATION. Nonspecific attachment of IgE, and at times IgG, antibodies to the surface of mast cells or basophils arms the cells for degranulation of histamine and other mediators of acute inflammation upon encounter of specific antigen. Antibodies adhering to mast cells and basophils are known as *cytotropic antibodies.* The attachment of antibody to these cells occurs through the Fc portion of the antibody.

Attachment of allergen to the specific antigen recognition sites of cytotropic antibody evokes cytoplasmic degranulation of mast cells and basophils. Degranulation takes place through cross-linkage of the Fab portions of antibodies bound to cell surface membrane receptors. Cross-linkage of the antibody receptors imparts a Ca^{++} influx across the cell membrane, acting as a signal for release of histamine, serotonin, bradykinin, and the other mediators of acute inflammation in allergic individuals.

IgE is the primary cytotropic antibody. The number of IgE molecules attached to a single mast cell is in the range of 3,000 to 4,000 in nonallergic individuals. Allergic individual cells may carry four to five times this number of IgE molecules.

Testing for allergies in vivo is carried out by injecting small amounts of allergen into the dermis. Individuals with IgE-mediated (cytotropic) allergy demonstrate the tertiary effects of primary reaction between antigen and antibody. Mast cell degranulation mediates the inflammatory response, and the injection site demonstrates an erythematous swollen area. These results may be correlated with results of an in vitro RIA method of testing for IgE antibody to allergen. The RAST (radioallergosorbent) test uses purified allergen attached to an immunoadsorbent such as cellulose particles or discs. Following exposure of the disc to patient serum, antibody to allergen is detected by washing the disc and then using radiolabeled antiIgE. Combined results of skin tests, RAST testing, and serum IgE quantitation have enhanced the diagnosis and treatment of common allergies.

Testing antigens and antibodies in vivo—observing the tertiary manifestations associated with humoral immunity—has had great application in immunology. Early descriptions of simple skin test reactions led to important discoveries concerning the nature of protective immune reactions and, later, immunological tissue damage in hypersensitivity diseases.

SCHULTZ-CHARLTON PHENOMENON. The Schultz-Charlton phenomenon was described in 1918. It derived from the observation that antibody to the erythrogenic toxin of scarlet fever blanched the scarlet rash at the site of skin injection of the antibody. Subsequently, the Dick test used this principle to detect susceptibility

Table 7-4 : The Arthus Reaction: Sequence

Antigen immunization

Reinjection of antigen at 2–3 weeks

Antibody-antigen complexes

Immune complex deposition in vessel walls

Complement fixation

Chemotaxis and inflammation

PMNs attracted—phagocytosis of complexes

PMN lysozyme-mediated necrosis

Vascular thrombosis
 Platelet release of vasoactive mediators
 Increased vascular permeability
 Continued inflammation

to the toxin of scarlet fever. In the Dick test, erythrogenic toxin obtained from a culture of a *Streptococcus* strain known to cause scarlet fever is injected into the dermis. Individuals with antibody to the toxin fail to develop the rash at the site of injection. Unprotected individuals develop a reaction upon injection. Unfortunately protection against the toxin does not assure immunity against streptococcal infections and the severe associated sequelae such as rheumatic fever.

The Schick test (1913) exploits an identical rash-related observation in diphtheria. Diphtheria toxin causes a skin rash, and individuals immunized against diphtheria fail to develop a localized rash upon injection of the toxin. Fortunately the antibody in this test does protect against the serious cardiotoxic effects of diphtheria.

ARTHUS REACTION. Following intradermal injection of antigen into certain preimmunized animals, a localized Ag-Ab reaction takes place. Formation of immune complexes promotes release of histamine and other mediators of acute inflammation. The reaction begins to show swelling and erythema. The sequence of events in this Arthus reaction is listed in Table 7-4.

In man the Arthus reaction is occasionally troublesome following injection of foreign material, such as drugs or other antigens, in individuals with previous exposure to the antigen. The Arthus reaction is an important manifestation of the potential of the immune mechanism for tissue damage.

Immune Mechanisms in Tissue Damage

Although immune reactions are basically protective to the host, the IgE-mediated and Arthus reactions are examples of harmful immune reactions. Pathogenetic immune reactions are occasionally even lethal.

The diseases of immunological origin have been classified according to the mechanism involved. The observed effects of many of these diseases are tertiary manifestations of primary Ag-Ab reactions. Immune mechanisms in tissue damage are reviewed more extensively in Chapter 13.

Bibliography

General

Gill, T. J. Methods for detecting antibody. *Immunochemistry* 7:997, 1970.

Kwapinski, J. B. G. *Methodology of Immunochemical and Immunological Research.* New York: Wiley-Interscience, 1972. P. 245.

Rose, N. R., and Bigazzi, P. E. (Eds.). *Methods in Immunodiagnosis.* New York: Wiley, 1973. P. 71.

Rose, N. R., and Friedman, H. (Eds.). *Manual of Clinical Immunology,* 2nd ed. Washington, D.C.: American Society of Microbiology, 1980.

Weir, D. M. (Ed.). *Handbook of Experimental Immunology.* Oxford: Blackwell, 1973.

Williams, C. A., and Chase, M. M. (Eds.). *Methods in Immunology and Immunochemistry,* Vol. IV. New York: Academic, 1970.

Primary Reactions

Capra, J. D., and Kehoe, J. M. *Hypervariable regions, idiotypy, and the antigen-combining site.* Adv. Immunol. 20:1, 1975.

Froese, A. Kinetic and equilibrium studies on 2, 4-dinitrophenyl hapten-antibody systems. *Immunochemistry* 5:253, 1968.

Kitagawa, M., Yagi, Y., and Pressman, D. The heterogeneity of combining sites of antibodies as determined by specific immunoabsorbants. *J. Immunol.* 95:446, 1965.

Pinckard, R. N. Equilibrium Dialysis and Preparation of Hapten Conjugates. In D. M. Weir (Ed.), *Handbook of Experimental Immunology.* Oxford: Blackwell, 1975. P. 17.1.

Wilson, S., and Miles, A. A. (Eds.). *Topley and Wilson's Principles of Bacteriology and Immunity.* Baltimore: Williams and Wilkins, 1965. Pp. 227–329.

Pressman, D., and Grossburg, A. L. *The Structural Basis of Antibody Specificity.* New York: Benjamin, 1968.

Immunofluorescence and Immunoenzyme Assays

Johnson, G. D., Holbrow, E. J., and Dorling, J. Immunofluorescence and Immunoenzyme Techniques. In D. M. Weir (Ed.), *Handbook of Experimental Immunology.* Oxford: Blackwell, 1973. P. 151.

Nakamura, R. M., Chisari, F. V., and Edgington, T. S. Laboratory Tests for Diagnosis of Autoimmune Diseases. In M. Stefannini (Ed.), *Progress in Clincal Pathology.* New York: Grune and Stratton, 1975. P. 177, Vol. VI.

Nakamura, R. M., and Tan, E. M. Recent progress in autoantibodies to nuclear antigens (ANA). *Hum. Pathol.* 9:85, 1978.

Park, C. W. Spectrofluorometric Methods. In D. M. Weir (Ed.), *Handbook of Experimental Immunology.* Oxford: Blackwell, 1973. P. 18.1.

Wisdom, G. B. Enzyme immunoassay. *Clin. Chem.* 22:1243, 1976.

Radioimmunoassay

Hunter, W. M. Radioimmunoassay. In D. M. Wier (Ed.), *Handbook of Experimental Immunology.* Oxford: Blackwell, 1973. P. 14.1.

Rodford, D., and Catt, K. J. Mathematical theory of radiological assays: The kinetics of separation of bound from free. *J. Steroid Biochem.* 3:255, 1972.

Immunoprecipitation   Cawley, L. P. *Electrophoresis and Immunoelectrophoresis.* Boston: Little, Brown, 1969.

Mancini, G., Carbonara, H. O., and Heremans, J. F. Immunoclinical quantitation of antigens by single radial immunodiffusion. *Immunochemistry* 2:235, 1965.

Ouchterlony, O. Diffusion-in-gel methods for immunological analysis. *Prog. Allergy* 6:30, 1962.

Ouchterlony, O., and Nilsson, L. A. Immunodiffusion and Immunoelectrophoresis. In D. M. Weir (Ed.), *Handbook of Experimental Immunology.* Oxford: Blackwell, 1975. P. 19.1.

Ritzmann, S. E., and Daniels, J. C. (Eds.). *Serum Protein Abnormalities: Diagnostic and Clinical Aspects,* Boston, Little, Brown 1975.

Agglutination   Coombs, R. R. A., Mourant, A. E., and Race, R. R. A new test for the detection of weak and "incomplete" Rh agglutinins. *Br. J. Exp. Pathol.* 26:255–266, 1945.

Herbert, W. J. Passive Hemagglutination with Special Reference to the Tanned Cell Technique. In D. M. Weir (Ed.), *Handbook of Experimental Immunology.* Oxford: Blackwell, 1973. P. 20.1.

Hirst, G. K. The quantitative determination of influenza virus and antibodies by means of red cell agglutination. *J. Exp. Med.* 75:49, 1942.

Jones, F., and Orcutt, M. The prozone phenomenon in specific bacterial agglutination. *J. Immunol.* 27:215, 1934.

Williams, C. A., and Chase, M. M. (Eds.). *Methods in Immunology and Immunochemistry,* Vol. IV. New York: Academic, 1970.

Complement   Austen, K. F. (Ed.). The immunobiology of complement. *Transplant. Proc.* 6:1, 1974.

Ruddy, S., Gigli, I., and Austen, K. F. The complement system of man (4 parts). *N. Engl. J. Med.* 287:489, 545, 592, 642, 1972.

Williams, C. A., and Chase, M. M. (Eds.). *Methods in Immunology and Immunochemistry,* Vol. IV. New York: Academic, 1970.

Miscellaneous   Dick, G. F., and Dick, G. H. A skin test for susceptibility to scarlet fever. *J.A.M.A.* 82:265, 1924.

Notkins, A. L. Viral infection: Mechanisms of immunologic defense and injury. *Hosp. Pract.* 9:65, 1974.

Smith, H. Mechanisms of virus pathogenicity. *Bacteriol. Rev.* 36:291, 1972.

Starr, S. E., and Allison, A. C. Role of T lymphocytes in recovery from murine cytomegalovirus infection. *Infect. Immunol.* 17:458, 1977.

Stossel, T. P. Phagocytosis (3 parts). *N. Engl. J. Med.* 290:717, 774, 883, 1974.

Waldman, R. H., and Ganguly, R. Immunity to infections on secretory surfaces. *J. Infect. Dis.* 130:419, 1974.

Williams, C. A., and Chase, M. M. (Eds.). *Methods in Immunology and Immunochemistry,* Vol. IV. New York: Academic, 1970.

Winkelstein, J. A. Opsonins: Their function, identity, and clinical significance. *J. Pediatr.* 82:747, 1973.

8 : Amplification and Ancillary Systems Associated with Immunity

The amplification and ancillary systems associated with host defense include, in addition to the complement system (see Chapter 9), the cellular elements (excluding the lymphocytes) of the peripheral blood and the cells of the reticuloendothelial system (RES). This chapter covers the nonspecific entities associated with host defense and discusses the morphological and physiological properties of the cellular constituents that work in association with the specific immune systems. The role of cellular elements in various types of inflammatory responses and the consequence of deficiency in these elements are also elucidated.

Cells Associated with Host Response to Injury

Chapter 9 deals with the contribution of the amplification and ancillary humoral systems to the exudation associated with inflammation and discusses the many biological peptides that stimulate emigration of the cells making up the exudates. This section briefly describes the pertinent morphological characteristics, functions, and deficiencies or dysfunctions of the cells involved in the amplification mechanism in humans.

Characteristics, Distribution, and Biological Functions

NEUTROPHILS. Polymorphonuclear neutrophilic leukocytes (PMNs) are granulocytes that possess a number of functional properties important to host resistance. These typical *inflammatory cells,* associated with acute inflammation, are essential for the pathogenesis of the acute, necrotic reactions of immunological diseases, such as the vasculitis of immune complex disease (serum sickness), the Arthus reaction, the severe glomerulonephritis of nephrotoxic nephritis, and many other immune complex diseases. PMNs are, nevertheless, primarily involved in the continuous defense against nonimmunologically related inflammatory infections caused by bacteria and other parasites. The major route by which PMNs exert their defenses is phagocytosis, which will be discussed in detail later.

Neutrophils vary in size from 10 to 15 μ in diameter. Figure 8-1 shows a peripheral neutrophil. Neutrophils are the major granulocytes in peripheral blood (2 to 3 $\times$ 10^{10} cells in the total blood volume and 1.5 to 3.0 $\times$ 10^{12} in bone marrow). A mature neutrophil has a half-life of 6.6 hours, as measured by ^{32}DFP-labeled PMN (DFP = diisopropyl fluorophosphate).

Fig. 8-1 : A. A peripheral blood neutrophil; and B. an electron micrograph (X7000).

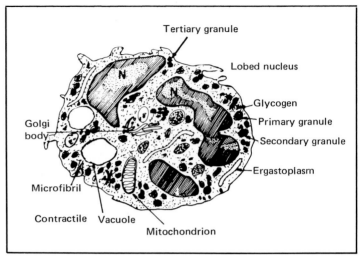

A

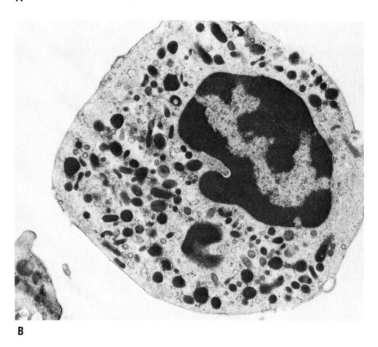

B

The nucleus of a neutrophil is multilobed, and in stained smears many pink-staining granules can be seen in the cytoplasm. Under the electron microscope these granules are of varying density and size and have been designated α, β, and γ. They constitute the major source of the enzymes in the killing of bacteria following phagocytosis. Some of the enzymes found in the cytoplasm of neutrophils are summarized in Table 8-1 and include hydrolases,

Table 8-1 : Some of the Enzymes Associated with Cytoplasmic Granules of Granulocytes, Macrophages (Monocytic Origin), Lymphocytes, and Platelets

Cell Type	Organelle	Enzymes
1. Granulocytes		
a. Neutrophil	Lysosome	Acid phosphatase, acid lipase, aryl sulfatases A and B, acid ribonucleases and deoxyribonucleases, cathepsin B, C, D, E, collagenase, phosphoprotein and phosphatidic acid phosphatases, phospholipase, organophosphate-resistant esterase, β-glucuronidase, β-galactosidase, β-N-acetylglucosaminidase, α-L-fucosidase, α-1,4-glucosidase, α-N-acetyl-galactosaminidase, hyaluronidase, lysozyme
	Peroxisome-related	D-amino acid oxidase, L-α-OH acid oxidase, catalase, myeloperoxidase
b. Eosinophil	Lysosome	Acid protease, βglucuronidase, aryl sulfatase, nucleases and phosphatase, peroxidase
c. Basophil (mast cell)	Lysosome	Proteases, phospholipase A, glucuronidase, acid and alkaline phosphatases, ATPase
	Granules	Histamine, serotonin, heparin, dopamine, acid mucopolysaccharides, (dopa, tryptophan, and histidine decarboxylases), heparin-synthesizing enzymes of cytoplasm. (Note that not all these substances are enzymes.)
2. Lymphocytes	Peroxisome-related	D-amino acid oxidase, L-α-OH acid oxidase, peroxidase, catalase
	Lysosome	Arylsulfatase, β-glucuronidase, β-galactosidase, N-acetyl-β-glucosaminidase, N-acetyl-α-galactosaminidase, α-mannosidase, α-arabinosidase, β-xylosidase, β-cellobiosidase, β-fucosidase, cathepsin D
3. Macrophages	Lysosome and cytoplasmic mitochondria	Acid phosphatase, β-glucuronidase, cathepsin, esterase, lysozyme, α-glycerolphosphate dehydrogenase, DPN- and TPN-diaphorases (isocitric, lactic, malic, succinic and deydrogenases), uridine diphosphate, glucose-glycogen transglycosylase
4. Platelets	Granules and cytoplasm	Trypsin and chymotrypsin-like cathepsin, elastase (from proelastase-activated by trypsin), ribonuclease (pH optimum synthesis), cyclooxygenase, peroxidase, isomerases, thromboxane synthetase

oxidases, and peroxidases. The Fc of IgG, as well as IgE and C3b receptors, has been demonstrated on the membrane of neutrophils.

EOSINOPHILS. The eosinophilic leukocytes (Figure 8–2) are similar in size and in nuclear structure to the neutrophils. The major distinguishing characteristic of eosinophils is their cytoplasmic granules (0.2 to 1.0 μ), which are much larger than neutrophilic granules and have a strong affinity for acidic aniline dyes such as eosin. The granules contain large quantities of stable peroxidase, lipids, and proteins. Crystalloid structures of various patterns can be seen in these granules by electron microscopic examination. In human eosinophils the crystalloid structures have various shapes (ovals, squares, two or more cores, etc.) and are generally localized in the central region of the granule. The crystalloids appear to stain strongly for peroxidase activity when analyzed by electron microscopic histochemical staining using 3, 3'-diaminobenzidine tetrachloride. Eosinophilic granules contain enzymes similar to those in neutrophils but appear to lack lysozyme and phagocytin: nevertheless, these granules are considered to be lysosomes.

Like the neutrophils, eosinophils have a short life span in the peripheral circulation. They constitute 2 to 5 percent of the total circulating leukocytes of peripheral blood. The bone marrow contains 200 times more eosinophils than the blood, and the tissues have 500 times more than the blood. The eosinophils of the tissues are primarily found in the intestinal walls, skin, external genitalia, and lungs. Blood eosinophils are regulated by the adrenal corticosteroids. An increase in these hormones due to stress or therapeutic administration of the adrenal corticosteroids results in decreased numbers of eosinophils in the circulating blood. The exact functions of eosinophils are unknown, but they do have limited phagocytic capabilities. When phagocytosis occurs, the cells can degranulate, and in this respect eosinophils appear to be similar to neutrophils. It has been demonstrated that eosinophils contain a factor(s) that neutralizes histamine, serotonin, and perhaps kinin. This could be the means by which these mediators of vascular change are controlled. This concept helps to explain the appearance of large numbers of eosinophils during an allergic manifestation due to an immediate type of hypersensitivity associated with the release of the vasoamines and SRS-A. For example, arylsulfatase of eosinophils has been implicated in the destruction or inactivation of SRS-A. Evidence for the existence of the neutralizing factor(s) has been shown recently. The pharmacologically active mediators released by basophil and eosinophil are discussed in the paragraphs that follow.

Fig. 8-2 : A. A peripheral blood eosinophil; and B. an electron microscopic photograph (X7800).

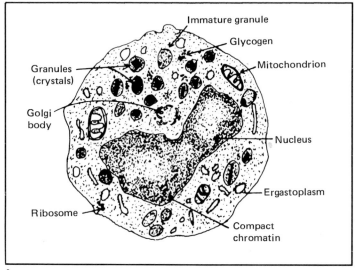

A

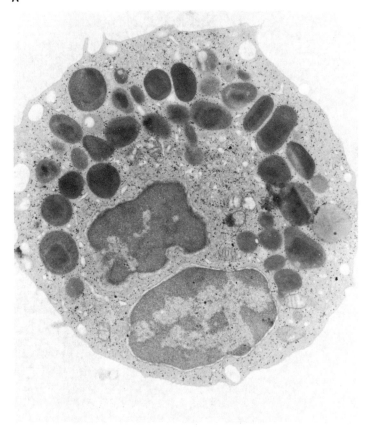

B

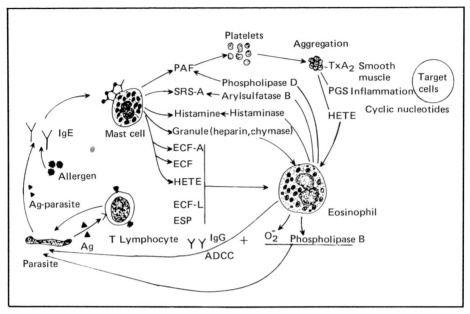

Fig. 8-3 : The eosinophil's response to factors released from a sensitized T lymphocyte or a mast cell. The mast cell response is mediated by allergen or parasitic antigens via interaction with IgE. PAF = platelet activating factor; SRS-A = slow-reacting substance of anaphylaxis; ECF-A, ECF-L = eosinophilic chemotactic factors from mast cells (ECF-A) and from lymphocytes (ECF-L); ESP = eosinophilic stimulation promoter (from lymphocytes); HETE = 12-L-hydroxyl-5.8.10.14-eicosatetraenoic acid, a product of arachidonate via lipooxygenase action, having chemotactic activity; O_2^--superoxide (free radical); ADCC = antibody dependent cytotoxic cell; TxA_2 = thromboxane A_2; PGs = prostaglandins.

The biological action of eosinophils is depicted in Figure 8-3. An allergic reaction mediated via IgE action on mast cells or basophils releases a variety of pharmacologically active compounds, which in turn activate eosinophils and release compounds neutralizing the active agents. In Figure 8-4, the killing action of eosinophils is shown against the schistosomula of *Schistosoma mansoni* treated with normal rabbit serum. This action is mediated via the C3 receptors of eosinophils, which react with the C3 fragment that coats the schistosomula surface. Eosinophils also can destroy parasites through specific immunoglobulins binding the parasites via the Fc receptor. The killing is mediated via O_2^- (superoxide anion) radicals and phospholipase elaborated by eosinophils (see Figures 8-3 and 8-4). The enzymes of eosinophils are summarized in Table 8-1. Fc and C3 receptors have been demonstrated in the membrane of eosinophils.

BASOPHILS. Basophils (Figure 8-5) are essentially noninflammatory cells that are chemically, structurally, and functionally

Fig. 8-4 : Eosin-
ophilic killing of a
parasite via the C3
receptor binding site
in the absence of
antibody.

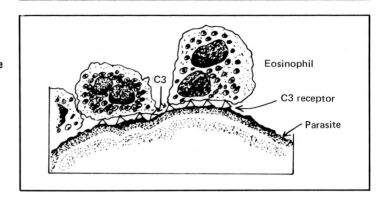

identical to the mast cells encountered in connective tissues.
These cells, together with platelets, probably play a significant
role in the release of vasoamines such as histamine and serotinin.
Basophils constitute 0.5 percent of the circulating blood leukocytes. They are characterized by large electron-dense cytoplasmic
granules having a predilection for basic aniline dyes, which
suggests that they contain acid mucopolysaccharides. It has been
known for some time that these granules contain heparin, which
is responsible for the metachromasia. Degranulation of mast
cells releases histamine in addition to heparin. In some species,
such as the rat, mast cells also contain serotonin (5-hydroxy-
tryptamine) in their cytoplasmic granules. About 30 percent of
the dry weight of mast cell granules is heparin, and approximately 35 percent is basic protein. The histamine content of
mast cell granules varies from species to species and from tissue
to tissue (7 to 40 ng per cell). Packed peritoneal mast cells of
the rat contain 630 to 700 μg serotonin per milliliter of cells.
It has been suggested that mast cell granules are composed of
polysaccharide protein-ion complexes to which vasoamines
(histamine, serotonin, dopamine) are bound electrostatically.
Other constituents of mast cell granules are summarized in
Table 8-1.

The following substance can initiate mast cell or basophil degranulation with the concomitant release of heparin and vasoactive amines: IgE-Ag complexes, anaphylatoxin (C3a, C5a),
basic protein (neutrophil lysosomal protein), and anti-mast cell
antibody plus complement; chemicals such as dextrans, poly-
vinylpyrrolidine, bee venom, and rose thorn; surface-active agents
such as bile salts, lysolecithin, 48/80, and Tween 20; and physical
agents (heat, ultraviolet radiation, x-rays, and radioisotopes).
The mechanisms by which these agents produce degranulation
differ, although vasoactive amines are released in all cases. The
degranulation process is an active one and requires energy. The
primary physiological functions of basophils and mast cells are

Fig. 8-5 : A. A peripheral blood basophil. B. Electron micrograph (X7000).

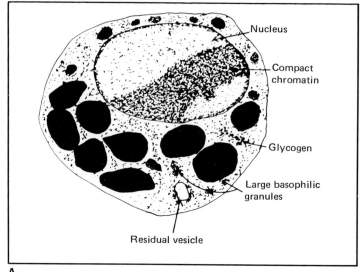

Nucleus

Compact chromatin

Glycogen

Large basophilic granules

Residual vesicle

A

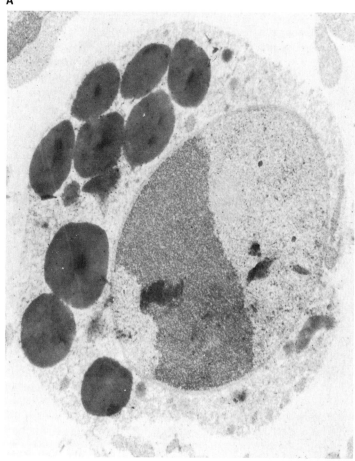

B

not clear. Their characteristic perivascular distributions suggest a possible role in the regulation of the permeability of the terminal vascular beds via the release of vasoactive amines. Abnormal release of the vasoactive amines by mast cells contributes to the inflammatory patterns observed in immediate and delayed hypersensitivities and in nonimmunological disorders. Receptors for the Fc portion of IgE and IgG have been demonstrated on membranes of mast cells and basophils. Eosinophilic chemotactic factors (ECF) and platelet-activating factor (PAF) are released also by activated mast cells or basophils. The factors released by basophils or mast cells and their relationship to eosinophils in an allergic phenomenon or parasitic infestation have been depicted in Figure 8-3.

MONOCYTES AND MACROPHAGES. Monocytes (Figure 8-6) of the peripheral blood measure 12 to 15 μ in diameter when examined in stained blood smears. The nucleus is generally kidney-shaped, and the cytoplasm stains grayish blue with aniline dyes such as crystal violet. The cytoplasm also contains azurophilic granules of reddish blue. Blood monocytes are considered immature macrophages, and their primary source is the bone marrow. There is general agreement that monocytes migrate from the circulation and mature into typical tissue and inflammatory macrophages at the site of the injury. This has been substantiated with radioautographic procedures using ^{3}H-thymidine. The source of macrophages in the lung, peritoneal cavity, and inflammatory exudate is the bone marrow. Macrophages may also arise by mobilization and proliferation of existing tissue macrophages, migration of Kupffer cells from the liver into the lungs, and (possibly) differentiation of specialized endothelial cells and septal cells of lung to macrophages. Differences and similarities are evident between macrophage cells from different tissue sites, as follows:

Source of Macrophage	Mitotic Rate	Adheres and Spreads on Glass
Sessile or fixed tissue (bone marrow, spleen, and liver)	High	Slowly
Alveolar tissue	High	Readily
Peritoneal and blood monocytes	Low	Readily

Tissue macrophages are larger than blood monocytes (15 to 80 μ), and the number of azurophilic granules in them varies. Macrophage nuclei vary in size and shape, and multinucleated forms

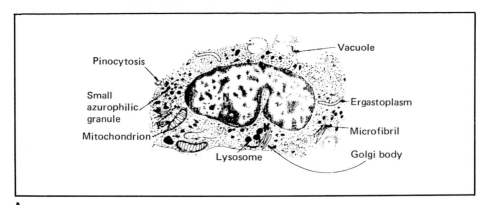

A

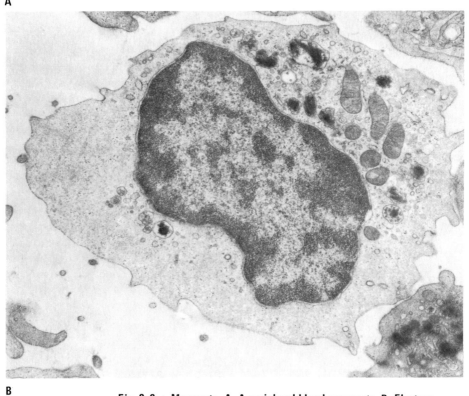

B

Fig. 8-6 : Monocyte. A. A peripheral blood monocyte. B. Electron micrograph (X7000).

may be present. The epithelioid cells of chronic inflammation (granulomatous) are macrophages with ovoid nuclei resembling epithelial cells. The presence of diffuse lipids in the cytoplasm gives these cells a pale appearance. Lipid droplets may also be shown in the cytoplasm of macrophages. Electron micrographs of monocytes and unstimulated peritoneal macrophages show great similarity. Unlike peripheral granulocytes, monocytes have a well-defined Golgi apparatus composed of flattened sacs, small vesicles, and a few granules; a moderate amount of rough endoplasmic reticulum; varying numbers of electron-dense granules; and many small vesicles in the cytoplasm.

The major functions of macrophages, as of neutrophils, are phagocytosis and degradation of ingested material. Significant numbers of neutrophils also are ingested by macrophages following tissue damage or an acute infection. The half-life of monocytes has been estimated to be 3 days. Some of the enzymes found in macrophages are listed in Table 8-1. Macrophages, like neutrophils, are influenced by complement factor (Ag-Ab-C1423 in immune adherence) and by sensitized T cell lymphokines such as MIF (migration inhibitory factor).

The ability of certain antibodies (IgG1 and IgG3) to adhere to the macrophage membrane (macrophage receptor, MR) permits the IgG to react with its antigen and may play a significant role in macrophage-mediated protection against certain infections. These macrophage-adherent immunoglobulins are known as *cytophilic antibodies.* Adherence occurs through the Fc portion of the IgG molecule. Similar binding of IgG to macrophages that react with erythrocytes (sheep RBC) gives the typical rosette appearance attributed to macrophages. The role of the macrophage as an accessory or auxiliary cell (A cell) in the processing of antigens (which is sometimes needed for T cell–B cell interactions) has been discussed (see Chapter 5). Complement fragments C3b and C3d have been shown to bind to the macrophage surface and act as opsonins. Peripherally activated monocytes have been shown to synthesize prostaglandins E_2 and $F_{2\alpha}$. These prostaglandins have been implicated in the modulation of the immune response (see Chapter 5) and in inflammatory processes.

KILLER CELLS (K CELLS). The K cell is a mononuclear cell associated with the null cell population, discussed briefly in Chapter 3. It possesses neither T cell nor B cell markers such as E-receptors (SRBC-receptors) nor immunoglobulins on its membrane. Nevertheless, killer cells have been recognized by their ability to bind to the Fc portion of immunoglobulins IgG and IgM. How they destroy target cells is unknown, but in order to do it, killer cells must either arm themselves with Ig or attach

Fig. 8-7 : K cell attaching itself to a target cell. Either (a) the Ig is attached to the K cell via its Fc receptor, and the armed K cell attacks target cell; or (b) the Ig binds to the antigenic receptors on the target cell, and the K cell is then attached via the Fc receptor.

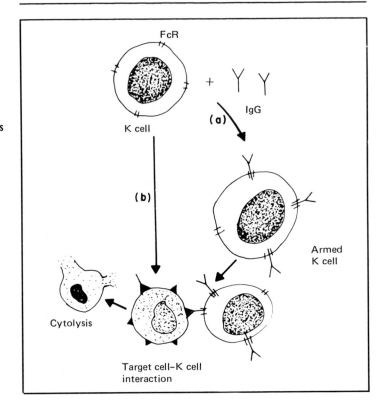

themselves to the Fc portion of the antibody attached to the target. This action of the cell is depicted in Figure 8-7. K cells have been designated as *antibody-dependent cytotoxic cells* (ADCC). They differ from the antibody-binding macrophages or monocytes. K cells have no adherence property and no battery of enzymes, e.g., the hydrolases associated with the lysosomes of macrophages. Further discussion of K cells is presented in Chapters 10, 13, and 16 under cell-mediated cytotoxic cells. The closely related natural killer cells are discussed in Chapters 3 and 16.

PLATELETS. The significance of platelets in the intrinsic pathway for coagulation of blood is well known. Platelets (Figure 8-8) are the fundamental formed elements involved in the creation of the hemostatic plug (thrombus) of flowing blood. The platelets of all mammals are small nonnucleated colorless bodies (corpuscles). They are oval or round biconcave disks, 2 to 4 μ in size, which when seen in profile appear as small plump spindles or rods. The shape of platelets and their granules is clearly seen electron microscopically (Figure 8-8). They are not uniform in size, and their numbers vary considerably in peripheral blood of individuals. The average number per cubic millimeter of blood is reported to be 2.5×10^5, although other, higher, mean values

Fig. 8-8 : Platelet.
A. A peripheral
blood platelet.
B. Electron micro-
graph (X7000).

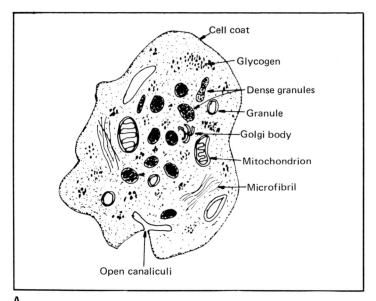

Cell coat

Glycogen

Dense granules

Granule

Golgi body

Mitochondrion

Microfibril

Open canaliculi

A

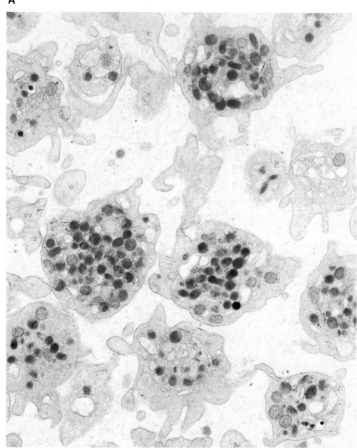

B

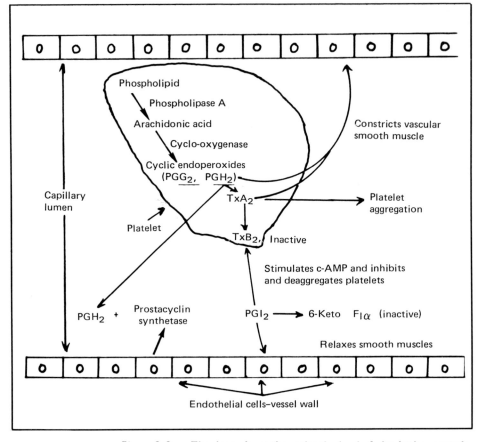

Figure 8-9 : The dynamics at the molecular level of platelet hemeostasis, and its relationship to the endothelial cell of the capillary wall.

have been reported. The actual numbers are difficult to assess because of platelets' ability to adhere readily to each other and to various surfaces.

The regulation of platelet hemostasis is summarized in Figures 8-9 and 8-10. The major biochemical pathway involves the synthesis of prostaglandin products from the precursor fatty acid arachidonate. The stimulus for activation enters via the surface-connected canalicular system (SCCS). The SCCS is made up of invaginations in the membrane surfaces of platelets. The stimulus within the proximity of the dense tubular system (DTS) activates the enzyme phospholipase A_2, releasing arachidonic acid (AA) within the DTS and causing the subsequent formation of AA products through the enzyme cyclooxygenase and through the major intermediary compound prostaglandin G_2 (PGG$_2$). PGG$_2$ is converted to thromboxane A_2 (TxA$_2$) by

Fig. 8-10 : Platelet
activation and the
interrelationship
between PGG$_2$,
TxA$_2$, c-AMP
c-GMP, and Ca^{++}.

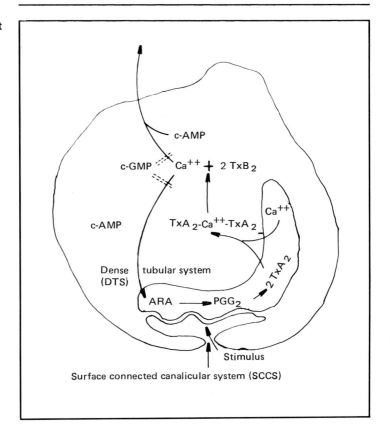

thromboxane synthetase enzymes. TxA$_2$ transports Ca^{++} from
DTS storage to the platelet cytoplasm, activating the actin and my-
osin proteins in the cytoplasm. The degree of contraction is modulated by the availability of Ca^{++} in DTS for the contractile proteins.

The cyclic nucleotides appear to modulate the action of Ca^{++} by
controlling the concentration in the cytoplasm in the proximity
of the contractile proteins. c-AMP appears to stimulate Ca^{++}
uptake by DTS and extrusion of Ca^{++} from the cell. Thus, c-GMP
would sustain contractility as long as Ca^{++} is available. On
the other hand, c-AMP appears to modulate the system to a normal status. Synthesis of prostaglandins D$_2$, E$_2$, and F$_{2\alpha}$ occurs
via the intermediary endoperoxides PGG$_2$ and PGH$_2$. The enzymes involved in the conversion of the short-lived endoperoxides
(half-life, 4 to 5 minutes) to prostaglandins are peroxidase, iso-
merase, and reductase, respectively, for PGE$_2$, PGD$_2$, and PGF$_{2\alpha}$.

Vasoactive amines are released following platelet activation by
Ag-Ab complexes in the presence of complement. This is especially pronounced in some species of animals. In the case of

the rabbit, the sequence of platelet activation and vasoactive amine release can be shown as follows:

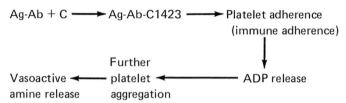

Neutrophils, eosinophils, and macrophages also adhere to the Ag-Ab-C1423 complex (immune adherence). The amines released by platelets are contained within granules distinct from lysosomes. Energy (presumably as ATP) is required for the release of the vasoactive amines, and platelet lysis does not usually accompany the release. Concentrations of vasoactive amines are lower in human platelets than in those of the rabbit. Also, instead of adhering to Ag-Ab-C1423 complexes, they aggregate directly with the antibody globulin of the Ag-Ab complexes. Thus, the release of ADP and vasoactive amines in man occurs without the intervention of complement. Platelets of ruminants and pigs are similar to those of man. Although the mechanisms are different in all the species mentioned here, the *end result* (release of vasoactive amines) is the same.

Collagen and several nonimmunological materials also can initiate release of vasoactive amines from platelets. Other factors that can trigger platelet release of amines include aggregated IgG, antigen plus sensitized leukocytes, antiplatelet antibody, the enzymes thrombin and trypsin, the catecholamines, arachidonic acid, and ristocetin. The latter substance is of unknown chemical structure and is isolated from *Nocardia lurida.* Ristocetin induces platelet aggregation in normal platelet-rich plasma (PRP), while individuals with von Willebrand's disease show abnormal aggregation due to deficiency in Factor VIII antigen, antihemophilic factor, and von Willebrand's factor in the platelets. Table 8–2 summarizes data for selected platelet functional defects.

Phagocytosis

Phagocytosis (Figure 8–11) is the process by which a phagocytic cell destroys invading bacteria. The major phagocytic cells are the neutrophils and the macrophages. Phagocytosis can be viewed as a sequence of three events. *Chemotaxis,* the attraction of the phagocytes to the site of injury, is the first event. It is related to the release of peptides during complement activation, kallikrein activation, and antigen reaction with specific sensitized T lymphocytes. In addition, chemotactic factors released by bacteria and from tissue breakdown products have been demonstrated. These seem to be small glycoprotein fragments and polysaccharide.

Fig. 8-11 : Phago-
cytosis of bacteria
by a PMN, forma-
tion of phagolyso-
some, digestion of
the bacteria, and
elimination (exo-
cytosis). N =
nucleus; M = mito-
chondrion; ER =
endoplasmic
reticulum.

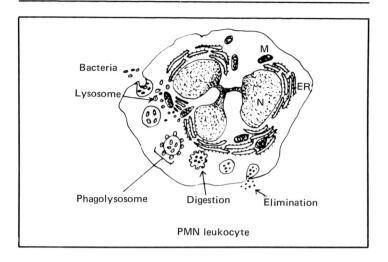

PMN leukocyte

Table 8-2 : Diseases with Platelet Defects as Determined with Various Platelet Inducers

Platelet Stimulus	Diseases		
	Thrombasthenia	Thrombopathia	von Willebrand's
ADP	Abnormal	Normal (first phase)	Normal
Epinephrine	Abnormal	Abnormal	Normal
Collagen	Abnormal	Abnormal	Normal
Ristocetin	Normal	Normal	Abnormal
Glass retention	—	—	Abnormal

The term *phagocytosis* is used both for the overall process and for
the second step, the *engulfment (ingestion)* of the bacteria.
This occurs when the outer cytoplasmic membrane of the cell
surrounds the bacteria, with the formation of a vacuole within
the cytoplasm of the phagocyte. Soon after engulfment, the
third step, the actual *killing* of the bacteria, begins. Lysosomal
(and perhaps peroxisomal) granules fuse with the vacuole and
release their enzymatic contents into it. Within the resultant
packet, now called a *phagolysosome* or *phagosome,* the killing
and digestion of the bacteria occur. The subunits or fragments
formed are egested (eliminated from the cell) and, in many
instances, passed on to the appropriate lymphocytes for cell-
mediated or humoral immune response. Those subunits or antigens coming from macrophages have been designated "super-
immunogens" by some investigators.

Phagocytosis is enhanced by naturally occurring opsonins (immunoglobulins) against bacteria and by specific antibody im-

munoglobulins. As mentioned earlier, these effects can be amplified through the participation of complement and the immune adherence phenomenon. Fibrin clots also assist phagocytosis by creating surfaces and by restricting bacterial migration, both of which make entrapment easier.

Pinocytosis is used to describe a process similar to phagocytosis. It involves the intake of soluble material (proteins) and colloidal suspensions (such as virus particles). Terms, such as *endocytosis and exocytosis,* have been used for ingestion and egestion, respectively, by phagocytic cells.

Biochemistry of Phagocytosis

The significant biochemical event associated with phagocytosis is an increase in anaerobic glycolysis (Embden-Meyerhof pathway). This increase is necessary for the ingestion step. Increases in glucose utilization occur following phagocytosis with the formation of lactic acid and hydrogen peroxide (H_2O_2). Energy increases of from 5 to 40 percent over those in a resting leukocyte have been shown to occur in a leukocyte that is actively ingesting bacteria. Suppression of glycolysis or of the hexose monophosphate pathway (HMP) will result in decreased ingestion of bacteria. H_2O_2 (which increases four to six times normal levels following active phagocytosis) plays a significant role in killing the ingested organisms. Hydrogen peroxide plus peroxidase and chloride ions or other appropriate hydrogen donors has been shown to play a significant role in the killing of ingested bacteria. In some instances halogenation involving Cl^-, H_2O_2, and peroxidase) of bacterial membrane results in the death of the organism. In other instances the aldehydes and ketones formed through peroxidatic action have been shown to be the toxic substances.

Hydrogen peroxide, in the presence of ascorbic acid, results in the formation of free radicals, which could alter membrane surfaces such as those of the ingested bacteria. This effect would increase the vulnerability of the bacterial surface to the lysosomal enzymes present in the phagolysosome. For example, it has been shown that H_2O_2 plus ascorbic acid can render *Salmonella* membrane surfaces susceptible to lysozyme attack by exposing the muramic acid (2-amino-3,o- (1-carboxyethyl-2-deoxy-D-glucose) residues previously protected by the membrane capsules of the bacteria. Evidently the free radicals formed depolymerize the protective covering of the plasma membrane, since any reducing chemical, such as thiosulfite, which inhibits free radical formation, reverses this phenomenon. In this context it is interesting to note that macrophages have a high ascorbic acid content.

Once the ingested bacteria are killed, complete destruction follows, catalyzed by the numerous hydrolases found in the lysosomes. The enzymes contained in the phagocytes have been summarized in Table 8-1. A congential absence of any of these enzymes causes one of the so-called *lysosomal disorders*. The synthesis of H_2O_2 in PMN leukocytes is presented in Figure 8-12; which illustrates a typical killing process carried out by a neutrophil. The oxidases (which produce H_2O_2 from O_2) and the peroxidases (which degrade it to H_2O) are probably the enzymes found in the peroxisomes. The aldehydes and ketones are perhaps formed by $NADP^+$-dependent deydrogenases, but this process, as it pertains to phagocytosis, is not well understood in man.

Leukocyte Deficiencies

Defects of the nonspecific immune system associated with neutrophils may be (1) quantitative, in which case there is a decrease in the number of neutrophils (neutropenia); and (2) qualitative, in which case there is a defect in some metabolic or biochemical function of these cells, but a normal morphological appearance and number.

Neutropenias, acquired and inherited, have been observed in association with decreased production of myeloid precursors due to bone marrow defects. The acquired types can be caused by drugs, pollutants, radiation, endotoxin, overwhelming infections, neoplasia, and disorders of the bone marrow and spleen. The inherited forms are x-linked recessive or autosomal dominant. Increased susceptibility to infections is common in both acquired and inherited neutropenias. *Micrococcus pyogenes* and *Diplococcus pneumoniae* are the common causes of infection in the neutropenic individual.

Qualitative changes in neutrophils have been associated with chronic granulomatous disease (CGD). Transmission is familial, presumably as an x-linked recessive trait. Both males and females have been affected, although at different ages. Defects in the biochemical pathways have been implicated in the inability to kill low-grade pathogens such as *Escherichia coli, Micrococcus pyogenes, Serratia marcescens, Paracolon hafnia,* and *Klebsiella enterobacter.* CGD has been associated with a deficiency of glucose-6-phosphate dehydrogenase, a deficient myeloperoxidase, and also with defects in the glutathione peroxidase and reductase systems. Since all these defects have not been found in any one patient, the defect in CGD has yet to be completely elucidated.

Myeloperoxidase deficiency disease is associated with an inability of neutrophilic leukocytes to kill ingested bacteria. Generation of H_2O_2 is severely diminished, and ability to break down H_2O_2 is defective. Deficiency of neutrophilic granules has been associated with myeloperoxidase deficiency disease and Chédiak-Higashi syndrome.

The Inflammatory Process

The inflammatory process involves interlocking networks of the complement, clotting, fibrinolysis, and kinin systems, and of the cellular elements. All these systems are dependent upon proteolytic

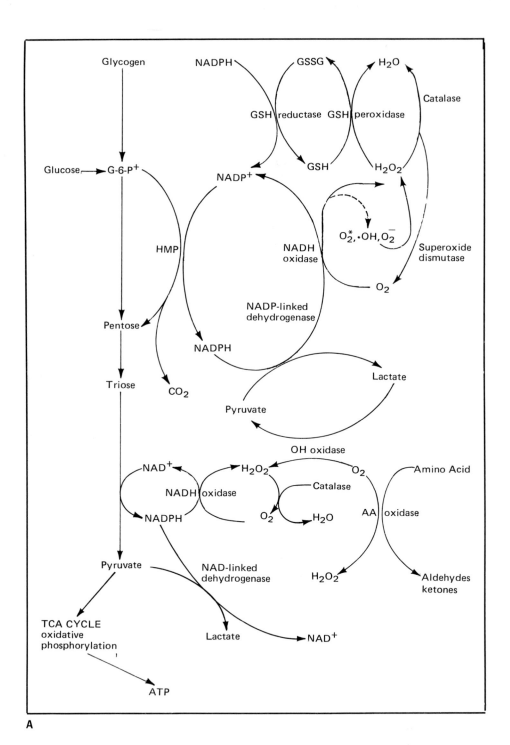

A

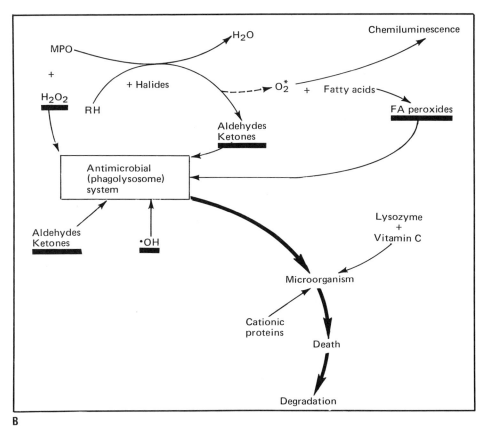

B

Fig. 8-12 : The biochemical pathway in the killing of microorganisms by neutrophils and possibly macrophages. This pathway has not been demonstrated for lymphocytes as yet. The glutathione system consists of the enzymes glutathione reductase and peroxidase. The system is important for generating $NADP^+$ for HMP and is closely associated with NADH oxidase (generates H_2O_2 for GSH peroxidase). The glutathione system is implicated in chronic granulomatous disease. A. The biochemical pathway. Agents associated with the antimicrobial effect include the major cʊ n-nent H_2O_2; the free radical O^*_2 (singlet oxygen), which generates the toxic fatty acid peroxides; OH (hydroxyl), which has a direct effect on the microorganism; O^-_2 (superoxide), which also generates the toxic FA peroxides, aldehydes, and ketones formed via amino acid oxidases; and the well-known MPO (myeloperoxidase) and halide system, which generates toxic aldehydes and ketones from low molecular weight H^+ donors such as amino acids and dehydroxy fatty acids. HMP (hexose monophosphate shunt) contributes significantly to the killing via generation of NADPH. G-6-P = glucose 6- phosphate. B. Phagocytosis within a PMN leukocyte. A. phagolysosome (vesical within the cytoplasm of the PMN) constitutes ingested microbes and the hydrolytic enzymes released by the granules. The microorganisms are killed and degraded within the phagolysosome. Cationic proteins, lysozymes, and vitamin C (free radicals) also contribute to the demise of the microorganism. The presence of catalase will readily destroy the H_2O_2 generated; thus in most pathological situations this enzyme is suppressed in tissues. At the same time there is a four- to tenfold increase in H_2O_2 generation. Therefore, the oxidases appear to play a major role in the generation of H_2O_2 and the free radicals.

and other enzymatic reactions, which are regulated by activation of inactive precursors by selective proteolysis, positive feedback, stoichiometric inhibition, multistep amplification, and enzymatic degradation of the active products. The inflammatory process is initiated in response to injury, and it is essential to the survival of the host. The inflammatory reaction often becomes part of the immune process and the final mediator of expression of immunological reactions (both deleterious and advantageous). The process comprises a series of biochemical and microanatomical changes of the terminal vascular bed and of the connective tissues. These changes are intended to eliminate the injurious agents and to repair the damaged tissues. Inflammation involves a great many host responses. This section will limit itself to a brief review of the biochemical events associated with coagulation, fibrinolysis, and kinin generation in their relationships to the inflammatory state. The complement system, a part of the inflammatory process, is discussed in Chapter 9. The inflammatory cells, peripheral blood leukocytes, and tissue macrophages have been discussed earlier in this chapter.

Acute Inflammation   Much progress in the study of inflammation has been made since the earlier description of the four basic symptoms in the first century AD: "Notae vero inflammatimis sunt quatuor: rubor et tumor uni calore et dolore." Since then it has been shown that inflammation can also lead to loss of function or death, in addition to the redness (rubor), swelling (tumor), heat (calore), and pain (dolore).

The sequence of events in the acute inflammatory response that is from tissue injury are as follows (Figure 8–13):

Tissue injury results in an increased permeability and dilation of blood vessels (erythema) in the injured region. Initiation of fibrin deposition via the clotting system occurs with the activation of Hageman factor (HF, clotting Factor XII).

The deposited fibrin aids in trapping the deleterious agents and platelets within the coagulum. This, in addition to the activity of the opsonins (heat-labile), also enhances phagocytosis by neutrophils and macrophages. HF subunits (formed by the action of plasmin on activated HF) activate prekallikrein by converting it to kallikrein (chemotaxic factor). This stimulates the emigration of blood leukocytes and plasma cells, and these cells contribute to phagocytosis and localized antibody synthesis. One of the hallmarks of acute inflammation is the infiltration and presence of polymorphonuclear cells in the vicinity of the injured site.

Increased blood plasma and tissue fluids at the injured site occurs (as shown by swelling edema) with elevation of the local levels of the bactericidal serum factors (specific antibody, complement factors, kinin, opsonins, etc.). At the same time, the increase in

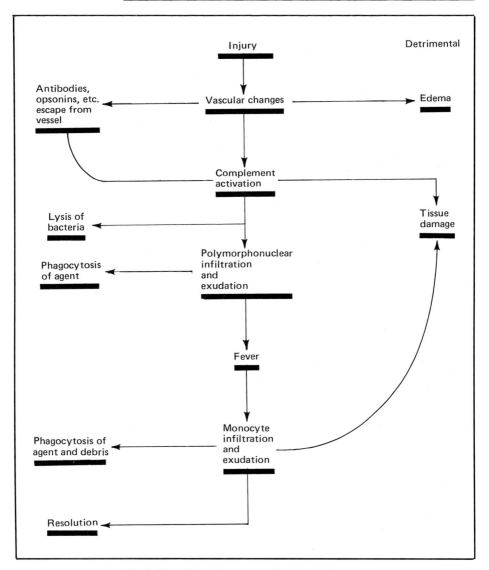

Fig. 8-13 : The major events of an acute inflammatory response may be beneficial (left), leading to resolution of the injury after destruction of the inciting agent; or detrimental (right), leading to edema and tissue damage.

fluids contributes to the dilution of the toxins formed. Increased prostaglandins and other degradation products from platelets, neutrophils, and monocytes also contribute to the process of inflammation.

Nonspecific acute phase serum such as C-reactive proteins may appear and may stimulate localized phagocytosis, activation of complement, and activation or suppression of lymphocytes.

The physiological and biochemical alterations (e.g., increased CO_2, decreased O_2, increased body temperature, and accumulation of organic acids) that occur at the site of injury may be deleterious to the invading bacteria.

Finally, resolution with tissue repair occurs following macrophage action, with the appearance of fibroblasts and deposition of collagen.

Chronic and Granulomatous Inflammation

Persistence of the deleterious agent following the initial acute inflammatory process can lead to a chronic inflammation. For example, persistence of foreign bodies such as silica or asbestos deposited in the lungs can lead to silicosis and asbestosis. Excessive sodium urate formed endogenously due to a disorder in purine metabolism can induce inflammation of the joints—gout. Crystals of urate may be found in the synovial fluid of joints of patients with gout. Persistence of the irritant can lead to tissue injury. In their effort to phagocytize and remove the irritant the leukocytes release hydrolases from the lysosomes, causing damage to the surrounding healthy tissue, particularly when the leukocytes die. This situation can lead to chronic immunological disorders. Chronic inflammation may eventually resolve, especially if the irritant can be removed or minimized.

Characteristic granulomas with resolution have been discussed in Chapter 3 (see Figure 3-1). Nonimmunological granulomas may also occur, involving nonantigenic foreign body irritants. The hallmark of a granulomatous inflammation is the involvement of the *mononuclear cells* (lymphocytes, monocytes, macrophages, and plasma and epitheloid cells). Granuloma is defined as an inflammation characterized by the presence of lymphocytes, monocytes, and plasma cells, and is a response to reactions identified by the presence of mononuclear phagocytes including epithelioid and giant cells. It is an organized collection of mature mononuclear phagocytes, which may or may not be accompanied by accessory features such as necrosis. Thus there can be *pure* and *complex* granulomas. Chronic inflammation is distinguished from granulomatous inflammation by the organization and activation of mononuclear phagocytes in the latter.

Granulomas develop in three stages: (1) infiltration of young mononuclear phagocytes; (2) maturation and aggregation of these cells into a mature granuloma; and (3) further maturation of these cells into an epithelioid granuloma. Giant cells (multinuclear) in some granulomas are presumably formed either by fusion of macrophages or division without cleavage or demarcation of cell membranes.

Granulomatous inflammation is highly effective in the destruc-

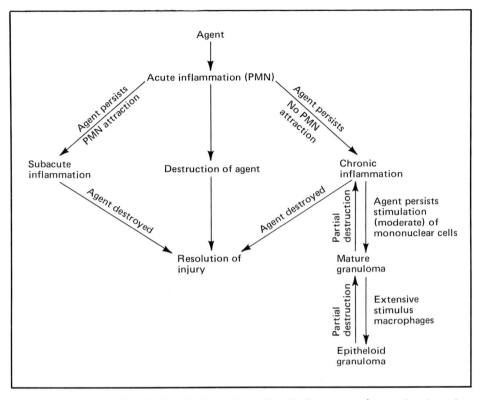

Fig. 8-14 : The interrelationship of inflammations (acute, chronic, and granulomatous) and their resolution.

tion and sequestration of pathogens, which are persistant, resistant, and intracellular parasites. Granulomas may also be involved in inducing immunity and taking part in the destruction of tumors.

The interrelationships of acute, subacute, chronic, and granulomatous inflammations are shown conceptually in Figure 8-14.

Summary

1. This chapter has discussed the cells associated with amplification of the immunological response, both in host defense and in host self-injury.

2. The cells involved in the nonspecific expansion of immunological injury include the following: neutrophils, eosinophils, basophils, monocytes and macrophages, K cells, and platelets of the peripheral blood.

3. Neutrophils are associated with acute inflammation, a short half-life (6.6 hours), a size of 10 to 15 μ, a multilobed nucleus (PMN), and a cytoplasm consisting of neutrophilic granules. The lysosomal granules contain hydrolases, and the peroxisome-like granules contain the myeloperoxidases and

oxidases. The major function of neutrophils appears to be phagocytosis of microorganisms and their destruction through the enzymes.

4. Eosinophils are similar in size to neutrophils and contain granules that bind acidic dyes (eosin). The granules contain a characteristic crystalline structure of various shapes in electron microscopic preparations. The granules consist of peroxidases, lipids, and proteins. These cells appear to be regulated by the adrenal corticosteroids. Eosinophils are characteristically found in patients with allergy and in parasitic infestation associated with allergy.

5. Basophils of the peripheral blood are few in number and are characterized by large cytoplasmic granules that bind to basophilic dyes. The granules contain acidic mucopolysaccharides, histamine, and basic proteins. Enzymes are also present in the granules, as are active pharmacological compounds.

6. Monocytes, considered to be premacrophages, measure 12 to 15 μ in size. The nucleus is generally kidney-shaped, and the cytoplasm shows essentially no granules characteristic of PMN. Monocytes do have lysosomal granules containing the hydrolases for the digestion of various substrates. When activated, monocytes are involved in phagocytosis and in the regulation of the immune response via the various factors they produce (monokines, Chapter 5). Monocytes are involved in the chronic and granulomatous inflammations and contribute to the resolution and repair of injured tissues.

7. Platelets are nonnucleated small colorless bodies (2 to 4 μ). They are involved in blood coagulation and release prostaglandins and vasoactive amines, which potentiate inflammation and changes in the capillaries and smooth muscles.

8. The killer cell is a mononuclear cell found in the null cell population. It has a receptor for the Fc portion of immunoglobulin IgM or IgG. Armed with immunoglobulins, the K cell can specifically attack a target cell to which the immunoglobulin has been stimulated.

9. Phagocytosis is the process of ingestion of agents by phagocytes. It follows the sequence (1) *chemotaxis,* attraction of the phagocyte to the agent or area of injury via the various chemotactic factors, e.g., C3a or C5a of the C system; (2) *ingestion* of the agent, the act of *phagocytosis;* (3) *destruction* of the ingested agent via the enzymes within the phagosome. *Pinocytosis* or *endocytosis* refers to the ingestion of molecules such as proteins by a similar process (ingestion of particulate matter). Antibodies, opsonins, fibrin and membrane surfaces enhance the phagocytosis by phagocytes.

10. Leukocytic deficiencies may be congenital or may be induced by drugs during chemotherapy (*iatrogenic* deficiency). Deficiency in the enzyme myeloperoxidase in neutrophils causes a serious situation in which the individual's PMNs lack the ability to kill ingested bacteria. Chronic granulomatous disease (CGD) is familial and probably x-linked recessive. Leukocytes (PMN) of affected individuals lack the ability to kill nonpathogenic bacteria, which are catalase negative producing strains. Catalase (an enzyme that breaks down H_2O_2) producing bacteria are generally pathogenic and resistant to phagocytic destruction, because these organisms can readily destroy the H_2O_2 produced by PMNs via the HMP. The defect of the leukocytes may be in the biochemical killing pathway demonstrated in PMNs. The disease is characterized by the persistence of the microorganism and the formation of granulomatous lesions.

11. Inflammation can be categorized as acute, chronic, or granulomatous. Acute inflammation is of short duration and involves a multitude of interactions and interrelationships between PMN, the coagulation and fibrinolytic systems, complement, and nonspecific humoral factors, with subsequent resolution when the deleterious agent is destroyed. Persistence of the deleterious agent results in chronic inflammation and subsequent granulomatous inflammation, with the involvement of mononuclear cells including lymphocytes, monocytes, macrophages, and epithelioid cells. Giant cells may be seen in some granulomatous inflammations.

12. The elements involved in the amplification systems discussed in this chapter and in Chapter 9 are necessary for the host defense against many deleterious factors, but they also contribute to the injury to "self," as discussed in Chapter 13.

Bibliography and Selected Reading

General

Cohen, S. The role of cell-mediated immunity in the induction of inflammatory responses. *Am. J. Pathol.* 88:502, 1977.

Douglas, S. D. Cells Involved in Immune Responses. In H. H. Fudenberg, D. P. Stites, J. L. Caldwell, and J. V. Wells (Eds.), *Basic and Clinical Immunology* (2nd ed.). Los Altos, Calif.: Lange, 1978. Pp. 78–95.

Hamashima, Y. (Ed.). *Immunohistopathology.* Philadelphia: Lippincott, 1976.

Movat, H. Z. (Ed.). *Inflammation, Immunity and Hypersensitivity. Cellular and Molecular Mechanism* (2nd ed). Hagerstown, Md.: Harper and Row, 1979.

Cells Associated with Host Response

Clark, R. A. F., Gallin, J. I., and Kaplan, A. P. Mediator release from basophil granulocytes in chronic myelogenous leukemia. *J. Allergy Clin. Immunol.* 58:623, 1976.

Cohn, Z. A. Macrophage physiology. *Fed. Proc.* 34:1725, 1975.

David, J. R. Macrophage activation by lymphocyte mediators. *Fed. Proc.* 34:1730, 1975.

Ehlenberger, A. G., and Mussenzweig, V. The role of membrane receptors for C3b and C3d in phagocytosis. *J. Exp. Med.* 145:357, 1977.

Goetzl, E. J., and Austen, K. F. Cellular characteristics of the eosinophil compatible with a dual role in host defense in parasitic infections. *Am. J. Trop. Med. Hyg.* 26:142. 1977.

Green, D., Chédiak, J. R. Von Willebrand's disease: Current concepts. *Am. J. Med.* 62:315, 1977.

Reddi, K. K. Human platelet RNAse. *Biochem. Biophys. Res. Commun.* 79:532, 1977.

Sher, A. Complement-dependent adherence of mast cells to schistosomula. *Nature* 263:334, 1976.

Snyderman, R., and Pike, M. C. Macrophage migratory dysfunction in cancer: A mechanism for subversion of surveillance. *Am. J. Pathol.* 88:727, 1977.

Stossel, T. P. Phagocytosis: Clinical disorders of recognition and ingestion. *Am. J. Pathol.* 88:741, 1977.

Ward, P. A., Johnson, K. J., and Kreutzer, D. L. Regulatory dysfunction in leukotaxis. *Am. J. Pathol.* 88:701, 1977.

Weiss, H. J. Platelets: Physiology and abnormalities of function (part I). *N. Engl. J. Med.* 293:531, 1975.

Weiss, H. J. Platelets: Physiology and abnormalities of function (part II). *N. Engl. J. Med.* 293:580, 1975.

Inflammation

Adams, D. O. The granulomatous inflammatory response. *Am. J. Pathol.* 84:164, 1977.

Ryan, G. B., and Mayno, G. Acute inflammation. *Am. J. Pathol.* 86:185, 1977.

Wilhelm, D. L. Inflammation and Healing. In W. A. D. Anderson and J. M. Kissane (Eds.), *Pathology,* Vol. 1. St. Louis: 1977. Pp. 25-89.

Willoughby, D. A. Inflammation. *Endeavour* 2:57, 1978.

9 : The Complement System

The amplification and ancillary systems associated with the specific immunological reactions include the complex humoral complement (C) system. Previous chapters (1-7) have encompassed the specific immune systems, antigens, and their interrelationship. This chapter covers the nonspecific humoral entities associated with host defense, in particular, the complement system. The C system functions in conjunction with the immune system and also with nonimmune systems that are activated by tissue injury. The C system amplifies and is ancillary to injury initiated by a variety of deleterious factors, including the specific immune reaction, and is also involved in "self" destruction in autoimmune and hypersensitivity diseases. In addition, the deficiency states of the components of complement may lead to serious consequences to the defense of the organism.

Introduction to the Complement System

Complement is an essential part of the normal host defense mechanism and functions as an effector pathway of the humoral immune and inflammatory process. As we will see, the complement system is involved in the phagocytosis and lysis of invading cells (e.g., virus, bacteria). The complement system has two possible activation pathways: the *classic* and the *alternative pathway.* The terminal reaction phase of the complement system is called the *membrane attack mechanism.*

Several of the complement components are found normally in plasma in an inactive form. The term *activation* is applied when these individually distinct complement components undergo chemical and physical processes to become a functional and integrated unit that has enzymatic or biological activity. The processes of activation may involve a limited proteolytic cleavage. The enzymes responsible for these limited proteolytic reactions are usually other complement molecules that have been activated by similar proteolytic reactions. C1r, C1s, C2, C3, C4, C5, and Factor B are all activated by a limited proteolytic reaction.

Another significant feature of the activation process involved in complement pathways is the formation of large multimolecular protein-protein complexes. Following initial proteolytic cleavage of one or more of the members of complement protein complex, there usually follows a regulated self-assembly mechanism. An example of such a complex is the C5b-9 complex, which has enzymatic activity and can disrupt lipid bilayer membranes.

The classic pathway consists of the reaction steps involving the first component of complement, C1 (C1q, C1r, C1s), as well as C4, C2, and C3. The classic pathway can be triggered *immunologically* by antibodies of the IgG or IgM classes or nonimmunologically by a number of agents, including DNA, various polyanions, C-reactive protein complexed to phospholipids, and certain lipids such as lipid A of gram-negative bacterial lipopolysaccharide.

The alternative or properdin complement activation pathway involves the following proteins: Factor B, Factor D, C3, properdin, C3b inactivator, and β1H. The alternative and classic pathways converge at the C3 step. The alternative pathway can be activated by the surface bacteria viruses, complex polysaccharides, or zymosan-aggregated IgA and transformed cells.

The membrane attack pathway is initiated by the C5 cleaving enzyme, activated by either the classic or the alternative pathway, and includes the reaction steps of C5, C6, C7, C8, and C9. The C5 to 9 complex is involved in the disruption and lysis of the lipid bilayer of membranes.

The activation of the alternative pathway is *not* necessarily dependent upon a specific antigen-antibody interaction and therefore may represent a natural defense system against the invading organisms in the *unimmunized host.*

The complement system is a double-edged sword. On the one hand it protects the host against the invading organism, and it is becoming increasingly apparent that various types of complement deficiency (acquired or hereditary) in man are associated with an enhanced predisposition to infection and certain diseases. On the other hand, in some instances the activation of the complement system by soluble antigen-antibody complexes can initiate a pathological process. The antibody may be directed against either a foreign antigen or a "self" antigen (an autoimmune process). In disorders of this type, known as *immune complex diseases,* the soluble antigen-antibody complexes are deposited on the surface of vascular endothelial cells. These deposits activate the complement system, leading to deleterious effects consisting of acute inflammation and intravascular coagulation (vasculitis).

The components of the complement system, together with control proteins, consist of a group of more than twenty plasma proteins. The activation process is similar to blood-clotting reactions, in that it involves a cascade of limited proteolytic reactions in which a series of activated enzymes are formed from their precursors. The cleavage products participate in a variety of biological reactions. One result of these reactions is to make binding sites available for other complement components, to allow assembly of the C components, leading to lysis, chemotaxis of leukocytes, enhancement of phagocytosis by opsonization, platelet aggregation, and increased vascular permeability.

This section will include discussions relative to the chemical composition of the components of the system, the molecular events of complement action leading to cytolysis, a brief mention of complement deficiencies, and their relationship to other inflammatory amplification systems.

Nomenclature and Terminology

The entire complement system, including the control proteins, consists of more than twenty plasma proteins. These proteins vary in molecular size from 25,000 to greater than 500,000 daltons and are immunochemically distinct proteins. The major components are designated numerically as C1, C2, C3, and C4. Some components are designated by letter names—Factor B or Factor D—or by terms such as properdin or β1H because of historical significance. The names of a few of the proteins are based on their functional role, e.g., C3b inactivator.

The individual polypeptide chains of complement proteins are designated by Greek letters, e.g., C3α and C3β. The low molecular weight fragments of complement components resulting from cleavage or activation by the enzymatically active components in the classic pathway are suffixed by lower case letters, e.g., C2a, C2γ, C4α, etc., *complement conversion,* and the fragments themselves are *conversion products.* A bar over the name or term of a complement component denotes an *active enzyme,* e.g., enzymatically active SAC1 is shown as SAC$\overline{1}$, SA being the surface (S) antigen and antibody (A).

The major components of the classic pathway are numbered C1 to C9. C1 consists of three subunits, designated C1q, C1r, and C1s. The alternative pathway has no universally recognized nomenclature but has a widely accepted terminology (Table 9-6).

Chemical and Physical Properties of the Clasic Pathway— C-proteins

The classic pathway includes a group of eleven distinct but functionally interrelated plasma proteins. These molecules are found in the fresh sera of animals of many species. Complement levels tend to fluctuate during certain diseases. In immunological diseases, complement is consumed, so that serum levels generally decrease. In some inflammatory states complement activity may increase. Differences in complement activity between species, which are attributable to the variation in concentrations of one or the other of the eleven components, have been demonstrated. Complement components of man have been linked to the major histocompatibility complex (see Chapter 12).

Examination of fresh serum has demonstrated that certain components of C are readily destroyed by oxidizing agents and by heat. Heat treatment of fresh serum at $56°C$ irreversibly inactivates C1 and C2 activities, while treatment of fresh serum with zymosan (a complex containing mostly protein and carbohydrate, prepared from yeast cell walls, also called anticomplementary factor) removes the C3 components. Dilute ammonium hydroxide treatment of fresh serum inactivates the C4 component.

With the advent of chromatographic procedures using anionic and cationic cellulose derivatives, gel filtration chromatography, and zonal electrophoresis, rapid advances in the characterization of many of the components have been achieved. The significant known physicochemical characteristics of the eleven components of C that participate in the classic pathway are shown in Table 9-1 and Figure 9-1. Molecular weights range from a low of 80,000 daltons (C1s and C9) to a high of 40,000 daltons (C1q). Concentrations of C components in fresh serum range from a low of 2.5 mg/dl (C2) to a high of 138 mg/dl (C3). In immunological assays by radial immunodiffusion, quantification of C3 and C4 levels in serum have been used for recognition of complement action in immunological diseases. Complement fixed to an antigen-antibody complex in tissue has been detected with fluorescence-labeled anti-C3 in immunofluorescence analysis using fluorescence microscopy. Complement component levels have been estimated by measuring the concentrations of C1, C2, C3, C4, and C5 in serum by radial immunodiffusion. The majority of the C components migrate in the β-globulin region in zonal electrophoresis, although C1q, C8, and C9 migrate in the γ, $\gamma1$, and α regions, respectively.

C1q is an interesting molecule containing large amounts of carbohydrate, hydroxyproline, hydroxylysine, and glycine. It appears to be chemically related to the collagenic proteins. C1q consists of three different peptide chains, as deduced from chemical reduction and alkylation. Each of the three peptides exhibits a collagen-like region, situated near the N-terminus, which is characterized by repeating X-Y-glycine triplets, often with hydroxyproline (X) and hydroxylysine (Y). This portion constitutes about 40 percent of the chain. The unique structure of C1q consists of six globular segments connected to six strands, which are attached to a single fibril-like central piece (see C1q in Figure 9-3), as shown by analysis of the purified C1q with the

Table 9-1 : Physicochemical Properties of the Major Components of Complement

| Properties | C1 | | | C4 | C2 | C3 | C5 | C6 | C7 | C8 | C9 |
	C1q	C1s	C1r								
Molecular weight (daltons)	400,000	90,000	170,000	206,000	120,000	180,000	180,000	90,000	110,000	163,000	80,000
Sedimentation coefficient ($S_{20,w}$)	11.1	4.0	7.0	10.0	5.5	9.5	8.7	5–6	5–6	8.0	4.5
Serum concentration (mg/dl)	19.0	11.0	20.0	60.0	2.5	138.0	8.0	7.5	5.5	5–10	5–10
Relative electrophoretic mobility	γ_2	α_1	β_1	β_1	β_1–α_2	β_2–β_1	β_1	β_2	β_2	γ_1	α_2
Carbohydrate content (%)	15.0	—	—	14.0	—	2.7	19.0	—	—	—	—
Functional sulfhydryl content (number of SH groups)	—	—	—	—	2	1.2	+	—	—	—	—

+ = present; — = unknown.

Fig. 9-1 : Two-dimensional diagram of the electrophoretic mobility patterns of the classic pathway components of complement.

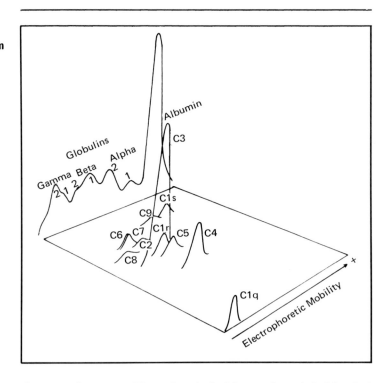

electron microscope. Thus, the whole C1q consists of six identical subunits, and each subunit is composed of three different polypeptide chains. The C-terminus regions of the three peptide chains constitute the globular region, whereas the collagen-like segment of the three chains forms a triple helix and constitutes the strands and the single central piece. The globular region of C1q constitutes the binding site for the antibody Fc portion in an Ag-Ab complex, and the central piece interacts with C1r and C1s subunits (Figure 9-3).

Biological Activation of Complement

CLASSIC PATHWAY. The classic pathway consists of eleven C components that interact sequentially in a cascade of limited proteolytic reactions leading to the conversion of precursors to activated enzymes. The classic C system is usually activated by the interaction of an antibody with its specific antigen (present either on a cell surface as an erythrocyte, parasitic cell, malignant cell, etc., or in an aqueous system as a soluble antigen). Table 9-2 lists some of the known activators of the C classic pathway. Note that the classic pathway can be triggered by a nonimmunological mechanism with agents such as DNA, other polyanions, C-reactive protein complexed to phospholipids, lipid A of lipopolysaccharides, and certain proteolytic enzymes such as plasmin and trypsin.

Table 9-2 : Activators of the Classic Complement Pathway

Activators

Antigen-antibody complexes
  IgG1, IgG3, and IgM
    Bind strongly
  IgG2
    Bind weakly
Aggregated immunoglobulins
Complexes
  Staphylococcal protein A–IgG
  Bovine conglutinin-conglutinogen
  C-reactive protein-phospholipids (residues containing phosphorylcholine,
    including C-polysaccharide of *Pneumococcus*)
Certain bacterial endotoxins (lipid A of lipopolysaccharides)
Polyinosinic acid–DNA
Plasmin and trypsin

The sequence of the classic pathway of complement by antibody activation is best illustrated by the lysis of sheep erythrocytes (SRBC-antigen) by their specific antibody (hemolysin), produced in rabbits by administration of SRBC. The general scheme of the complement reactions is shown in Figures 9-2 and 9-3. The classic pathway has been divided into three functional units: (1) the *recognition unit* (the interaction of the C1 complex with the antibody), (2) the *activation unit* (involves C4, C2, and C3), and (3) the *membrane attack unit* (consists of C5b, C6, C7, C8, and C9 and is involved in cytolysis).

The Recognition Unit. The recognition unit, the C1 component (a trimolecular complex), consists of three subunits, the C1q, C1r, and C1s, which are held together by calcium ions. The specific sites are located on the C1q for combining with specific receptors, C_H2 for IgG and C_H4 for IgM, on the Fc portion of the antibody molecules (IgG1, IgG2, IgG3 and IgM), which have aggregated on the surface of the antigen-containing cells. Specific antibodies, when complexed to antigen residing on the cell surface, fix and activate C1q (it undergoes conformational change). The change in C1q unmasks an enzymatic activity in C1r, which in turn cleaves a peptide from C1s, exposing its active site and thereby creating the first major enzyme of the system (known as C1 esterase). The activated complex is shown as $\overline{C1}$. The initial activation of C1q requires at least two binding sites, which are provided by two Fc portions of the antibody molecules. Thus, two IgG molecules or one IgM molecule are essential for activation. Note that IgM, a pentamer, can provide up to five Fc binding sites.

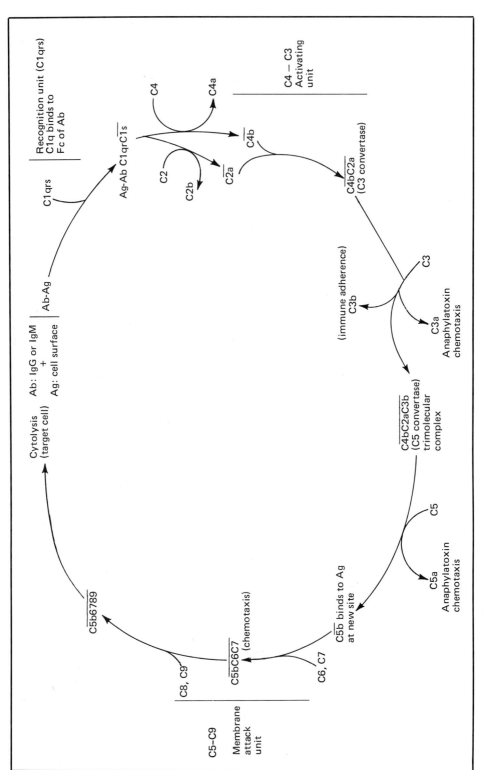

Fig. 9-2 : The classic pathway of complement action.

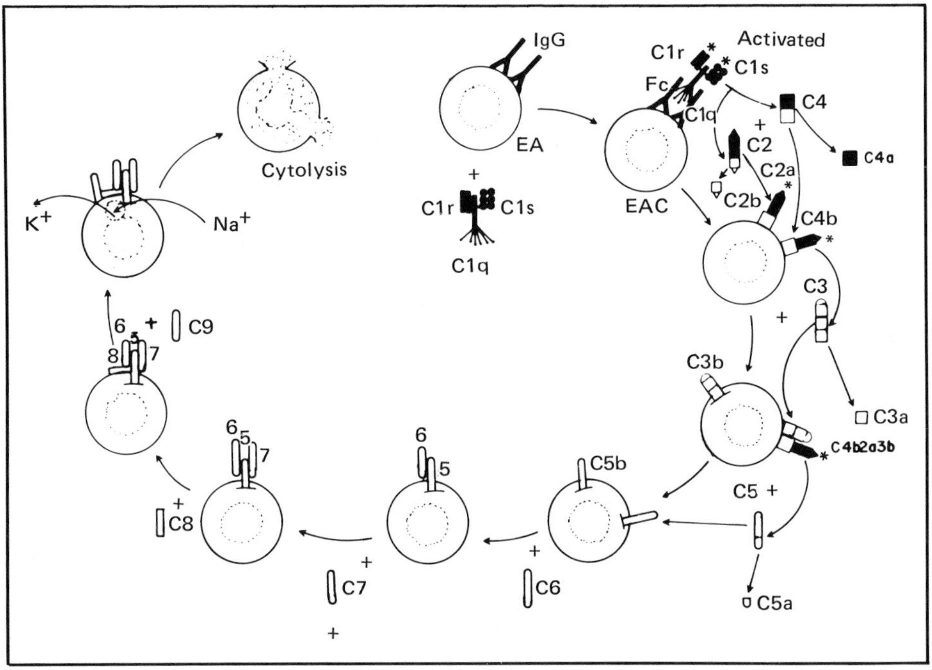

Fig. 9-3 : The classic complement pathway of activation. Asterisk-active enzyme. The recognition unit, a trimolecular complex of C1q, C1r, and C1s, fits to the Fc receptors of two IgG molecules (EAC). The IgG molecules are attached to the red blood cell surface (EA). The attachment of the C1 trimolecular complex initiates C pathway activation. The change in configuration of C1q following attachment activates C1r, which enzymatically acts on C1s. C1s is subsequently activated to the well-known esterase. The C activation unit is assembled following cleavage of C4 and C2 in that order. C4b and C2a form the active enzyme C3 convertase, following attachment via C4b to another site on the antigen's surface. The bimolecular enzymatic complex subsequently cleaves C3 to give C3b and C3a. The latter is anaphylatoxin. C3b forms a trimolecular complex with C4bC2aC3b and acts as C5 convertase. In addition, C3b binds to other sites on the surface of the antigen and acts in the immune adherence phenomenon (adherence of platelets, monocytes, macrophages, and PMNs). The trimolecular complex C4bC2aC3b cleaves C5 and forms C5b and C5a. The latter, like C3a, is an anaphylatoxin. C5b attaches to another site on the antigen's surface and initiates the membrane attack complex. Fusion of C6 and C7 to sites on C5b occurs following attachment of C5b on antigen surface, and another trimolecular complex is formed (C567). C8 and C9 then join the trimolecular complex. C8 is believed to act on the membrane to open a channel to the interior of the cell. Sufficient changes in permeability result to allow water and Na^+ to enter and $K+$ to leave the cell. The cell expands and disruption results. Macromolecules escape, and cell lysis is complete.

In humans, C1 function is controlled by a serum protease inhibitor, C1 inactivator ($\overline{C1}$INA).

The Activation Unit. Activation is initiated by $\overline{C1}$, which cleaves C4 and then C2 (the adsorption of C2 is promoted by Mg^{++}) into their major cleavage products, C4b and C2a. $\overline{C1}$ amplifies the cleavage process and produces a shower of these fragments. Subsequent reactions occur only with those fragments bound to the cell membrane, however. The C4b and C2a form a bimolecular complex ($\overline{C4b2a}$) on the cell membrane, which exhibits an enzymatic activity toward C3. $\overline{C4b2a}$, also known as C3 convertase, splits the C3 into C3a (smaller fragment) and C3b (larger fragment). The attachment of C3b to $\overline{C4b2a}$ leads to a trimolecular complex ($\overline{C4b2a3b}$), which has enzymatic activity toward C5. The C3a released into the fluid (aqueous) phase is an anaphylatoxin and functions in the inflammatory processes. Solid phase refers to the cell surface. The C3b fragment, in addition to its role in the enzyme complex $\overline{C4b2a3b}$, promotes phagocytosis by PMN leukocytes, monocytes, and macrophages by binding to several sites on the cell membrane.

The Membrane Attack System. The $\overline{C4b2a3b}$ trimolecular complex (also known as C5 convertase) catalyzes the cleavage of C5 into C5a and C5b. C5a is an anaphylatoxin and participates in the inflammatory process like C3a. The C5b attaches to a new site on the cell membrane alongside the C4b2a3b complex which decays rapidly. Following the binding of C5b, the remainder of the terminal components of the sequence are self-assembled on the membrane. Initially a trimolecular complex (C5b67) is formed, then C8 and C9 are attached to the complex. These processes are nonenzymatic. The actual cytolysis of the target cell is initiated by C8 and C9, but the exact mechanism is not understood. Electron microscopic observations have revealed "hole-like" (doughnut) lesions on the membrane surface of the target cell. It has been suggested that the terminal complement components C8 and C9 enter the bimolecular cell membrane and, through physical and chemical interaction with the membrane proteins, phospholipids, and fatty acids, create hole-like channels that permit electrolytes to enter and leave the cell. Through these channels K^+ leaves the cell, and water and Na^+ enter the cell, eventually resulting in osmotic lysis.

As already noted, the complement system not only mediates cytolysis but also participates in the inflammatory process. The biological activities of various complement components are indicated in Figure 9–2 and Table 9–3. The cells possessing receptors for complement components are shown in Table 9–4.

Presently the nature of the receptors in the sequence of complement activation of each component, e.g., the residue on C4 that

Table 9-3 : Biological Action of the Complement Components and Activated Products

Complement Component	Biological Activity
C2 and C4	Virus neutralization
C2b	Increases vascular permeability (kinin-like)
C3a and C3b	Enhances phagocytosis of PMN leukocytes, with lysosomal release, immune adherence
C3a, C5a, and C5b67	Increases chemotaxis; C3a exhibits kinin-like activity
C3 fragment	Mobilization of leukocytes from bone marrow
C3a and C5a	Anaphylatoxins release histamine from mast cells; C5a causes lysosomal enzyme release
C1–7	Facilitate lymphocytotoxicity
C1–9	Cytotoxic to specific sensitized target cell or adjacent cells; activate tissue lysosomal enzymes

Table 9-4 : Cells Possessing Receptors for Complement Fragments

Cells with Receptors	Complement Component
B lymphocytes	C3b, C4b
Neutrophils	C3b
Monocytes	C3b, C3d, C4b
Macrophages	C3b, C4b
Erythrocytes (primates)	C3b, C4b
Platelets	C3b, C4b

is the site of attack by $\overline{C1}$, is unknown. Recent studies have shown that the sugar residues of glucose, mannose, lactose, or galactose may play a significant role in the functional activity of human and guinea pig C1, C4, and C2. This was determined by the use of lectins such as castor bean type II, wheat germ agglutinin, soy bean, phytohemagglutinin, and leukoagglutinin. These compounds react with specific sugar residues and thus inhibit complement activity in the classic pathway in the hemolytic assay. Castor bean type II proved to be effective in the inhibition of C1, C4, and C2. Wheat germ agglutinin, soy bean and PHA inhibited human and guinea pig C1.

ALTERNATIVE PATHWAY OF C ACTIVATION. As noted earlier, the alternative pathway can be activated by bacterial polysaccharides, endotoxin, aggregated IgA, cobra venom, and other factors (see Table 9-5). This pathway is considered a phylogenetically older system in C activation. Some of the reported

Table 9-5 : Activators of the Alternative Complement Pathway

Substances	Specifically Identified Components
1. Immunoglobulins (aggregated)	IgG1, IgG2, IgG3, IgG4, IgA1, IgA2, IgD
2. Polysaccharides	Endotoxin, lipopolysaccharides of gram-negative organisms, zymosan, inulin, and agar
3. Others	Cobra venom factor (CVF), trypsin, plasmin, B lymphocytes and carcinoma cells, Epstein-Barr virus, infected B cells, (all react via C3P)

properties of the alternative pathway C components are presented in Table 9-6; a schematic representation of the pathway is given in Figure 9-4.

The activation of the alternative pathway consists of *initiation* and *amplification.* Initiation is nonspecific and does not require an immunoglobulin or an antibody-like recognition factor. Initiation invokes two steps: (1) random binding of C3b through its labile binding site (S1) to an activator; and (2) discriminatory interaction of the bound C3b with surrounding surface structures. The random event is triggered by C3 convertase, which is a fluid-phase enzyme. This native C3 and factor B form a reversible complex, which, when activated by factor D, becomes the initial C3-cleaving enzyme $\overline{C3bBb}$ (C3 convertase). The amount of C3b deposition is minimal, since the amount of the enzyme produced at a given time is low and the efficiency of binding characteristic of C3b deposition during the fluid phase is low. The discriminatory phase occurs after the binding of C3b* (Figure 9-4). In the normal control situation C3b* binds to a nonactivator and is able to combine with β1H (cofactor for C3bINA) and become inactivated via the effects of C3bINA (C3 inactivator) and β1H. Inactivation of C3b* will also occur in the fluid phase if no binding takes place with either a nonactivator or an activator.

When C3b* binds to the surface of activators, the C3b is protected from degradation by the control proteins β1H and C3bINA. In the discriminatory phase of activation, the protected C3b on the surface of the activator interacts with factors B and D and forms a proteolytic enzyme, $\overline{C3bB}$, which has C3 convertase activity analogous to $\overline{C42}$ of the classic pathway.

Thus when C3b* binds to an activator, the control of C3b* by β1H and C3INA is restricted, since the binding to β1H is decreased. In the discriminatory phase of initiation, C3 convertase is formed on the activator, and amplification via the solid phase

Table 9-6 : Terminology Used for Components of the Alternative Pathway and Their Physical and Chemical Characteristics

Name	Synonym	MW	Electro-phoretic Mobility	Concentration mg/liter	Fragments
C3	—	180,000	β_2	1600	C3a, b, c, d
Factor B	C3 proactivator C3PA, GBG	80,000	β	225	Ba, Bb
Factor Bb	C3 activator	60,000	γ	—	—
Factor Ba		20,000	β	—	Ba
Factor D	C3 proactivator convertase C3 pase	24,000	α	2	ND*
β1H	Cofactor C3bINA	150,000	α	13	ND*
C3b inactivator C3bINA	—	88,000	β	3.5	β1 38,000 α1 50,000 } reduction
Native properdin (NP)	—	230,000	β—agar α_2—agarose	25	ND* —

*ND = not determined.

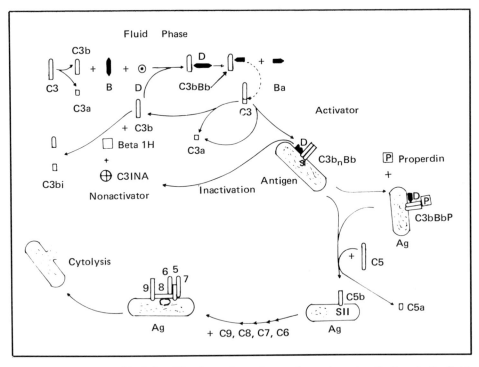

Fig. 9-4 : The alternative pathway of complement activation. In the fluid phase C3 is cleaved and C3b attaches to the surface of either an activator or a nonactivator. Factor Be (C3PA) will associate with C3b following cleavage by factor D (C3PA convertase); and if C3b is bound to a nonactivator surface, β1H cleaves Bb, rendering the C3b$\overline{\text{Bb}}$ (C3 convertase) inactive and rendering C3b vulnerable to cleavage by C3b inactivator (C3bINA) to give nonactive C3bi. Ba from cleavage of B has shown chemotaxis for PMN, while Bb activates macrophages and spreading of monocytes. Attachment of C3b to an activator via site 1 (S1) results in the generation of more C3 convertase (C3b$_n$Bb) following addition of properdin (P), which stabilizes the complex. Both C3b$_n$b and C3b$_n$BbP act on C5; and the subsequent C lytic function leading to cytolysis of an antigen (bacteria) is similar to that of the classic pathway involving C6, C7, C8, and C9. The initiation and amplification require five proteins, C3, Factors B and D, β1H, and C3INA. Properdin is not required for initiation or amplification, but contributes to the stabilization of the C3 and C5 convertase functions of C3bBb$_n$.

C3 convertase begins. The ability of bound C3b to distinguish between a nonactivator and an activator is an important function of C3b and confers a discriminatory ability on the alternative C pathway. Amplification of the alternative pathway mechanism occurs when the C3 convertase C3b$\overline{\text{Bb}}$ cleaves and activates more native C3 molecules, leading to the formation of a C5 convertase (S1-C3b$_n$Bbn). The formation of C5 convertase initiates the membrane attack unit of the C pathway (S1$_n$–C5b-9), as illustrated in Figure 9-4. Properdin (NP), which is essentially not necessary in this pathway, nevertheless can contribute by its complexing with S1-$\overline{C3b_n Bb_n}$ to give S1-C3b$_n$ Bb$_n$ P. Properdin appears to enhance the enzymatic activity by decreasing the spontaneous rate of decay of the polymolecular complex S1-C3b$_n$ Bb$_n$. The control reaction of S1-$\overline{C3bBb_n}$ and S1-C3b$_n$ Bb$_n$ P is restricted via β1H and C3bINA to give S1-C3bi and S1-C3biP products, respectively. S1-C3bi is further degraded by protease to C3c and S1-C3d, while S1-C3biP is converted further to inactive P + S1C3d.

Biological Activities Associated with C Pathways

Complement participates in a number of ways in the biological system that is associated with inflammation and tissue injury. The most widely known effector mechanism is the lytic effect on cell membrane and consequent increase in cellular permeability. This is accomplished via the classic or alternative pathways by the C5 to C9 complex. Of greater importance are the other biological activities that depend on interaction with the cellular complement *conversion product* receptors that are present on a wide variety of cells (Table 9-4). The specialized cellular functions that are evoked by the complement fragments depend on the innate physiological properties of the cell. The same complement fragment causes widely differing responses in cells with differing functional properties, e.g., C3b binding to C3b receptors on B cells elicits different physiological responses from C3b binding to platelets. The effects on the various target cells by the complement fragments are numerous and varied.

C2 and C4. The C2 and C4 components of complement have been associated with virus neutralization. *C2b* is a kinin-like substance that directly causes an increase in vascular permeability and is released during the action of $\overline{C1s}$ on C2.

C3a and C5a. C3a and C5a are anaphylatoxins and elicit release of histamine from leukocytes, mast cells, and platelets, initiating smooth muscle contraction and increasing the permeability of capillaries. Thus they enable further complement and antibody, polymorphonuclear leukocytes, lymphocytes, and other cellular elements (platelets) to enter tissues in which an immune reaction is occurring.

The infiltration of platelets indicates aggregation of these cellular elements and intravascular coagulation. C3a and C5a are inactivated by serum carboxypeptidase B (anaphylatoxin inactivator). The enzyme counterbalances the excessive action of these complement polypeptides.

C3a, C5a, and C5b67. These complement fragments are associated with *chemotactic activation* of certain leukocytes, especially the polymorphonuclear leukocytes of the peripheral blood, causing cells to accumulate at the injured site. Thus C3a and C5a, in addition to being anaphylatoxins, also possess chemotactic properties. Recently C5a has been found to be the major component of complement that is chemotactic for polymorphonuclear leukocytes.

C3b, C3d, and C4b. These complement fragments have been associated with *immune adherence.* Membrane receptors for C3b, C3d, and C4b have been demonstrated on certain leukocytes, macrophages, platelets, and lymphocytes of B cell lineage (Table 9-4). These receptors cause such cells to adhere to other cells or particles bearing these C fragments on their surfaces. This phenomenon, known as *immune adherence,* is particularly important in facilitating phagocytosis by cells having C3b receptors. These receptors on B cells may be important also in localizing antigen-antibody complexes in the germinal centers of lymph nodes. Thus, these C fragments with the phagocytic cells appear to act as *opsonins.*

C3 Fragments. A C3 fragment appears to be responsible for mobilizing leukocytes from the bone marrow.

Regulation of the Complement System

The complement system is regulated by (1) the presence of specific inhibitors (or inactivators) of the enzymes that participate in the complement system and (2) the instability of some complexes that are produced in the sequential reactions.

$\overline{C1}$-inhibitor ($\overline{C1}$INH) (105,000 daltons) is an α_2-globulin and inhibits the enzymatic activities of $\overline{C1}$ activity by combining with the enzyme in stoichiometric proportions. A congenital deficiency of $\overline{C1}$INH, known as *hereditary angioedema,* gives rise to recurrent episodes of subepithelial edema of the skin and the upper respiratory and gastrointestinal tracts. It is inherited as an autosomal dominant trait.

The inactivation of C3b (the active fragment of C3 that attaches to C4b2, giving $\overline{C4b2a3b}$) is accomplished by an enzyme (also known as C3 inactivator) that catalyzes the cleavage of C3b into two fragments, C3c and C3d.

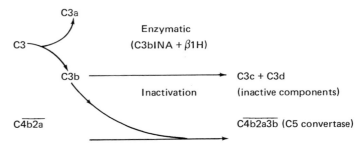

A deficiency of C3 enzyme inactivator has been observed in some subjects. The clinical manifestations in this disorder are due to the accumulation of C3b, which causes *activation of the alternative pathway* (discussed earlier) with severe depletion of factors B and C3, which may be responsible for the recurrent pyogenic infections seen in affected patients. Increased production of C3a may also be responsible for the observed allergic reactions. Infusion of purified C3 inactivator (or fresh plasma) can ameliorate the symptoms by inhibiting C3 hypercatabolism.

Inactivation of C3a and C5a (anaphylatoxins) is done by cleavage of the carboxyl-terminal arginine from these molecules by carboxypeptidases (300,000 daltons, α-globulin). Formation of unstable complexes, which undergo spontaneous decay, also provides a control mechanism by preventing the accumulation of intermediates. A protein substance (β_1-globulin) has been isolated that inactivates C6.

Site of Synthesis of C Proteins

Advances in the purification and isolation of each individual complement component of the classic pathway C1 to C9 have contributed to the delineation of the sites of synthesis of these proteins. Recent developments in cell and organ cultures have added to our knowledge of complement biosynthesis in tissues.

Table 9-7 summarizes the organ and cell types that have been implicated in the biosynthesis of the various components of complement of man. Sites of synthesis of all the complement components in humans have been established with the exception of some of the membrane attack components C6, C7, C8, and C9. Sites of synthesis for complement components C6, C8, and C9 have been demonstrated in the rabbit, pig, and rat, respectively. C6 and C9 have been synthesized in the liver of these animals, while C8 has shown wide tissue distribution.

Complement Deficiency and its Role in Diseases

Inherited abnormalities of the complement system of man have been described for nine of the eleven classic components and two inhibitors. Table 9-8 summarizes the information available regarding hereditary complement deficiencies. There are also *acquired* abnormalities that lead to alterations in the serum complement levels. Elevated levels may be observed in many acute inflammatory states or infections. These disorders may be found in association with diabetes, amyloidosis, thyroiditis, pregnancy, ulcerative colitis, polyarteritis, rheumatoid arthritis, rheumatic fever, spondylitis, hepatic disease, surgery, myocardial infarction, cancer, sarcoidosis, etc. Low levels are seen in immune complex disorders such as systemic lupus erythematosus, rheumatoid arthritis, acute post-streptococcal nephritis, serum sickness, and cryoglobulinemia.

Table 9-7 : Sites of Synthesis of Human Complement Proteins

Component	Tissue	Cell
C1	Intestine, genito-urinary tract (GU) (not kidney)	Epithelial (columnar and transitional), fibroblast, macrophage
C1q	"	"
C1r	"	"
C1s	"	Epithelial (columnar and transitional)
C2	Wide distribution	Macrophage/monocyte
C3	Liver	Parenchymal
C4	Wide distribution	Macrophage/monocyte
C5	Wide distribution	Macrophage/monocyte
C6, C7, C8, C9	?	?
C1 inhibitor	Liver	Parenchymal

Table 9-8 : Hereditary Complement and C-Inhibitor Deficiencies and Associated Clinical Findings

Component	Associated Disorders and Diseases
Deficiency in	
C1q	Systemic lupus erythematosus (SLE), other immunodeficiency; classic agammaglobulinemia (X-linked)— increased metabolism of C1q
C1r	Rheumatoid disease, renal disease, SLE, recurrent infections
C1s	SLE
C2	Nephritis, susceptibility to infection, arthralgia, SLE, discoid LE, chronic vasculitis, and polymyositis
C3	Recurrent infections
C4	SLE
C5	SLE, Leiner's disease, repeated infections, defect in opsonization
C6	Infections
C7	Raynaud's phenomenon, rheumatoid arthritis
C8	Gonorrhea, SLE
CI inactivator (also known as C1 esterase inhibitor)	Hereditary angioedema, SLE
C3b inactivator	Recurrent infections

Assessment of Concentration and Complement Activity

All of the classic pathway components can be measured both immunochemically and functionally. The conversion products of C3 and C4, the major C components in serum, can be detected and quantified. Factor B (C3 proactivator) of the alternative pathway and its activated form can be quantified by radial immunodiffusion and the activation assessed by immunoelectrophoresis. C3PA, factor B, when activated in sera, will give two immunoelectrophoretic components: (1) a β-mobility protein (Ba) of 20,000 daltons and (2) a γ-mobility protein (Bb) of 60,000 daltons (See Table 9-6). In the detection of complement activation or consumption, the most sensitive changes occur in C1, C4, and C3 for classic pathway activation and in factor B (C3PA) and C3 for alternative pathway activation. Since the concentrations in serum of later-acting C components (C5, C6, C7, C8, C9) are generally lower, their measurements are variable. Activation of the alternative pathway is evidenced by a decrease in C3 and appearance of conversion products (Bb, Ba) of factor B in the presence of normal levels of C124 and absence of C4 conversion products.

The classic measurement of complement function is via the hemolytic assay complement fixation test (Figure 9-5). The test system uses sheep erythrocytes (SRBC), rabbit anti-SRBC (hemolysin), and fresh serum as a complement source (guinea pig, human, etc.). The lytic value is indicated as CH_{50} units of C activity (This is the 50 percent lysis unit of complement). This procedure, however, does not assess the function or concentration of each individual component. The concentration of the individual components in serum is generally assessed by immunochemical means, which include quantitative radial immunodiffusion, crossed immunoelectrophoresis, and immunofluorescence for identification in tissues (see Chapter 7).

The assessment of complement levels in disease, particularly autoimmune disease, plays a significant role in diagnosis and has been effectively utilized.

Interrelationship of C and Other Biological Functions and Systems

The Blood Clotting Process

The clotting process consists of the sequential conversion of inactive enzymes into active form. Table 9-9 summarizes some of the properties of the blood clotting factors. There are two coagulation pathways: intrinsic and extrinsic. The intrinsic pathway derives all its factors from plasma, whereas the extrinsic system depends on factors derived from plasma as well as tissue extracts.

The coagulation factors are all proteins with the exception of Ca^{++} (also labeled as a factor), which is *required* in a number

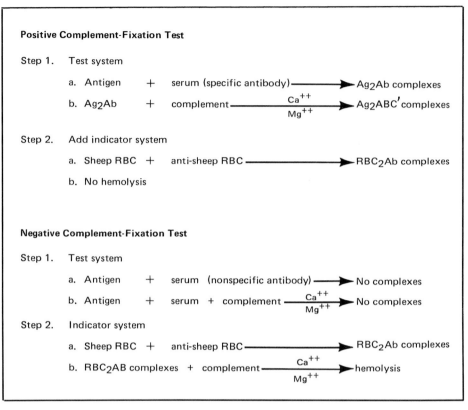

Positive Complement-Fixation Test

Step 1.   Test system

    a. Antigen   +   serum (specific antibody) ⟶ Ag_2Ab complexes

    b. Ag_2Ab +   complement $\xrightarrow[Mg^{++}]{Ca^{++}}$ Ag_2ABC' complexes

Step 2.   Add indicator system

    a. Sheep RBC + anti-sheep RBC ⟶ RBC_2Ab complexes

    b. No hemolysis

Negative Complement-Fixation Test

Step 1.   Test system

    a. Antigen   +   serum (nonspecific antibody) ⟶ No complexes

    b. Antigen   +   serum + complement $\xrightarrow[Mg^{++}]{Ca^{++}}$ No complexes

Step 2.   Indicator system

    a. Sheep RBC + anti-sheep RBC ⟶ RBC_2Ab complexes

    b. RBC_2AB complexes + complement $\xrightarrow[Mg^{++}]{Ca^{++}}$ hemolysis

Fig. 9-5 : Analysis of complement activation using the sheep RBC and rabbit anti-sheep RBC (hemolysin) system (the <u>complement-fixation</u> test [CFT]). Ag_2 Ab = Antigen$_2$ antibody$_1$, Ag_2AbC = Antigen$_2$ antibody$_1$ Complement, and RBC_2Ab = Red blood cell$_2$ antibody$_1$.

of reactions. The various steps involved in both intrinsic and extrinsic pathways are shown in Figure 9-6. The intrinsic system begins with the activation of Factor XII. This activation is assumed to occur due to the interaction of Factor XII with collagen (exposed when the endothelium is injured). Activated factor XII (XIIa) also mediates the conversion of prekallikrein to kallikrein and the eventual formation of kinins (discussed later). The eventual formation of a clot results from the conversion of soluble fibrinogen by the action of thrombin (a serine protease) into insoluble gel fibrin. The fibrin peptides undergo polymerization by forming a linkage between glutamine side chains in one fibrin monomer and a lysine side chain of another fibrin molecule. This reaction is catalyzed by factor XIIIa.

There are a number of inherited deficiencies of clotting factors that lead to excessive or uncontrolled bleeding. Some examples of these are hemophilia A (deficiency of factor VIII), hemophilia

Table 9-9 : Nomenclature and Some Physicochemical Properties of the Blood Coagulation Factors and Members of the Kinin System

International Classification (Number)	Synonyms	Molecular Weight		Electrophoretic Mobility
		Bovine	Human	
Factor I	Fibrinogen	340,000	341,000	β_1
Factor II	Prothrombin	68,500	69,000	α_2
Factor IIa	Thrombin	33,700	35,000	β
Factor III	Tissue thromboplastin	1.7×10^7	—	—
Factor IV	Calcium	—	—	—
Factor V	Ac-globulin, labile factor, proaccelerin prothrombin accelerator	290,000	70,000–350,000	β_2, β
Factor VII	Stable factor, autoprothrombin I	35,000–63,000	50,000–100,000	β, α
Factor VIII	Antihemophilic globulin	180,000	300,000–400,000	β_2, β
Factor IX	Christmas factor, autoprothrombin II, plasma thromboplastin component	49,900	100,000–200,000	β
Factor X	Stuart-Prower factor	86,000	—	α
Factor XI	Plasma thromboplastin antecedent	—	100,000–200,000	$\beta\text{-}\alpha$
Factor XII	Hageman factor	—	60,000–100,000	γ_1
Factor XII (activated)	—	—	100,000	—
Factor XII (fragments; subunits)	Prekallikrein activators (PKA)	—	30,000–70,000	Prealbumin
Factor XIII	Fibrin-stabilizing factor	—	350,000	Globulin
Prekallikrein	Fletcher factor	—	127,000	γ_2
Kallikrein	—	—	108,000	γ_2
Plasminogen	Profibrinolysin	—	81,000	β
Plasmin	Fibrinolysin	—	75,400	β
Kininogen	α_2-globulin	—	50,000–200,000	β
Bradykinin	Kallidin I	—	1,060	Pretransferrin
Kininases	Peptidases	—	—	—

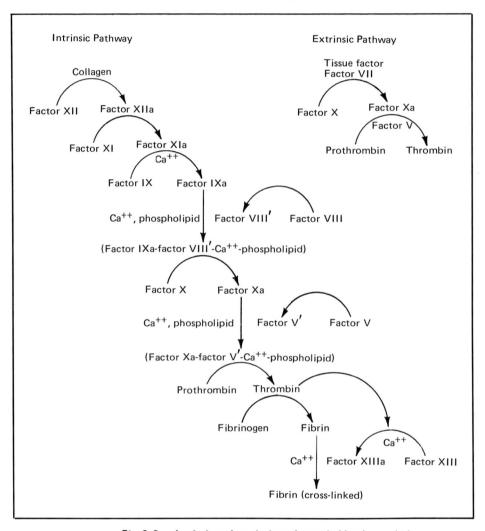

Fig. 9-6 : Intrinsic and extrinsic pathways in blood coagulation.

B (deficiency of factor IX), hemophilia C (deficiency of factor XI), congenital parahemophilia (deficiency of factor V), afibrinogenemia, and dysfibrinogenemia.

The Fibrinolytic System

Lysis of a fibrin clot, part of the tissue repair process, is mediated by the plasminogen-plasmin system. Plasmin, a proteolytic enzyme, degrades fibrin (and fibrinogen) to polypeptides, the fibrinogen degradation products (FDP) of varying molecular weights. The reactions that lead to the generation of plasmin are as follows:

Proactivator $\xrightarrow{\text{Kinases}}$

Plasminogen $\xrightarrow{\text{Activator}}$ Plasmin

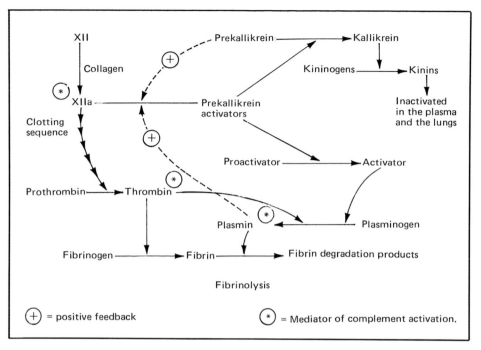

Fig. 9-7 : The kinin-generating system and its interrelationship with blood coagulation, fibrinolysis, and the complement system.

The plasminogen conversion to plasmin can be catalyzed by thrombin, by enzymes found in certain bacteria (e.g., streptokinase and staphylokinase), or by urokinase. The proactivator is converted to an activator by proteolytic fragments of factor XIIa, known as prekallikrein activator (PKA). PKA itself is generated from XIIa by the action of plasmin (an example of positive feedback). These interrelationships are shown in Figure 9-7.

The Kinin System The kinins are a group of highly active peptides and are derived from plasma precursors known as *kininogens.* Kinins are implicated in most of the signs seen in acute inflammation. These include generalized dilatation of the peripheral arterioles, increased capillary permeability, the production of pain, and the migration of leukocytes to the injured area. These highly potent biological substances are rapidly inactivated in plasma and in the lungs. There are two enzymes (kininases) that catalyze the inactivation of kinins. Kininase I is a carboxypeptidase, and kininase II is a dipeptidyl carboxypeptidase. It is of interest that kininase II also catalyzes the conversion of angiotensin I to angiotensin II by the removal of terminal histidylleucine moiety. Angiotensin II is a powerful vasoconstrictor; thus kininase II, while inactivating powerful vasodilators (the kinins), is also able to generate a potent vasoconstrictor.

The major kinins are bradykinin (a nonapeptide; H-Arg-Pro-Pro-Gly-Phe-Ser-Pro-Phe-Arg-OH), lysylbradykinin (known as kallidin), and methionyllysylbradykinin.

The kinin-forming system and its relationship to blood coagulation, complement, and fibrinolytic processes is shown in Figure 9-7. Note the central role played by factor XIIa and the positive feedback of plasmin and kallikrein in the conversion of XIIa to prekallikrein activators (PKA). The PKAs are proteases that convert prekallikrein to kallikrein and proactivator to activator.

Kallikrein, the proteolytic enzyme responsible for the conversion of kininogen to kinin, is inhibited by two serum factors: $\overline{C1}$ inhibitor (C1INA) and α_2-macroglobulin. In hereditary angioneurotic edema the $\overline{C1}$ inhibitor is deficient. A subject with this disorder exhibits problems due to uncontrolled complement activation as well as excessive production of kinins. Other severe disorders due to excessive generation of kinins are gram-negative septicemia, carcinoid syndrome, coronary artery disease, inflammatory joint disease, certain transfusion reactions, and dumping syndrome.

Summary

1. Complement comprises an important and complex group of proteins involved in the amplification of host nonspecific and specific immune responses to deleterious agents.
2. Eleven major proteins are involved in the classic pathway. These include, in order of activation, C1qrs (C1), C4, C2, C3, C5, C6, C7, C8 and C9. Their physiochemical properties are presented in Table 9-1.
3. C1 consists of three components, C1q, C1s, and C1r. C1q is the recognition unit that attaches to the Fc portion of the Ag-Ab complex. Two IgG antibodies or one IgM antibody is required for C1q binding.
4. As a consequence of C1q binding, C1r is activated and converts the proenzyme C1s into its activated form, C1 esterase ($\overline{C1}$). The activated $\overline{C1}$ catalyzes the cleavage of C4 and C2. Fragments C4b and C2a form the $\overline{C4bC2a}$ complex (C3 convertase), which catalyzes the cleavage of C3.
5. The $\overline{C4b2a3b}$ complex (C5 convertase) splits C5 into C5a and C5b.
6. Up to this point the complement activation sequence is referred to as the *activating unit*.
7. The final *membrane attack unit* involves the sequential activation of C6, C7, and finally C8 and C9, leading to cell lysis.
8. In addition to C3 to C9, five other proteins are involved in the alternative pathway of C activation. These are $\beta 1H$ and

C3bINA, which are modulating factors for control of C3b levels; factor B (C3 proactivator), which is activated to Bb (C3 activator) via factor D (C3 proactivator convertase); and native properdin (NP). Properdin is not necessary but can contribute to the stabilization of the C5 convertase $(S1\text{-}C\overline{3b_n\,B_n})$.

9. The biologically active components generated in the classic sequence have been shown to have the following functions: C2 and C4 bring about virus neutralization; C2b increases vascular permeability (kinin-like); C3a and C3b enhance phagocytosis of PMN with release of lysosomal enzymes, immune adherence, and anaphylatoxin activity; C3a, C5a, and $C\overline{5b67}$ increase chemotaxis; C3 fragment mobilizes leukocytes from bone marrow; C3a and C5a, anaphylatoxins, release histamine from mast cells, and C5a induces lysosomal enzyme release; C1 to 7 facilitates lymphocytotoxicity; and C1 to 9 is cytotoxic to specific sensitized target cells, adjacent cells, and activates tissue lysosomal enzymes.

10. The activation sequence of the alternative C pathway is summarized in Figure 9-4. A variety of agents, which are summarized in Table 9-5, can initiate this pathway.

11. C sequence consists of several regulatory factors. $\overline{C1}$-inhibitor is an α_2-globulin present in serum. The presence of a C3-inactivator has also been demonstrated. C3-inactivator neutralizes the action of C3b by cleavage to C3c and C3d. The latter two fragments cannot bind to the C4b2a and thus stop the C activation. C3-inactivator requires $\beta1H$ as cofactor.

12. Other inactivators include the enzyme carboxypeptidase, which inactivates C3a and C5a, and a β_1-globulin, which inactivates C6.

13. Many sites of C component synthesis are known (Table 9-7).

14. Most of the complement components can be quantitated by radial immunodiffusion with their specific corresponding antibodies. Functionally the components can be assessed by the classic complement fixation test.

15. Complement deficiencies are associated with various diseases (briefly summarized in Table 9-8).

16. Complement, blood clotting, and fibrinolytic systems are interrelated.

Bibliography and Selected Reading

General

Agnello, V. Complement deficiency states. *Medicine* 57:1, 1978.

Colten, H. R. Biosynthesis of Complement. In F. J. Dixon and H. G. Kunkel (Eds.), *Advances in Immunology,* Vol. 22. New York: Academic, 1976. Pp. 67–118.

Cooper, N.R., and Ziccardi, R. J. The Nature and Reactions of Complement Enzymes. In D. W. Ribbons and K. Brew (Eds.), *Proteolysis and Physiological Regulation.* New York: Academic, 1976. P. 167.

Mayer, M. M. The complement system. *Sci. Am.* 229:54, 1973.

Müller-Eberhard, H. J. Complement. *Annu. Rev. Biochem.* 44:697, 1975.

Müller-Eberhard, H. J. Chemistry and function of the complement system. *Hosp. Pract.* 12:33, 1977.

Müller-Eberhard, H. J. Complement abnormalities in human disease. *Hosp. Pract.* 13:75, 1978.

Classical and Alternative Pathways

Bagler, M. D. P., Langone, J. J., and Borsos, T. T. Effect of lectins on the hemolytic activity of complement components. *Immunochemistry.* 15:465, 1978.

Bruns, G. A. P. Complement genes on chromosome 6. *N. Engl. J. Med.* 296:510, 1977.

Ehlenberger, A. G., and Nussenzweig, V. The role of membrane receptors for C3b and C3d in phagocytosis. *J. Exp. Med.* 145:357, 1977.

Götze, O., and Müller-Eberhard, H. J. The alternative pathway of complement activation. *Adv. Immunol.* 24:1, 1976.

Pangburn, M. K., Schreiber, R. D., and Müller-Eberhard, H. J. Human complement C3b inactivator: Isolation, characterization, and demonstration of an absolute requirement for the serum protein β1H for cleavage of C3b and C4b in solution. *J. Exp. Med.* 146:257, 1977.

Schreiber, R. D., and Müller-Eberhard, H. J. Assembly of the cytolytic alternative pathway of complement from eleven isolated plasma proteins. *J. Exp. Med.* 148:1722, 1978.

Schreiber, R. D., Pangburn, M. K., Lesavre, P. H., and Müller-Eberhard, H. J. Initiation of the alternate pathway of complement: Recognition of activators by bound C3b and assembly of the entire pathway from six isolated proteins. *Proc. Natl. Acad. Sci. USA* 75:3948, 1978.

Whaley, K., and Ruddy, S. Modulation of the alternative complement pathway by β1H globulin. *J. Exp. Med.* 144:1147, 1976.

Whicher, J. T. The value of complement assays in clinical chemistry. *Clin. Chem.* 24:7, 1978.

Ziccardi, R. J., and Cooper, N. R. Demonstration and quantitation of activation of the first component of complement in human serum. *J. Exp. Med.* 147:385, 1978.

Complement and Other Biological Factors

Coleman, R. W. Formation of human plasma kinins. *N. Engl. J. Med.* 291:509, 1974.

David, E. W., and Fujikawa, R. Basic mechanisms in blood coagulation. *Annu. Rev. Biochem.* 44:799, 1975.

Graham, J. B. Genetic counselling in classic hemophilia A. *N. Engl. J. Med.* 296:966, 1977.

Griffin, J. H., and Cochrane, C. G. Mechanisms for involvement of high molecular weight kininogen in surface dependent reactions of Hageman factor coagulation (Factor XII). *Proc. Natl. Acad. Sci. USA* 73:2554, 1976.

Holmberg, L., and Nilsson, I. M. Von Willebrand's disease. *Annu. Rev. Med.* 26:33, 1975.

Hugli, T. E., and Müller-Eberhard, H. J. Anaphylatoxins: C3a and C5a. *Adv. Immunol.* 26:1, 1978.

Jaffe, E. A. Endothelial cells and the biology of Factor VIII. *N. Engl. J. Med.* 296:377, 1977.

Johnston, R. B., and Stroud, R. M. Complement and host defense against infection. *J. Pediatr.* 90:169, 1977.

Klein, H. G. Detection of carrier state of classic hemophilia. *N. Engl. J. Med.* 296:959, 1977.

Muller, W., Hanauski-Abel, H., and Lods, M. Reversible inhibition of C1q release from guinea pig macrophages by 2, 2' − dipyridyl. *FEBS Lett.* 90:218, 1978.

Ramalho-Pinto, F. J., McLaren, D. J., and Smithers, S. R. Complement mediated killing of Schistosomula of *Schistosoma mansoni* by rat eosinophils in vitro. *J. Exp. Med.* 147:147, 1978.

Zimmerman, T. S., and Edgington, T. S. Molecular immunology of Factor VIII. *Annu. Rev. Med.* 25:303, 1974.

10 : Immunobiology

The administration of an antigen to an animal activates a series of complex cellular biochemical processes involving several cell types of the host immune system (Chapters 3 and 5). Obviously these complex processes must involve genetic modulation at several regions of the immune response. These genetic controls include (1) recognition and processing of antigen; (2) synthesis, and elaboration of the specific antibody and (3) control of the function of the specific effector T cell.

Genetic regulation of the specific immune response has been examined (1) by structural analysis of the products of the specific immune response, that is, the antibodies or immunoglobulins (see Chapter 2); and (2) by examination and analysis of the genetic control of the animal's ability to recognize and respond to specific structurally defined synthetic immunogens.

Structural analysis of the immunoglobulins of normal individuals and myeloma patients and of specific antibodies has yielded a wealth of information on the genetic basis of antibody structure but not a clear picture of the basis of antibody diversity and specificity. Nevertheless, results of the structural analysis of immunoglobulins have demonstrated that both the light and heavy chains have an N-terminal variable region and a C-terminal constant region and that these regions are coded for by separate structural genes (*allotypic Ir genes*) (Figure 10-1). This has been deduced from structural analyses of rabbit and human immuno-globulins, the latter especially from monoclonal gammopathy (myeloma-B cell bone marrow malignancy).

The genetic control of the diversity and specificity of antibodies, however, is presently unclear. Two general explanations have been postulated: (1) the existence of a large pool of germline genes, each of which codes for a particular sequence in the V region (germline theory); and (2) a high degree of somatic varia-bility resulting from recombination or somatic mutation (somatic mutation theory). These theories were discussed in Chapter 2. Presently there is no convincing evidence for one or the other postulations. It is possible that both may contribute to antibody diversity.

Fig. 10-1 : Allo-typic Ir genes coding for the structural specificity of immuno-globulins.

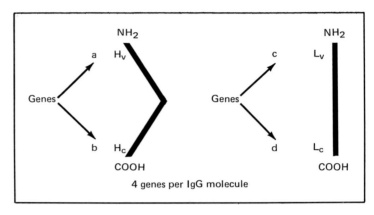

4 genes per IgG molecule

Ultimate understanding of genetic control of the specific immune response may require genetic analysis of the inheritance of the ability of a species to recognize antigenic determinants and to synthesize antibodies to them. In this regard the discovery of responders and nonresponders in several species of animals has been of great significance. These studies, which used specific immunogens, suggest that ability to respond to specific antigens and their unique configurations is under direct genetic control (see Benacerraf, 1975). The immunogens used in these studies were (1) weakly immunogenic alloantigens, (2) low doses of the complex soluble protein antigens conjugated to defined haptens such as dinitrophenol (DNP) and 3-iodo-4-hydroxy-5-nitrophenyl-acetic acid (NIP), and (3) defined synthetic antigens such as the D- and L- amino acid copolymers.

This chapter is concerned with the major histocompatilibity complex (MHC) of the mouse and especially with the H-2 complex, as associated with genetic control of the immune response. For all species thus far examined, *the ability to respond to a specific antigen appears to be regulated by autosomal dominant genes* in the MHC.

Immunogenetics

Understanding of the genetics of the immune responses requires knowledge of the major histocompatibility complex (MHC) genes and the products of their regulation.

Major Histocompatibility Complex (MHC)

MHC have been recognized in ten species of animals, including amphibians (*Xenopus laevis*), chickens, and several species of mammals. MHC occurs early in evolutionary development, as evidenced by its presence in amphibians and its probable occur-rence in all higher vertebrates in one form or another. Table 10–1 lists the species that have exhibited defined MHC.

Functional constituents associated with the MHC in all those spe-cies are (1) principal transplantation antigens; (2) serologically

Table 10-1 : Species Having Defined Major Histocompatibility Complexes (MHC)

Species	MHC
Man	HLA
Chimpanzee	ChLA
Rhesus	RhLA
Dog	DLA
Pig	SLA
Rabbit	RLA
Guinea pig	GPLA
Mouse	H-2
Rat	AgB
Chicken	B
Xenopus laevis	—

defined (SD) antigens of lymphocytes, although the SD antigens are broadly distributed on other tissues; (3) location of the immune response (Ir) genes (role in resistance or susceptibility to disease); (4) major constituents regulating the mixed leukocyte reaction (MLR), the lymphocyte-defined (LD) antigens; (5) graft-versus-host reaction (GVHR); (6) multiple phenotypic traits or functions controlled by tight clusters of multiple genetic loci; and (7) extensive genetic polymorphism at many loci in the MHC.

This chapter emphasizes the mouse MHC and its role in the modulation of the immune response. The MHC of man is discussed in Chapter 12.

Definitions

HLA (human leukocyte antigen): Gene complex that defines the species regional or system designation and is assigned locus symbols A, B, C, and D. Numbers 1, 2, 3, etc., identify specificities within each locus; and the prefix w between locus symbol and specificity number indicates provisional specificity. For example, HLA-Bw17 is the histocompatibility leukocyte antigen with locus B and workshop (w) specificity number 17.

MLC (mixed leukocyte culture reactions) (also referred to as MLR): Assayed by analysis of ^{3}H-thymidine incorporation by lymphocytes (responder) stimulated by allogeneic lymphocytes (stimulator) in vitro. The stimulator lymphocyte DNA synthesis is rendered inactive by treatment with mitomycin C.

CML (cell-mediated lympholysis): Destruction of target allogeneic lymphocytes by specific effector lymphocytes. The active cytotoxic lymphocytes are designated CTLs or Tc. In the mouse these T cells carry the Ly-2+3+ differentiation antigens.

Recombinant: An animal that has experienced a recombinational event *during meiosis.* This consists of a cross-over and recombination of portions of two chromosomes.

Congenic (originally *congenic resistant*): Referring to a lineage of mice identical or nearly identical with other inbred strains except for the substitution of at least one histocompatibility locus of a foreign allele, introduced by an appropriate cross with a second inbred strain. Congenic resistant mice are homozygous mice containing all the genes of one strain, except for a specific locus or group of closely linked genes derived from another strain.

MHC (major histocompatibility complex): Designated HLA in man and H-2 in the mouse (see Table 10–1 for other species). The genes included in this complex modulate the strongest major transplantation antigens, although not exclusively.

SD (the first or initial serologically defined HLA antigens): The classic HLA-A, -B, and -C loci of the MHC in man and of H-2K and H-2D in the mouse. These antigens are the primary target of cytotoxic lymphocytes, although other evidence suggests that other antigens not related to the SD-designated antigens (defined as CD-cytotoxic determinants) are the targets for T cytotoxic lymphocytes (Tc).

LD (lymphocyte-defined): (the first or initial) HLA antigens defined by the lymphocyte response in the MLC; the lymphocyte antigenic determinants of the MHC. These strong antigens are modulated by the HLA-D locus in man and the LD-1 locus in the mouse. Helper T lymphocytes respond to LD antigens (HLA-D) and thus correspond to the responder T cell in the MLC reaction. The Tc lymphocyte also proliferates in the MLC, but the majority of the responding cells are T helper cells.

Ia (immune response–associated): the immune response gene region in the MHC; also, the associated antigens, which are found in the B cells, macrophages, epidermal cells, and sperm and are modulated by the H-2I locus in the mouse. In man, the antigen is designated as *Ia-like* or B cell antigen.

Ir (immune response): The Ir immune locus controls the ability of the animal to respond immunologically to a variety of antigens. It is a constituent of the MHC.

GVHR (graft-versus-host reaction): The immune response of the transplanted tissue graft to the unrelated histocompatibility antigens of the recipient (host). It is exhibited principally in bone marrow or lymphocyte transplantation.

Haplotype: The HLA chromosomal region, including all the loci of that region. An individual has two haplotypes, one inherited from each parent.

Genotype: The genes carried by an individual.

Phenotype: The antigens expressed and detected on the cells of an individual, that is, antigens modulated by the genotypic makeup of the individual.

PLT: (primed LD typing): Lymphocytes are primed in a 10-day MLC to detect certain MHC-controlled HLA-D antigens. Such primed lymphocytes (responders) from the MLC reaction can be used to test whether the cells of any one individual have the LD antigens that were used to prime the T lymphocytes. The PLT cell is used for the detection of HLA-D antigens. An increase in ^{3}H-thymidine incorporation will occur when a PLT cell is added to an unknown that has the same HLA-D as the original stimulator or the original known priming cells.

Private and Public Specificities: Private specificities designate antigenic specificities coded by alleles in each locus unique for specific haplotypes. *Public specificities* designate antigenic specificities that are shared among different H-2 alleles. The "short" HLA specificities in humans are analogous to the private antigenic specificities of the mouse. In both species, private specificities represent antigenic specificities that are characteristic for specific histocompatibility alleles.

Mouse H-2 Complex   The major histocompatibility complex of the mouse is found on chromosome 17. It is referred to as the histocompatibility-2 (H-2) complex (see Figure 10–2). It consists of five major regions, K, I, S, G, and D, with subregions in I designated I-A, I-B, I-J, I-E, and I-C. The MHC in the mouse has been located to the right of the centromere; and there are linked markers on both sides of the MHC: the T and tf regions to the left of K, and T1 and thf to the right of D. At present, nine distinct marker loci have been defined in the H-2 complex. These are H-2K, Ir-1A (Ia-1), Ir-1B, Ia-4, Ia-5, Ia-3, Ss, H-2G, and H-2D. The basic methods for recognition of these gene marker loci of the H-2 complex are reagents obtained from planned immunization of inbred, congenic, and recombinant mice strains and from CML studies. Each of the gene marker loci controls a distinct function and expressed product (antigen).

Properties of the H-2 complex as summaried in Table 10–2 show that many diverse traits are associated with the MHC and that these have been localized to specific regions of the MHC through analysis of appropriate intra-H-2 recombinants. A *region* can be

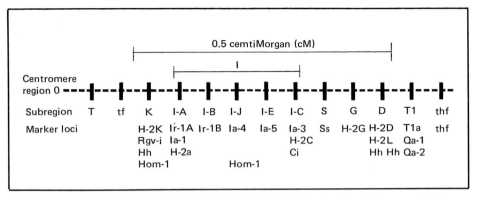

Fig. 10-2 : The major histocompatibility complex of the mouse (H-2 gene complex), situated on chromosome 17.

defined as the segment of chromosome demarcated by intra-H-2 cross-overs that have separated a specific locus from its neighboring loci. Thus, the G region is restricted by the positions of the cross-overs that separate the H-2G locus from the Ss locus on the left and the H-2D locus on the right (Figure 10-2). The regions defined so far may contain multiple genes (polymorphism), since it is not known whether all loci of the MHC have as yet been identified. Present studies suggest that the H-2 complex could encompass as many as 500 genes. If this is the case, then an average H-2 region might contain 50 to 60 discrete loci. Thus, the assignment of several traits to the same region, for example, T1a T-antigens and H-2D (T1a) transplantation antigens to the T1 region, does not mean that these different traits are regulated by the same gene.

As indicated in Table 10-2, two general characteristics of traits appear to dominate the MHC: (1) traits involving the mechanisms of immune response recognition and ancillary functions (complement); and (2) traits involving control of polymorphic cell surface structures (alloantigens). Obviously much more work is required for the resolution of such questions as: (1) the number of discrete genes and their specific regulation; (2) the nature of the gene products; and (3) whether a single gene action regulates different expressed traits.

The detection of SD and LD antigens in the MHC can be assayed by the MLR and CML procedures. Earlier studies indicated that the LD antigens were not detectable by the CML procedures. It has been demonstrated, however, that the H-2K and H-2D regions in the mouse can be measured by SD and CML (even with one amino-acid difference on the target antigen; therefore K and D regions are considered strong antigens).

**Table 10-2 : Gene Marker Loci and Their Associated
Functional Components in the Mouse MHC**

Components (Functions)	Gene Marker Locus	Region (MHC)
Complement (C1, C2, C3, C4)	Ss	S
Ss protein, SLp (serum protein variants)	Ss	S
Transplantation antigen	H-2K, Ir-1A, Ir-1B H-2D (T1a)	K, I, D (T1)
CML target antigen (LD, detected)	H-2K H-2A, H-2C H-2D, H-2L Qa-1, Qa-2	K I D T1
Serologically detected H-2	H-2K, H-2D	K, D
Immune response	H-2K, Ir-1A, Ir-1B	K, I
Ia lymphocyte antigen	Ir-1A, Ir-1B, Ia-4, Ia-5, Ia-3	I
Ir-Thy-1	H-2K	K
MLR, GVH stimulation	H-2K, Ir-1A, Ir-1B, Ia-4, Ia-5, Ia-3 H-2D	K, I D
Immune surveillance	H-2K, H-2D	K, D
T helper	Ir-1A	I (I-A)
T suppressor	Ia-4	I (I-J)
Thymus leukemia alloantigen	T1a	T1
Erythrocyte antigen	H-2G	G
Virus susceptibility	Rgv-1	K-1
T- and B-cell interaction	Ci, Ir-1A, Ir-1B, Ia-4, Ia-5, Ia-3	I
Hemopoietic histocompatibility	Hh	K, D, T1
Testosterone level	Hom-1	K, I
Macrophage-T relationship	H-2K, H-2D Ir-1A, Ir-1B, Ia-4, Ia-5, Ia-3	K, D I

*IR Genes and the
Immune Response*

GUINEA PIG. Evidence for the specific control of the immune response in guinea pigs has been found in inbred strains 2 and 13 and in random-bred lines. The genetic control of specific responsiveness depends heavily on the nature of the *antigens* used in the study. The synthetic antigens, homopolymers and copolymers, have contributed immensely to the understanding of gene regulation in the immune response. Some of these important synthetic antigens are listed in Table 10-3.

Table 10-3 : Synthetic Polypeptide Antigens Used in the Examination of the Genetic Control of Specific Immune Responsiveness in Guinea Pigs

Polymers	Acronym	Ratio
Homopolymers		
Poly-L-lysine	PLL	
Poly-L-arginine	PLA	
Copolymers		
L-glutamyl-L-alanyl	GA	6 : 4
L-glutamyl-L-tyrosyl	GT	1 : 1
L-glutamyl-L-alanyl-L-tryosyl	GAT	6 : 3 : 1
Hapten conjugates		
2,4-Dinitrophenyl-poly-L-lysine	DNP–PLL	
2,4-Dinitrophenyl-poly-L-glutamyl-L-lysine	DNP–GL	

Table 10-4 : The Immune Response Expressed by Strain 2 (Responder) and Strain 13 (Nonresponder) Guinea Pigs to Homopolymers and Copolymers

Strain	Gene	Polymers	Immune Response
2 Responder	PLL gene	PLL PLA PLO GL Hapten-polymers	(a) DTH, (MIF, blastogenesis) (b) Specific anti-body
13 Nonresponder	No PLL gene	PLL PLA PLO GL Hapten-polymers	None " " " "

The initial specific immune response (Ir) gene found in guinea pigs was induced by the positively charged homopolymer, poly-L-lysine (PLL). This is referred to as the *PLL gene* and is found in all strain 2 and some Hartley guinea pigs. This PLL gene is lacking in strain 13 guinea pigs. The PLL gene controls responsiveness to the positively charged homopolymers PLL, PLA, and poly-L-ornithine (PLO); to the copolymer L-glutamyl-L-lysine (GL); and to the hapten conjugates of the polymers (see Table 10-3).

Table 10-4 lists the humoral and cell-mediated immune responses of strain 2 guinea pigs to various synthetic polymers. Strain 13 guinea pigs show none of the immune responses noted for strain 2 to these same synthetic polymers. These responses are under

Fig. 10-3 : The immune response of offspring of guinea pigs to synthetic polypeptides.
A. Responder (R) X responder.
B. Nonresponder (NR) X nonresponder. C. NR X R. Ag = antigen, Ab = antibody, F₁ = offspring (first generation).

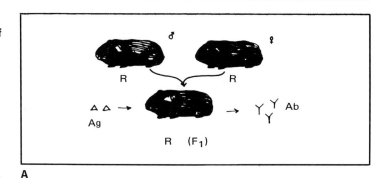

A

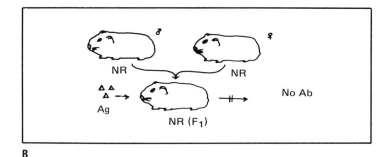

B

C

the control of the H-linked Ir genes (PLL gene). The PLL gene in guinea pigs appears to be responsible for the qualitative differences between responder and nonresponder animals. Earlier studies (see reference, Benacerraf, 1975) with random-bred strains of Hartley guinea pigs immunized with DNP-PLL separated the animals into nonresponders and responders. As shown in Figure 10-3, mating studies demonstrated that (1) mating of responders to responders or nonresponders to nonresponders gave offspring in the F_1 generation of responders and nonresponders, respectively; and (2) mating of nonresponders to responders gave F_1 offspring of all responders. Thus these studies indicated that responsiveness to these synthetic polymers is inherited as an autosomal dominant trait. Further studies with strains 2 and 13 inbred guinea pigs exhibited similar findings and indicated that immune responses to these synthetic polymeric antigens are inherited according to strict mendelian genetics and modulated by distinct dominant Ir genes. In the inbred guinea pig strains, the response to the synthetic antigens appears to be controlled by the same gene or by very closely linked genes. Similar conclusions can be drawn for some guinea pigs of the random-bred Hartley strains for the synthetic antigens, PLL, PLA, PLO, and GL, in which responsiveness is controlled by a single gene or by closely related linked genes. On the other hand, some Hartley strains appear to have distinct nonallelic genes controlling responsiveness to the synthetic polymers PLL, GA, GT, DNP-GA, and low-dose BSA.

MOUSE. Specific Ir genes controlling responsiveness to synthetic antigens and to low doses of protein antigens have also been demonstrated in mice. In addition, H-linked Ir responders have been shown to alloantigens in mice.

Several factors have contributed significantly to the use of the mouse for examination of the genetic control of immune responses: (1) availability of well-characterized inbred strains developed by transplantation investigators; (2) availability of congenic resistant strains that differ only in the H-2 complex; (3) documentation of recombinant events in mice within the H-2 complex precisely in the region of the Ir genes; and (4) the fact that the end results assayed are antibody synthesis, which is much more readily defined than DTH response. The mouse is a poor DTH responder. Nevertheless, the DTH is also regulated by the Ir genes, as shown by the use of antigens such as (T, G)-A--L.

As with guinea pigs, the immune response in mice to copolymers (Table 10–5) has been shown to be under dominant H-linked Ir gene control at a locus designated Ir-1. The ability of mice to respond to the various antigens listed in Table 10–5 is a quantitative genetic trait. Depending on the nature of the synthetic polypeptide antigen, the antibody responses of inbred mice are similar to those of guinea pigs in that they are all-or-none responses. A few mice strains with their haplotypes and their capacity to respond to the various antigens listed in Table 10–5 are summarized in Table 10–6. A few examples of recombinant mice and their detailed gene structure in the H-2 complex are given in Table 10–7.

The significant findings from studies of mice can be summarized as follows: (1) immune responses are controlled by dominant H-linked Ir genes; (2) many, if not all, of the genes have been mapped in the Ir region; (3) the Ir genes concerned with the

Table 10-5 : The Antigens That Have Been Used to Assess the H-linked Immune Response Genes in Mice

1. Random linear copolymers of L-amino acids

    GLA^5 $(Glu^{57}$-L-Lys^{38}-L-$Ala^5)_n$

    GLA^{10} $(Glu^{57}$-L-Lys^{38}-L-$Ala^{10})_n$

    GAT^{10} $(Glu^{60}$-L-Ala^{30}-L-$Tyr^{10})_n$

    GA $(Glu^{60}$-L-$Ala^{40})_n$

    $GL Pro^5$ $(Glu^{57}$-L-Lys^{38}-L-$Pro^5)_n$

2. Branched copolymers of L-amino acids
    (T, G)-A--L [(Tyr, Glu)-L-Ala-Lys]
    (H, G)-A--L [(His, Glu)-L-Ala-Lys]

3. Murine alloantigens
    IgG (allotypic determinants on BALB/c IgG myeloma)
    IgA (allotypic determinants on BALB/c IgA myeloma)
    Thy-I.1 (mouse θ antigen, thymocyte)
    Ea.1 (mouse RBC)
    Thyroglobulin, mouse

4. Foreign proteins
    Nase (staphylococcal nuclease)
    RE (Ragweed extract antigens)
    LDH_B (Porcine lactic dehydrogenase B)
    Bovine γ-globulin (BGG) (in low dose)
    Ovalbumin (1-OVA)

control of most of these responses are distinct; and (4) genetic control of the responses to synthetic polypeptide antigens is *specific*. As also found in guinea pig studies, some antigens appear to require two gene loci for expression of responsiveness to the antigen. In others, a single gene locus appears to regulate several closely related copolymers. In some instances the presence of tyrosine in the synthetic polypeptide tended to induce T suppressor function in some mice and thus unresponsiveness to the antigen.

The genetic explanation for the control by the I-region genes in responder and nonresponder mice to the polypeptide antigen, GAT, is schematically represented in Figures 10-4 and 10-5. The mechanisms of the complex interaction of macrophages and T and B cells may be true of H-linked I-region genetic modulation of all T-dependent antigens.

In the responder animal (Figure 10-4) GAT is presented in the immunogenic form by the antigen-presenting macrophage with specific Ia molecules. This results in the stimulation of the T helper ($Ly-1^+$) cells, which are Ia-restricted in specificity. The Th $Ly-1^+$ cell then stimulates the B cell to blastogenesis and antibody synthesis. GAT may also stimulate, but to a lesser extent in the responder mouse, T suppressor cells (Ts): first the

Table 10-6 : A Few Examples of Inbred Mice, Their Defined Haplotypes and Markers of Genetic Fine Structure (Table 10-7), and Their Capacity to Respond to Various Antigens (Table 10-5)

	Strain (Haplotype)				
Antigen	B10.A (a)	B10.BR (k)	C57BL/10 (b)	B10.D2 (d)	A.Sw (s)
GLA^5	+	+	±	++	++
GLA^{10}	+	+	±	++	++
GA	++	++	++	++	++
GAT^{10}	++	++	++	++	±
GL Pro^5	±	±	±	±	++
GLT^5	±	±	±	++	±
(T, G)-A--L	±	±	++	+	±
(H, G)-A--L	++	++	±	+	±
IgA	++	++	±	±	++
IgG	±	±	++	±	++
Thy-I.1	++	++	±	±	ND
RE	++	++	±	++	ND
Nase	++	++	±	++	++
1-BGG	++	++	++	±	ND
1-OVA	±	±	++	++	+
LDHB	±	±	±	++	++

++, +, and ± represent strong responders, intermediate responders, and low to negative responders, respectively. ND = not determined.

cyclophosphamide-sensitive pre-T suppressor 1, Ly-1$^+$, 2$^+$, 3$^+$; then T suppressor 1 (Ts1). The Ts1 cell elaborates T suppressor factor 1 (TsF$_1$), which acts on pre-T suppressor 2, a cyclophosphamide-resistant T cell with Ly-1$^+$, 2$^+$, 3$^+$ markers. The latter is transformed to Ts2 Ly-2$^+$, 3$^+$ cell which elaborate Ts2F$_2$. Ts2F$_2$ acts primarily by suppression of the Th Ly-1$^+$ cell (T helper), which acts on the B cell. Ts2F$_2$ may also act on the B cell directly or on Th1 "feedback inducer" Ly-1$^+$ cell, which then acts to suppress the B cell and stimulate pre-Ts1. The Ts1 and Ts2 cells are restricted by the I-J$^+$ subregion or Ia-4 marker locus genes.

In the nonresponder animal (Figure 10-5), the macrophage presents the antigen to the pre-Ts1 and also, via the Th1 Ly1$^+$, I-J$^+$ cell, induces the T suppressor pathway to such an extent that antibody synthesis is suppressed by virtue of the T suppressor

Table 10-7 : A Few Examples of the Detail Structure of the Intra-H-2 Recombinant Strains and Their Haplotypes

Strain	H-2 Haplotype	K	I-A	I-B	I-J	I-E	I-C	S	G	D
					H-2 Regions					
B10.A or A/J	a	k	k	k	k	k	d	d	d	d
B10.D2	d	d	d	d	d	d	d	d	d	d
C57BL/10	b	b	b	b	b	b	b	b	b	b
B10.BR	k	k	k	k	k	k	k	k	k	k
A.SW	s	s	s	s	s	s	s	s	s	s
B10.A (5R)	i5	b	b	b	k	k	d	d	d	d

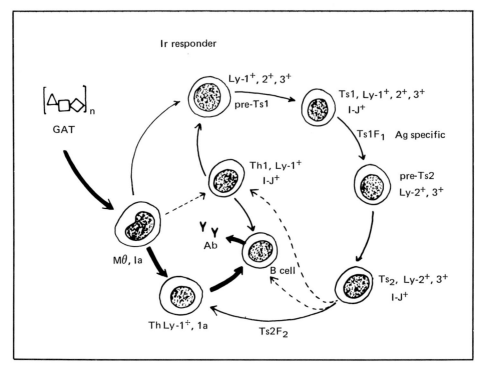

Fig. 10–4 : Mθ, Ts, Th, and B cell interaction in a responder mouse following antigen (GAT) administration. Heavy lines represent the major initial pathway, lighter lines represent the minor pathway, and broken lines represent possible pathways of action. Mθ = macrophage; Th Ly-1+ = T helper cell with Ly-1+, Ia-restricted gene product; Th1 Ly-1+, I-J+ = T helper cell 1 with Ly1+, I-J+-restricted gene product; pre-Ts1 = pre-T suppressor cell 1; Ts1 = T suppressor cell 1; Ts1F$_1$, I-J+ = T suppressor factor produced by Ts1F$_1$, I-J+ = restricted gene product; pre-Ts2 = precursor T suppressor 2, Ly-2+, 3+, I-J+ = restricted gene product; Ts2, Ly-2+, 3+, I-J+ = T suppressor 2, Ly-2+, 3+ markers, I-J+ restricted gene product.

cell augmentation. It has also been demonstrated that a possible gene defect in the macrophage that presents the antigen to Th cells results in transmission of the antigenic signal to the Ts pathway, thus inducing suppression of antibody synthesis. Figure 10–5 summarizes the nonresponder pathway following GAT stimulation.

Nonresponder animals possess B cells, in numbers comparable to those found in a responder animal, that are capable of binding antigens to which they are genetically unable to respond. Nonresponders may lack carrier-specific T helper cells and thus fail

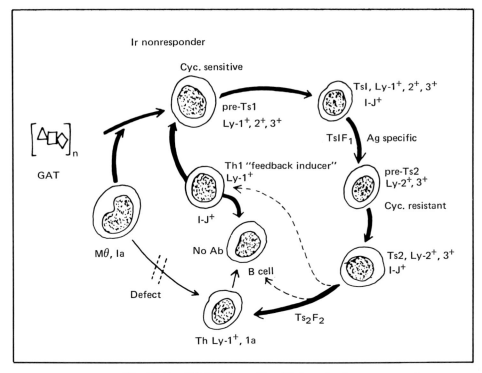

Fig. 10-5 : Mθ, Ts, Th, and B cell interaction in a nonresponder mouse following antigen (GAT) stimulation. (See Fig. 10-4 for explanation of abbreviations.)

to have the appropriate Ir gene product to initiate the carrier effect (Figure 10-6B).

The high specificity of the immune response controlled by the H-linked Ir genes can be exhibited by use of DNP-bovine insulin and DNP-pig insulin antigens. In both hormones, the DNP is attached to the B-chain of insulin at the amino acid 29 position. The two insulin hormones differ only by two amino acids, at the A-8 and A-10 positions of the A-chains and in the loop region of A-6 and A-11 at the disulfide linkages. Injection of DNP-insulin conjugates into three strains of mice with different haplotypes gave the results shown in Table 10-8. The responses to the two haptenic insulin antigens varied among the three different haplotypes. Although the anti-DNP antibodies from mouse $H-2^d$ and $H-2^b$ were indistinguishable, the antibodies to bovine insulin and pig insulin within the same strain, $H-2^d$, differentiated between the two antigens. Thus the antibodies exhibited remarkable specificity to distinguish the differences in the two amino acids in the A-chain.

Fig. 10-6 : A nonresponder animal with a normal number of B cells but deficient T helper cells.
A. Normal reaction between T and B cells (responder). Specific immuno-determinant receptor on B cell with associated recognition from T helper cell results in antibody synthesis by B cell. B. Same B cell. Lack of associated recognition T helper cell results in no antibody synthesis (nonresponder).

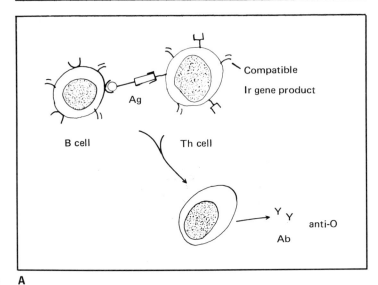

A

B

Table 10-8 : Mice with Differences in Their Haplotypes Immunized with DNP-Insulin (Bovine and Pig) Show Variable but Highly Specific Antibody Responses

		Antigen			
		Bovine DNP-Insulin		Pig DNP-Insulin	
Strain of Mice	Haplotype	Anti-DNP	Anti-BI	Anti-DNP	Anti-PI
BALB/c	H-2^d	++	++	+++	+++
C57BL	H-2^b	++	++	—	—
C57BR	H-2^k	—	—	—	—

*Other Aspects
of the H-linked
Ir Genes*

MAPPING IR GENES. The responsiveness of an inbred mouse to (T,G)-A--L, (H,G)-A--L, and (Phe, G)-A--L synthetic polymers is determined by its H-2 haplotype. The locus modulating this response is designated Ir-1. Studies with recombinant strains showed that the Ir gene is situated between the K and S loci (see Figure 10-2) and that this region is distinct from the K, S, and D regions. All known mouse Ir genes which could be mapped precisely have been localized in the I region. This region is distinct from the serological specificities of the histocompatibility complex modulated by the K and D regions. With the availability of strains with documented recombinant events in the I region between distinct Ir genes or between the K and S regions, the I region has been further expanded and subdivided into five subregions. These are designated I-A, I-B, I-J, I-E, and I-C, with genetic locus markers Ir-1A, Ir-1B, Ia-4, Ia-5, and Ia-3, respectively (see Figure 10-2). Table 10-2 summarizes the functions controlled by these gene loci. In addition to the recombinant strains, the use of the antigens listed in Table 10-5 have contributed to the analysis and examination of the I region.

GENETIC CONTROL OF CELLULAR INTERACTIONS. It is clearly recognized that the gene products of the I region of the MHC play a significant role in the interactions between T lymphocytes and antigen-pulsed macrophages (Mθ) and between T lymphocytes and B cells. At first it was thought that these cellular interrelationships depended primarily on the fact that these cells, T, B, and Mθ, share the same allelic forms at the I subregions. Recent evidence suggests, however, that this is not entirely the case. The I-region gene products have a critical function in cellular interactions, although their role is not to be a means for *self recognition* per se. The present contemporary concept can be schematically represented as shown in Figure 10-7. The antigen-specific T lymphocytes can recognize both the antigen presented by the self-macrophage or B lymphocyte and the compatible I-region gene product expressed by the B cell and macrophage. In the unprimed state, evidently T lymphocytes (subsets) capable of recognizing antigen and self I-region gene products (Figure 10-7A) are present, together with T lymphocytes capable of recognizing the same antigen gene products (Figure 10-7B). During conventional priming, the pool of T and self I-region gene products will be selectively expanded, leading to I-region restrictions on cellular interaction in the secondary responses.

IMMUNE RESPONSE FACTORS MODULATING CELL–CELL INTERACTIONS. *T Cell Factors.* One of the major areas of study has been the search for the various biological factors or substances

Fig. 10-7 : The genetic restrictions between T, B cells and macrophages (Mθ) to specific antigens in the cellular interactions between T lymphocytes and I-region gene products of Mθ and B lymphocytes of allogeneic (A) and xenogeneic (B) mice, A and Z, respectively.

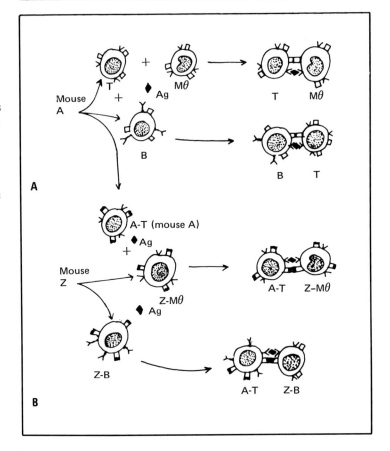

that are involved in the regulation of the T and B cell interactions. The *antigen-specific* T cell substances expressed as Ir gene products include both suppressor and enhancer factors. The antigen-specific T suppressor factor appears to act on the T helper cells but may also act on the pre-T helper cell to become a functionally active helper cell or may direct its action to the B cell. The limited information available on specific factors and the nonspecific allogeneic effect factor (AEF) is summarized in Table 10-9. The allogeneic effect factor has been shown to replace the T helper cell function and can stimulate B cells, as shown in in vitro immune responses.

A T cell suppressor factor (TsF) specific for the synthetic antigen GAT has been described as follows: (1) It consists in part of proteins with 45,000 daltons; (2) it binds specifically to GAT and is produced by Ly-2$^+$, 3$^+$ cells; (3) it is regulated by the I-J locus of the H-2 complex; (4) it does not have immunoglobulin properties; and (5) it possesses all the characteristics of an Ir gene product. It is highly possible that many analogous factors (family

Table 10-9 : Suppressor and Enhancer Factors, Associated with T Cells, Which Act on T Helper Cells and Subsequent B Cell Stimulation

Factors	MW	Property
T Cell		
Antigen-specific factor—enhancer	100,000 to 200,000	1. Enhances IgE response 2. Is anti-Fab anti-μ reactive 3. Has specific I region control (I-A)
Antigen-specific factor—suppressor (GAT, TsF)	45,000 to 50,000	1. Has suppressor activity 2. Does not react with anti-Ig 3. Has specific I region control (I-J) 4. Acts on Th cells 5. Produced by Ly-2^+, 3^+ cell
(T, G)-A--L specific enhancing factor		1. Enhances 2. Is reactive with anti-Ia serum 3. Does not react with anti-Ig
Nonspecific allogeneic effector factor	30,000 to 45,000	1. Acts on B cells 2. Consists of heavy and light (β_2-microglobulin) chains 3. Reacts with some anti-H-2 4. Reacts with anti-Ia
Macrophage		
Genetically related macrophage factor (GRF)		1. Is generated by macrophages incubated with soluble antigen and T cells, I-A subregion–restricted, Mθ-T cells 2. Generates T helper cells
Nonspecific macrophage factor (NMF)		1. From macrophages in culture without antigens 2. Replaces Mθ as T helper only when antigen is particulate 3. Not I region–restricted

of TsF) will be found for each specific group of closely related antigens.

Macrophage Factors. The induction of helper cell action on soluble or particulate antigens in vitro requires the cooperation of macrophages in many situations. The interaction between macrophages and T cells need not be direct cellular contact; but, like T cells, macrophages can elaborate factors that affect T helper cells. These, as indicated in Table 10-9, can be I-region gene-restricted such as the genetically regulated macrophage factor (GRF) and the nonrestricted nonspecific macrophage factor (NMF). Both of these factors modulate the T helper cells. GRF appears to function with Th cells with soluble antigens, whereas NMF affects Th cells in the presence of particulate antigens.

DISTINCTION BETWEEN H-LINKED Ir GENES AND ALLOTYPE-LINKED Ir GENES. Evidence to date suggests that the H-linked

**Table 10-10 : The Distinction Between the H-linked
Ir Genes and the Allotype-linked Ir Genes**

Genes	Properties
H-linked Ir genes	1. Associated with the MHC 2. Mode of analysis: ability of animals to respond to specific antigens; responders and nonresponders 3. Linked to T cell function 4. Modulate immune response 5. Regulate macrophages and T and B cells
Allotype-linked Ir genes	1. Code for immunoglobulin specificity; C and V regions; H- and L-chains 2. Mode of analysis: immunoglobulin structural analysis; specific antigen-antibody reactions 3. Not associated with MHC 4. Associated with B cell

Ir genes modulating responsiveness or nonresponsiveness to various antigens discussed in the preceding section are not synonymous with the allotype-linked Ir genes that code for the specificity of the antibody molecule. The distinction between the H-linked Ir genes and the allotype-linked genes is summarized in Table 10-10.

**Immunological
Tolerance**

Immunological tolerance is a physiological state or condition in which an animal is unable to respond immunologically to a given immunogen. The state of immune unresponsiveness can be exhibited in both cellular and humoral systems. It may be congenital (Immunodeficiency, Chapter 15) or acquired, the latter via immunosuppression by the variety of modalities discussed in Chapter 6.

True tolerant animals not only lack circulating antibodies to a particular antigen(s), but also have no cells synthesizing these antibodies, as shown by plaque-forming cell assays, examination of isolated cells, or direct immunofluorescence analysis for presence of intracellular antibodies. Thus, a valid proof of tolerance of an animal for an immunogen is the absence of synthesis of the corresponding antibodies.

Pseudotolerance may occur with a certain dosage of immunogen, generally just beneath a high dosage level that can induce true tolerance. In this case, circulating immunogen levels are sufficiently high that the antibodies synthesized form complexes with the immunogen and thus become undetectable when examined for circulating antibodies. Examination of the cells by immunofluorescence or plaque-forming assay, however, will exhibit cells synthesizing antibodies. Ultimately, circulating antibodies will emerge, with antigen clearance from the peripheral blood. In essence this phenomenon represents abnormal immune complex elimination: the antigen dose given maintains the antibody at a level where it is sequestered rather than rapidly cleared as is to be expected with lower antigen levels.

Conditions Associated with Tolerance

ANTIGEN. A major consideration in the induction of tolerance is the *nature* or *physical characteristics* of the antigen. In Chapter 4, the term *tolerogen* was used to define antigens that induce tolerance or immune unresponsiveness when given to an animal. Apparently tolerogens are monomeric or nonaggregated forms of antigen, and the tolerogenic effect is related to their inability to trigger the necessary signal for induction of the immune process; a polymer or aggregated form of the same antigen, on the other hand, can trigger the signal necessary for the induction of synthesis. An example is aggregated (polymeric) and nonaggregated (monomeric) human IgG. The former is immunogenic, and the latter is tolerogenic. These forms can be separated by ultracentrifugation, as obviously they differ in molecular weight. Monomeric tolerogens of all types of antigens exist.

ROUTE OF ADMINISTRATION. The route of administration of the antigen is important in the induction of tolerance. An antigen given with adjuvant subcutaneously tends to induce antibody synthesis. On the other hand, intravenous administration of the same antigen alone may have a tolerogenic effect, especially if a certain concentration of antigen is maintained.

DOSE. The *concentration* or dose of antigen also is important. For example, bovine γ-globulin (BGG) can induce specific unresponsiveness when given at high levels (high zone tolerance) exceeding the immunogenic level, but also by subimmunogenic doses just below the threshold levels for induction of antibody synthesis (low zone tolerance). Many, but not all, antigens could induce low and high dose tolerance and the concentration of antigen used could vary. The typical hypothetical curve for low and high zones of tolerance is shown in Figure 10-8.

An animal pretreated with subimmunogenic amounts of antigen, (pneumococcal polysaccharide, type III [S3]) responds poorly when challenged several days or weeks later with an optimal immunizing dose of the same antigen. This low-dose paralysis or tolerance is thought to be mediated by the S3-specific T suppressor cells triggered by the initial low dose. This concept is based on earlier evidence that low-dose paralysis for S3 is not inducible in congenital thymic (nude) mice and in T cell–depleted normal mice. T cell abrogation was carried out by treatment with T-depleting agents such as antilymphocyte globulin and specific virus (lactic dehydrogenase virus). This and other studies

Fig. 10-8 : The generally antici-pated curve of low-zone and high-zone tolerance of an animal to an antigen.

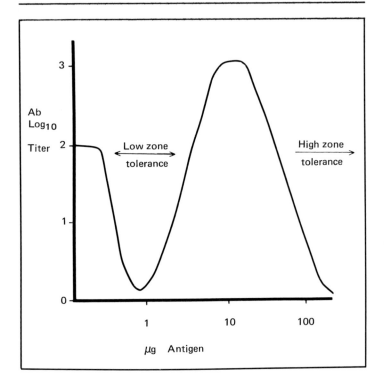

(see reference, Coutinho and Möller, 1975) provide good evidence for the T suppressor role in low-dose paralysis. However, the manner in which T suppressor cells limit the extent to which B cells generate antibody to S3 is not clear (see Figure 10-5). The T suppressor cells may act directly on the B cells or indirectly on the amplifier T cells (T helper cells). Evidence from other studies suggest that T suppressor cells act on T helper cells to suppress the helper effect on B cells and thus the humoral response.

A classic study of high zone tolerance was done by Felton and co-workers (1955). Mice injected with 1.0 mg of type II pneumo-coccal polysaccharide failed to become resistant to the challenge of the viable corresponding organism and also to synthesize detectable antibodies. This *immune paralysis* or unresponsiveness was persistent and specific. That is, these mice responded nor-mally to other immunogenic doses of other antigens, including other types of capsular polysaccharide. Doses of 0.01 to 1.0 μg of the same capsular pneumococcal polysaccharide resulted in resistance to the challenge from the viable strain and the presence of detectable circulating antibodies.

Tolerance can be established for any immunogens that can induce antibody synthesis. These include proteins, carbohydrates, synthetic immunogens, haptens, and others. However, particulate antigens such as bacteria, viruses, fungi, parasites, cells and aggregated proteins, which comprise complex and numerous immunodeterminants per particle, being excellent immunogens, have very poor tolerogenic qualities.

The immunological specificity of tolerance is remarkable. For example, if tolerance is induced to determinant Y, a portion of a molecule composed of X and Y, and the animal subsequently is challenged with the complete molecule (X and Y), then no anti-Y is formed (tolerant state), but antibody to X (anti-X) is induced in the animal tolerant to component Y.

MAINTENANCE. Induction of tolerance generally requires large concentrations of the antigen. The stability and persistence of tolerance are variable. High zone tolerance may be followed by a burst of antibody synthesis and rapid removal of antigen (immune clearance) and hence loss of tolerance. Maintenance of tolerance requires persistence of at least low levels of the antigen in the peripheral circulation. It is generally easier to maintain than to induce tolerance, but this depends on the particular antigen. Tolerance can be abrogated by cross-reacting antigens. For example, tolerance induced in newborn rabbits against native bovine serum albumin (by giving a high dose at birth), when challenged with BSA altered by addition of haptenic groups or by denaturation, is abrogated.

Newborn versus Adult Tolerance

Adequate amounts of heterologous immunogen given in fetal life or to a newborn can induce tolerance readily. The same dose or quantity given to an adult will induce an immune response. This difference in immune status appears to be one of degree of maturation and quantitative numbers of immunocompetent cells. Immunosuppression with x-irradiation and drugs such as cyclophosphamide, which, when given with antigen, depletes immunocompetent cells, can render an adult tolerant to the immunogen readily. Thus, the immune system of the adult becomes comparable to that of the newborn when depleted by immunosuppressive agents. Nevertheless, it is difficult to establish tolerance in individuals once antibody synthesis has been initiated.

The ease of establishment of tolerance in the fetus and neonate may be associated with the gradual development of self-antigens to the levels required for perpetuation of tolerance during adult life. Thus, the intrinsic ability of the fetus and neonate to respond to their own antigens gradually changes to an unresponsive state toward self-antigens as the levels required for maintenance of tolerance are achieved and stabilized in the child and adult; and this transformation is part of the development of self–non-self discrimination. Evidence presented suggests that self-tolerance is acquired and not coded genetically, as genetic coding of the self–non-self discrimination would necessitate germline structural genes coded only for antibody molecules with specificity against foreign antigens. This would be contrary to the evolutionary process, since any mutation affecting any self-antigen would result in an autoimmune reaction. Furthermore the genetic coding concept lacks the support of available experimental studies.

T and B Cells In Tolerance

Figure 10-9 presents a classic experiment that demonstrates several significant points in the immune response: (1) Intact T and B cells are necessary to the response to aggregated γ-globulin; (2) with T-dependent antigen, only one of the cell systems needs to be made tolerant to render the animal unresponsive to the antigen; (3) both T and B cells can be rendered tolerant; (4) T cells are rendered tolerant within the first few days (4 to 5) of administration of the tolerogen, with the maximum unresponsive state achieved in about 7 days, while T cell unresponsiveness persists as long as 23 weeks; and (5) B cell unresponsiveness appears in 9 days, with the maximum at about 18 days. Loss of B cell unresponsiveness occurred on about the forty-ninth day after injection of the tolerogen. Both B and T cells can be rendered unresponsive. T cells appear to be more sensitive to tolerogen, however. Other evidence shows that T cells are affected at lower doses of antigen and, hence, are related to low-zone paralysis. B cells, on the other hand, being less susceptible to tolerogen, appear to require larger antigen doses and thus are associated with high-zone paralysis.

Mechanism of Tolerance

The cellular basis for induction of tolerance or paralysis is depicted in Figures 10-10 and 10-11 for two-signal and one-signal concepts, respectively, of induction of antibody synthesis.

The two-signal concept of the immune response has been postulated and formulated on the basis of interpretation of the experimental findings in the attempts to understand induction and paralysis. The antigen-sensitive cell (B cell) has *specific antibody receptors,* which bind their specific antigenic determinant. This reaction leads to the presentation of signal 1. If the antigen is monomeric or haptenic or is T-independent without mitogenic property, then the cell becomes paralyzed (Figure 10,10-A).

The one-signal hypothesis considers the antigen binding to the antibody receptor of antigen-sensitive cell as nonreactive, that is, no signal is transmitted and the B cell is merely in a resting stage. Then the message transmitted via the mitogenic receptor on the B cell is considered as signal 1 (Figure 10-11,A), leading to

Fig. 10-9 : The roles of T and B lymphocytes in immunological tolerance, an in vivo study. HGG = monomeric human gamma-globulin; a, b, c, and d designate the source of cells: a = T cells; b = B cells (tolerant mice); c = T cell; d = B cell (immuno-competent mice).

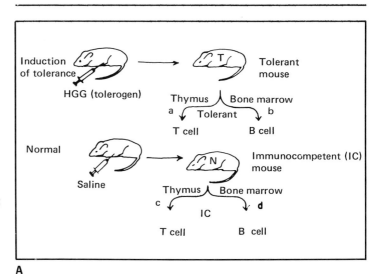

A

X-irradiated mouse	Cell mixture		HGG immunogen	Antibody synthesis
+	a	T	+ HGG ⟶	no
	b	B		
+	a	T	+ HGG ⟶	no
	d	B		
+	d	T	+ HGG ⟶	no
	c	T		
+	b	B	+ HGG ⟶	no
	c	T		
+	b	B	+ HGG ⟶	no
	d	B		
+	c	T	+ HGG ⟶	yes
	d	B		

B

antibody induction. Tolerance to T-independent antigens occurs when signal 1 exceeds the immunogenic level (Figure 10–11,B).

A T-independent antigen with mitogenic property would transmit signal 2 via the antigen-sensitive cell mitogenic receptor and hence induce antibody synthesis (Figure 10–10,B). The antigen-sensitive cells bound by T-independent antigens *lacking mitogenic*

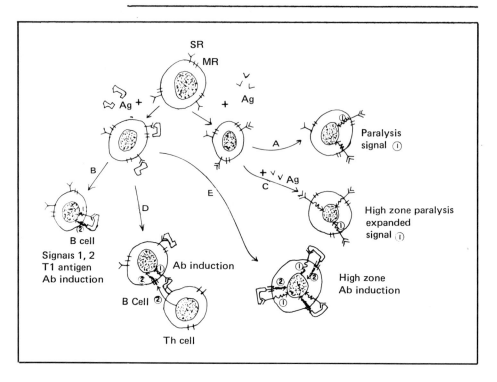

Fig. 10-10 : Immune paralysis based on the two-signal concept for the induction of antibody synthesis. A = paralysis; B = induction with T-independent (Ti) antigen; C = high-zone paralysis; D = induction in T-dependent (Td) antigen with Th-cell; E = high-zone antibody induction with Ti antigen. SR and MR are specific antigen and mitogen receptors, respectively.

property may be activated to antibody induction by macrophages or their factors or nonspecifically by mercaptoethanol. The action of mercaptoethanol is still unclear. With T-dependent antigens, the second signal—the triggering of antibody induction—is transmitted by the T helper or cooperating cell following the activation of their *associated recognition receptor* by the antigen (Figure 10-10,D). According to the one-signal concept, Figure 10-11,C, antibody induction occurs when signal 1 is transmitted by the T helper or cooperating cell via the mitogenic receptors of the antigen-sensitive cell (B cell) following the binding of the antigen to the associated recognition receptor.

In the two-signal system, high zone paralysis occurs when the antibody receptors of the antigen-sensitive cells (B cells) are saturated with the corresponding antigens and the expanded signal 1 induces paralysis (Figure 10-10,C). On the other hand, it has been suggested that saturation of the cooperating cell or T helper cells via the associated recognition receptors would cause

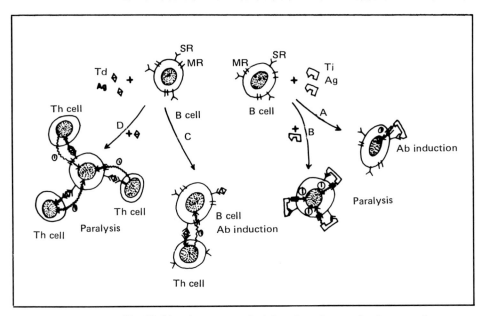

Fig. 10-11 : Immune paralysis based on the one-signal concept for the induction of antibody synthesis. A = T-independent (Ti) antigen-antibody induction; B = paralysis with Ti antigen; C = induction of antibody synthesis with T-dependent (Td) antigen; D = Td antigen paralysis. SR and MR are specific antigen and mitogenic receptors, respectively.

high-zone antibody induction (synthesis) (Figure 10-10,E). Expansion of the signal 1 mechanism by the T helper cell with the T-dependent antigen would cause paralysis, as indicated in Figure 10-11,D.

The signal 1 and signal 2 concepts of the cellular mechanism of induction and paralysis can each be supported by evidence in the literature. The answer to whether one signal or two signals is correct depends on the "resolution of the existence of functionally viable versus paralyzed self-reactive B cells, and receptor-blocked (resting B cells) versus paralyzed B cells in the T-dependent unresponsiveness." (See Cohn and Blomberg, 1975.)

The role of T suppressor cells in the regulation of antibody synthesis was presented in Chapter 5. T suppressor cells can contribute to paralysis in the following ways: (1) They may displace T helper function by binding to the associated recognition portion of the antigen; they may (2) interact with B cells directly or through release of appropriate inhibitory lymphokines; and (3) they may react with T helper cells directly. The latter action of Ts on Th cells has been demonstrated in nonresponder mice to the synthetic antigen, glutamyl-alanyl-tyrosine (GAT) (see Figure 10-5). Recent evidence, however, has shown that T suppressor cells do not play an active role in the maintenance of tolerance. Nevertheless, that T suppressor cells play a significant role in regulation of humoral antibody synthesis has been exhibited in the autoimmune diseases, such as systemic lupus erythematosus (SLE). Affected patients appear to have either a deficiency (lack of the correct number) of T suppressor cells or a functional incapacity to regulate the humoral immune response to self-antigens. This has been readily demonstrated in New Zealand Black mice (NZB), which in all cases develop a disease similar to SLE (See Chapter 14) with age (14 to 18 months). These animals also produce high levels of antibody to S3 polysaccharide with aging, and these levels can be depressed by passive administration of T cells from young NZB mice (8-10 months). Thus, loss of T suppressor regulatory function has been attributed in part to autoimmune disease. Whether it is common in natural self-tolerance for suppressor T cells to block antibody synthesis to self-antigens, or for blocking antibodies to interfere with effector T cell reactions against self-antigens, is still unclear, although these inhibitions have been demonstrated in many immune responses associated with disease processes. Through evolution, a variety of fail-safe regulatory mechanisms have developed to safeguard against the destructive antiself immune reactions. An overly effective mechanism for self-tolerance, leading to lack of protection against potentially damaging self-effects (autoimmunity) by the immune responses, would probably outweigh the protective benefits of the immune system.

Summary

1. The major histocompatibility complex (MHC) has been defined in man, chimpanzee, rhesus monkey, dog, pig, rabbit, guinea pig, mouse, rat, chicken, and *Xenopus laevis.*
2. This chapter emphasizes the histocompatibility complex (H-2) of the mouse and its role in the immune response.
3. The common functional features of all MHC demonstrated in all species are (1) principal transplantation antigens; (2) serologically defined (SD) antigen; (3) Ir genes; (4) MLR, the LD-defined antigens; (5) graft-versus-host reaction; and (6) extensive genetic polymorphism at many loci of the MHC (see Table 10-2).
4. The H-2 complex of the mouse is situated in chromosome 17 and consists of regions K, I, S, G, and D and of subregions of I, designated I-A, I-B, I-J, I-E, and I-C. The fine details of some inbred strains are included in Table 10-7.
5. The H-linked Ir genes (I region genes) control the ability of an animal to respond to a specific antigen. Nonresponders do not respond to a given specific antigen.
6. The antigens used for Ir gene studies are primarily synthetic polymers and copolymers of L-amino acids (L-glutamic acid, L-tyrosine, L-lysine, and L-alanine).

7. In both guinea pigs and mice, nonresponders (NR) and responders (R) have been demonstrated for a given antigen.
8. Mating studies of R × R, NR × NR, and NR × R have shown that the H-linked Ir gene is inherited as an autosomal dominant trait.
9. The H-linked Ir genes appear to be associated with the T-lymphocytes and T-dependent antigens.
10. T cell–macrophage interactions, T cell–B cell interactions, and macrophage–B cell interactions are all generally I region-restrictive. T suppressor cells are controlled by I-J subregion.
11. Cellular interactions are controlled by factors released by the cells. These factors are I-region gene products. T cell factors include (1) T suppressor factor(s) (TsF), which act(s) on T helper cells (causes suppression); and (2) an enhancing factor that also acts on T helper cells (stimulation). These factors may also act directly on responder cells.
12. A nonspecific allogeneic effector factor (AEF) is also elaborated by T cells and acts on B cells. It consists of a heavy and a light chain (β_2-M), total molecular weight, 45,000.
13. Macrophages elaborate a specific genetically regulated factor (GRF) and a nonspecific macrophage factor (NMF). The former is associated with soluble and the latter with particulate antigens.
14. The cytotoxic lymphocyte response in virus infections is highly I region–restrictive and immunologically specific.
15. H-linked Ir genes are distinct from allotype-linked Ir genes. The former are associated with the MHC and the T lymphocyte system. The latter are not associated with the MHC and appear to be associated with B cells and control of Ig synthesis.
16. Immunological intolerance is a state of unresponsiveness, either cell-mediated or humoral, to a given antigen. Induction of tolerance in an animal is dependent on the antigen, route of administration, antigenic dose, and maintenance of antigen levels.
17. Low zone tolerance occurs when Ts cells increase following low-dose antigen administration. High-dose tolerance results when excessive amounts of antigen are given to an animal, especially a newborn or an x-irradiated adult animal. Tolerance can be induced to all antigens but is much more difficult to attain with particulate and complex antigens (bacteria, virus, etc). It is difficult to induce tolerance in an animal previously exposed to the antigen (secondary response).
18. Both T and B cells can be rendered tolerant to an antigen. With T-dependent antigens, either T or B cells rendered unresponsive would make the animal tolerant to the antigen. T cells can be rendered tolerant more readily and for a longer time than B cells.

19. Thus far, one-signal and two-signal concepts of immune induction can explain equally well the mode of tolerance to an antigen.

20. This chapter covers areas in which much research is presently being undertaken; therefore the concepts presented may change rapidly.

Bibliography and Selected Reading

General

Benacerraf, B. *Immunogenetics and Immunodeficiency.* Baltimore: University Park, 1975.

Gill, T. J., III, Cramer, D. V., and Kunz, H. W. The major histocompatibility complex—comparison in the mouse, man, and the rat. *Am. J. Pathol.* 90:737, 1978.

Katz, D. H., and Benacerraf, B. The Regulatory Influence of Activated T Cells on B Cell Responses to Antigen. In F. J. Dixon and H. G. Kunkel (Eds.), *Advances in Immunology,* Vol. 15. New York: Academic, 1972. P. 2.

McDevitt, H. O., and Benacerraf, B. Genetic Control of Specific Immune Responses. In F. J. Dixon and H. G. Kunkel (Eds.), *Advances in Immunology,* Vol. 11. New York: Academic, 1979. P. 31.

McDevitt, H. O. (Ed.). *Ir Genes and Ia Antigens.* New York: Academic, 1978.

Seidman, J. G., Leder, A., Nan, M., Norman, B., and Leder, P. Antibody diversity. The structure of cloned immunoglobulin genes suggests a mechanism for generating new sequences. *Science* 202:11, 1978.

Major Histocompatibility Complex

Benacerraf, B., and McDevitt, H. O. The histocompatibility-linked immune response genes. *Science* 175:273, 1971.

Benacerraf, B., and Katz, D. H. The Nature and Function of Histocompatibility-Linked Immune Response Genes. In B. Benacerraf (Ed.), *Immunogenetics and Immunodeficiency.* Baltimore: University Park, 1975. P. 117.

Caldwell, J. L. Genetic Regulation of Immune Responses. In H. H. Fudenberg, D. P. Stites, J. L. Caldwell, and J. V. Well (Eds.), *Basic and Clinical Immunology* (2nd ed.). Los Altos, Calif.: Lange, 1978. P. 155.

Cantor, H., and Gershon, R. K. Immunological circuits: Cellular composition. *Fed. Proc.* 38:2058, 1979.

Frelinger, J. A., and Shreffler, D. C. The Major Histocompatibility Complexes. In B. Benacerraf (Ed.), *Immunogenetics and Immunodeficiency.* Baltimore: University Park, 1975. P. 81.

Ir Genes and Immune Response

Benacerraf, B., and Germain, R. N. Specific suppressor responses to antigen under I region control. *Fed. Proc.* 38:2053, 1979.

Erb, P., and Feldman, M. The role of macrophages in the generation of T helper cells. III. Influence of macrophage-derived factors in helper induction. *Eur. J. Immunol.* 5:759, 1975.

Germain, R. N., and Benacerraf, B. Antigen specific T cell mediated suppression. III. Induction of antigen specific suppressor T cells (Ts2) in L-glutamic acid^{60}-L-alanine^{30}-L-tyrosine^{10} (GAT) responder mice by non-responder derived GAT suppressor factor (GAT-TsF). *J. Immunol.* 121:608, 1978.

Hayes, C. E., and Bach, F. H. T cell specific murine Ia antigens: Serology of I-J and I-E subregion specificities. *J. Exp. Med.* 148:692, 1978.

Katz, D. H. Adaptive differentiation of murine lymphocytes: Implications for mechanisms of cell-cell recognition and the regulation of immune responses. *Fed. Proc.* 38:2065, 1979.

Kishimoto, T., and Ishizaka, K. Regulation of antibody response in vitro. IX. Induction of secondary anti-hapten IgG antibody response by anti-immunoglobulin enhancing soluble factor. *J. Immunol.* 114:585, 1975.

Klein, J. Genetics of Cell-Mediated Lymphocytotoxicity in the Mouse. In B. Benacerraf (Ed.), *Immunogenetics I,* Springer Seminars in Immunopathology, Vol. 1. New York: Springer, 1978. P. 31.

McDevitt, H. O., Deak, B. D., Shreffler, D. C., Klein, J., Stimpfling, J. H., and Snell, G. D. Genetic control of the immune response. Mapping of the Ir-1 locus. *J. Exp. Med.* 135:1259, 1972.

Murphy, D. G., Herzenberg, L. A., Okumura, K., and McDevitt, H. O. A new I subregion (I-J) marked by a locus (Ia-4) controlling surface determinants on suppressor T lymphocytes. *J. Exp. Med.* 144:699, 1976.

Schwartz, R. H. A clonal deletion model for Ir gene control of the immune response. *Scand. J. Immunol.* 7:3, 1978.

Tada, T., Taniguchi, M., and David, C. S. Suppressive and Enhancing T Cell Factors as I Region Gene Products: Properties and Subregion Assignment. In *Origins of Lymphocyte Diversity,* Cold Spring Harbor Symposium on Quantitative Biology, Cold Spring Harbor Laboratory of Quantitative Biology, Cold Spring Harbor, L. I., New York, 1977. Pp. 119-127, Vol. XLI.

Williams, R. M., and Benacerraf, B. Genetic control of thymus-derived cell function. I. In vitro DNA synthesis response of normal mouse spleen cells stimulated by mitogens concanavalin A and phytohemagglutinin. *J. Exp. Med.* 135:1279, 1972.

Immunological Tolerance

Anderson, B. Induction of immunity and immunologic paralysis in mice against polyvinyl pyrrholidone. *J. Immunol.* 102:1309, 1969.

Braley-Mullen, H. Selective suppression of primary IgM responses by induction of low dose paralysis to type II pneumococcal polysaccharide. *Cell. Immunol.* 37:77, 1978.

Chiller, J. M., Habicht, G. S., and Weigle, W. O. Kinetic differences in unresponsiveness of thymus and bone marrow cells. *Science* 171:813, 1971.

Cohn, M., and Blomberg, B. The self-nonself discrimination: A one or two signal mechanism? *Scand. J. Immunol.* 4:24, 1975.

Coutinho, A., and Möller, G. Immune activation of B cells. Evidence for one nonspecific triggering signal not delivered by the Ig receptors. *Scand. J. Immunol.* 3:133, 1974.

Coutinho, A., and Möller, G. The self-nonself discrimination: A one signal mechanism. *Scand. J. Immunol.* 4:99, 1975.

Coutinho, A., and Moller, G. Thymus-Independent B Cell Induction and Paralysis. In F. J. Dixon and H. G. Kunkel (Eds.), *Advances in Immunology,* Vol. 21. New York: Academic, 1975. P. 113.

Felton, L. D., Dauffmann, G., Prescott, B., and Ottinger, B. Studies on the mechanism of the immunological paralysis induced in mice by pneumococcal polysaccharides. *J. Immunol.* 74:17, 1955.

Morimoto, C. Loss of suppressor T lymphocyte function in patients with systemic lupus erythematosus (SLE). *Clin. Exp. Immunol.* 32:125, 1978.

Watson, J., Trenker, S., and Cohn, M. The use of bacterial lipopolysaccharides shows that two signals are required for the induction of antibody synthesis. *J. Exp. Med.* 138:699, 1973.

11 : Blood Group Antigens

The blood group systems encompass the important isoantigens in humans that are primarily involved in blood transfusions and organ transplants. Similar systems are also recognized in other species of mammals. The isoantigens in humans include the antigens of the ABO, Lewis, and Rh systems as well as twelve other antigenic groups recognized in erythrocytes, tissues, and body fluids. The isoantigens of erythrocytes and leukocytes are not restricted to the cells alone but can be found as part of the membrane structure in many other tissues. Some of the tissues that have isoantigens of the blood groups are listed in Table 11-1.

The isoantigens of erythrocytes play a significant role in blood transfusion and in transplantation of organs and tissues between allogeneic individuals and in certain immunological disorders.

The genetic aspects, structural nature, and role of these isoantigens in clinical medicine will be considered in this chapter.

Blood Group Antigens

The isoantigens of the ABO, Lewis, Ii, and Rh groups are recognized as part of the structural membrane of the erythrocytes. The antigenic specificities of the ABO and Lewis groups have been identified. The antigenic determinants are carbohydrates attached to proteins through the amino acids threonine or serine (Figure 11-1). Isoantigens are expressions of different alleles that occur at a single genetic locus within different individuals of one interbreeding population (genetic polymorphism). Isoantigens can be considered as the factors that make a person's tissues and blood cells immunologically unique (i.e., unlike those found in another individual).

ABO and Lewis Blood Groups

In man, the ABO isoantigens are medically important in blood transfusion and in tissue transplantation. They are found on the surface of red blood cell membranes and on various cells (especially those of epithelial origin) scattered throughout the body (Table 11-1). ABO antigens are also structurally related to bacterial and plant antigens (A, B, and H isoantigens). The bacterial antigens, particularly, with the precursor molecules of blood group isoantigens, include pneumococcal Type IV and the

Table 11-1 : Distribution of Erythrocyte Blood Group Antigens in Human Tissues

Blood Groups	Nature of Antigen	Tissue
ABO	Glycolipids in membranes soluble glycoproteins	Erythrocyted, leukocytes, platelets, epidermal cells, capillary endo-thelium, splenic sinusoids, gut epithelium, various body secre-tions, as well as certain plants and bacteria
Lewis	Glycoproteins	Serum, saliva, adsorbed onto erythrocytes
I-i	Glycolipids	Erythrocytes, leukocytes, lympho-cytes, secretions in breast milk and saliva
Rh	Primarily proteins	Confined to erythrocytes

somatic lipopolysaccharides of gram-negative bacteria. The geno-types and phenotypes of the ABO isoantigens are summarized in Table 11-2. The ABO isoantigens have reciprocal antibodies called *isohemagglutinins,* which are present in plasma. These appear soon after birth (2 to 3 months) and are primarily of the IgM class, although they often include some IgG and IgA sub-classes also. The frequency of ABO phenotypes occurring in three ethnic groups in the United States is presented in Table 11-2. The Lewis isoantigens are defined by two major antigens, Le^a and Le^b. They are glycoproteins and are present in serum and secreted in saliva. The erythrocytes acquire the Lewis pheno-type by absorbing Lewis substance from the serum.

GENETICS AND CHEMICAL NATURE. Four independent but closely related gene systems, ABO, Hh, Le and Se, determine the synthesis and specificities of five blood group isoantigens A, B, H, Le^a, and Le^b (Table 11-3). The ABO blood group is geneti-cally controlled by three alleles at one genetic locus (three allelic genes). These are the A, B, and O alleles, where O is an amorph. The O allele is expressed as the *absence* of the A and B alleles and is also involved in the expression of the H isoantigen. Sub-groups (notably A_1 and A_2) have been demonstrated in the A group. The secretory gene, Se, determines the capacity of an individual to secrete A, B, and/or H isoantigens. The Le pheno-type is closely related to the secretor status of the individual.

The ABO and Le isoantigens are glycolipids and glycoproteins on the erythrocyte membrane. Recent evidence indicates that blood group A and I (see Ii Blood Group) antigenic sites are

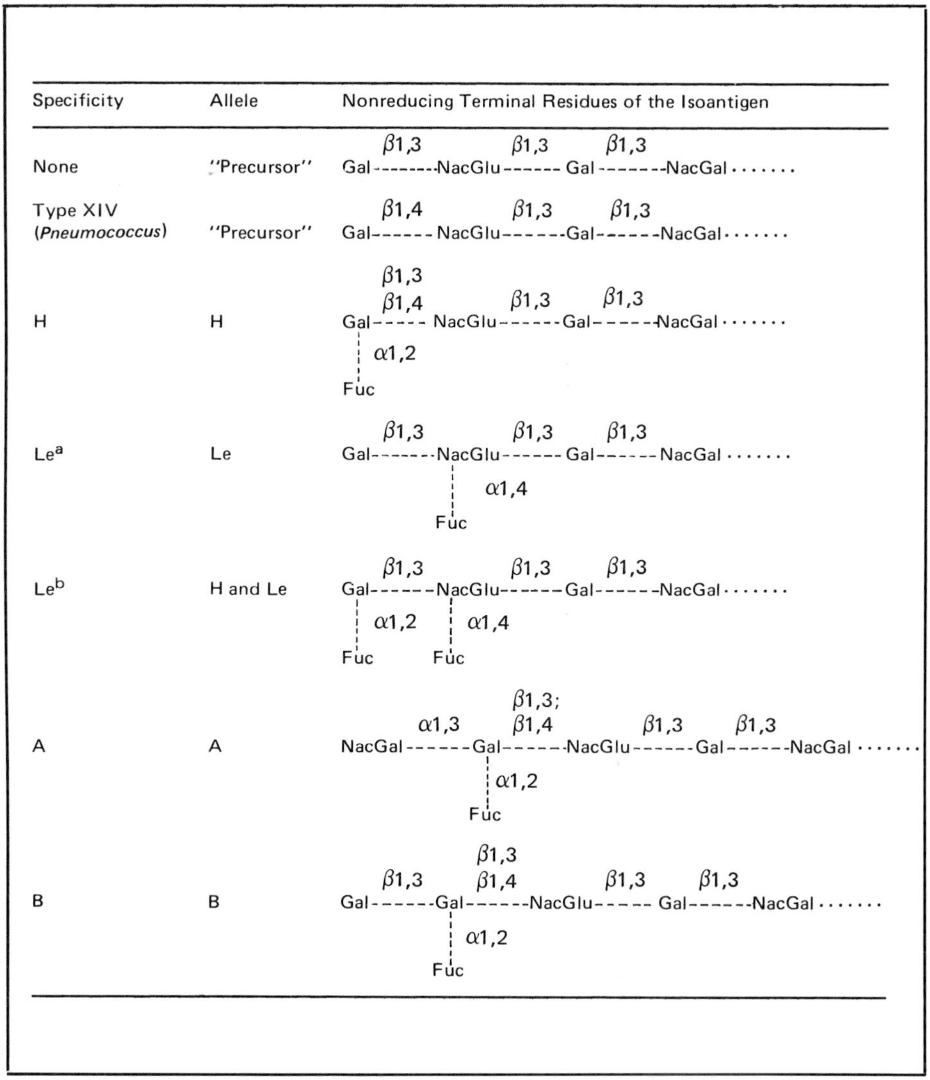

Specificity	Allele	Nonreducing Terminal Residues of the Isoantigen
None	"Precursor"	$\beta1,3$ ⟶ $\beta1,3$ ⟶ $\beta1,3$ Gal-------NacGlu------Gal------NacGal·······
Type XIV (*Pneumococcus*)	"Precursor"	$\beta1,4$ ⟶ $\beta1,3$ ⟶ $\beta1,3$ Gal------NacGlu------Gal------NacGal·······
H	H	$\beta1,3$ $\beta1,4$ ⟶ $\beta1,3$ ⟶ $\beta1,3$ Gal------NacGlu------Gal------NacGal······· ┊ $\alpha1,2$ Fuc
Le^a	Le	$\beta1,3$ ⟶ $\beta1,3$ ⟶ $\beta1,3$ Gal------NacGlu------Gal------NacGal······· ┊ $\alpha1,4$ Fuc
Le^b	H and Le	$\beta1,3$ ⟶ $\beta1,3$ ⟶ $\beta1,3$ Gal------NacGlu------Gal------NacGal······· ┊ $\alpha1,2$ ┊ $\alpha1,4$ Fuc Fuc
A	A	$\beta1,3$; $\alpha1,3$ $\beta1,4$ $\beta1,3$ $\beta1,3$ NacGal------Gal------NacGlu------Gal------NacGal······· ┊ $\alpha1,2$ Fuc
B	B	$\beta1,3$ $\beta1,3$ $\beta1,4$ $\beta1,3$ $\beta1,3$ Gal------Gal------NacGlu------Gal------NacGal······· ┊ $\alpha1,2$ Fuc

Fig. 11-1 : Antigenic determinants of the ABO and Lewis blood groups.

Note: 1. The first two isoantigens, labeled "precursor," are the basic carbohydrate sequences to which are added specific residues to form the ABO antigenic determinants. The first one is nonspecific while the second one is, as indicated, related to Type XIV (*Pneumococcus*) antigen.
2. Le^a and Le^b are the Lewis blood group isoantigens. They were discovered after the original ABO grouping was formed but are chemically closely related to the ABO isoantigens.
3. Gal = galactose; NacGlu = *N*-acetylglucosamine; NacGal = *N*-acetylgalactosamine; Fuc = fucose (6-deoxy-L-galactose).
4. When more than one type of linkage ($\beta1,3; \beta1,4$) is shown, both are known to occur without altering the antigenic specificity.

Table 11-2 : ABO Blood Groups

Genotype	Phenotype	Isoantigen in Red Cells	Isohemagglutinin Present in Plasma	Frequency, United States (%)		
				Caucasians	Negroes	Chinese
A_1O	A_1	A and A_1	Anti-B	27.6	—	—
A_1A_1				4.4	—	—
A_1A_2				2.9	—	—
A_2A_2	A_2	A	Anti-B	0.5	—	—
A_2O				9.2	—	—
Totals				44.6	27.0	28.0
BO	B	B	Anti-A and anti-A_1	8.05	—	—
BB				0.37	—	—
Totals				8.42	21.0	23.0
OO	O	H	Anti-A and anti-B	45.0	48.0	36.0
A_1B	A_1B	A_1 and B	None	2.54	—	—
A_2B	A_2B	A_2 and B	None	0.85	—	—
Totals				3.39	4.0	13.0

(—) Figures are not available for the phenotypes of these subgroups.

Table 11-3 : The Erythrocytic Phenotype and Antigenic Specificities Found in Secretions and the Probable Genotype of Each

Erythrocyte			Antigens Secreted			
ABH	Le^a	Le^b	ABH	Le^a	Le^b	Genotype
—	—	—	—	—	—	ABO, hh, lele (Se or sese)
—	3+	—	—	3+	—	ABO, hh, Le (Se or sese)
3+	—	—	—	—	—	ABO, H, sese, lele
3+	—	—	3+	—	—	ABO, H, Se, lele
3+	3+	—	—	3+	—	ABO, H, sese, Le
3+	—	2+	3+	+	2+	ABO, H, Se, Le

— = absences; numbers represent degree of antigenicity.
Source: W. M. Watkins, *Science* 152:172, 1966.

exclusively localized on the external surface of erythrocyte membranes. In secretions, such as saliva, the blood group iso-antigens are primarily glycoprotein in nature.

The antigenic specificity of the ABH and Le isoantigens is determined by the manner in which the four sugars D-galactose, L-fucose, N-acetyl-D-galactosamine, and N-acetylglucosamine are linked to two types of backbone precursor molecules (type 1 and 2 chains: see Figure 11-1). The two chains differ in their mode of linkage between D-galactose and N-acetylglucosamine. Type 1 precursor has no specificity and has $\beta1,3$ linkage, while Type 2 is similar in specificity to pneumococcal antigen (XIV) and has $\beta1,4$ linkage. However, Type 1 also cross-reacts with anti-pneumococcal XIV antiserum. The ABH and Le genes regulate the synthesis of the specific enzyme glycosyl transferases. These enzymes in turn are responsible for the mode of linkage of the sugars to specific positions on type 1 or 2 chains. Thus the conversion of precursor substances to specific H substance is done via the influence of the H gene, which adds L-fucose to D-galactose through an $\alpha1,2$ linkage. In turn, the H substance is a precursor of the A and B isoantigens. The A and B genes regulate the glycosyl transferase that modulates the addition of N-acetylgalactosamine and D-galactose in $\alpha1,3$ linkage to the H substance. N-acetylgalactosamine determines the A antigenic specificity. The B antigenic specificity is determined by D-galactose.

The secretor gene (Se) regulates the secretion or availability of the unaltered precursors (Type 1 or 2) or Le^a substance in secretor fluids, such as saliva to the glycosyl transferases, which are controlled by the ABH genes. The secretor gene (Se) does not elaborate a specific substance. Thus, the precursors and the Le^a substance are the substrates for the H gene (Figure 11-1). Individuals with genotypes sese are nonsecretors, that is, the A, B, or H substances are not found in saliva. However, these individuals have A, B, or H on their erythrocyte membranes (Table 11-3). It has been demonstrated that about 20 percent of Europeans are genotypically sese, i.e., nonsecretors.

The expression of the Le phenotype is regulated by the Se gene, although the Le and Se genes are inherited independently. Individuals having the Le gene (LeLe or Lele genotypes) elaborate the fucosyl transferase that attaches L-fucose to N-acetyl-D-glucosamine in an α1,4 linkage to precursor type 1 chain. This specifies the Le^a isoantigen. In those individuals with A, B, and H genes but lacking the secretor gene (genotype sese), the precursor and Le^a substance are acted upon by the A, B, and H enzymes. These individuals have Le^a glycolipid adsorbed to the erythrocyte membrane surface and Le^a glycoprotein in the saliva. The presence of SeSe or Sese genotypes in individuals with A, B, and H gene products converts the precursor and the Le^a substance (presence of Le genotype) to H and Le^b substances, respectively, by addition of L-fucose to the precursor (H substance) and a second L-fucose to Le^a to give Le^b. The Le^a substance on erythrocyte membrane is conspicuously absent in these individuals. Thus, the Le^b phenotype is due to the product of the interaction of H, Le, and Se genes. Le^b phenotypic individuals have trace amounts of Le^a, plus large amounts of H and Le^b in their saliva, and the erythrocytes contain only adsorbed Le^b (see Figure 11-1 and Table 11-3).

A rare instance of individuals with an absence of H gene (hh) has been observed in Bombay. These individuals ("Bombay" phenotype), have demonstrated circulating anti-A, and anti-B, and potent anti-H antibodies in their sera. Being hh genotype, they are unable to form H substance (precursor for the A, B, and Le^b substances) and thus also unable to form A and B substances, even in the presence of A and B genes.

The Ii group is similar to the isoantigens of the ABO groups. Adult erythrocytes possess mostly I isoantigens, with lesser amounts of i, whereas the inverse is demonstrated for newborn erothrocytes. Adult phenotype patterns of Ii appear after 18 months of age. These antigens are associated with serological specificities of cold-reacting antibodies. Multiple antigens to anti-I and anti-i have been detected in human ovarian cyst fluids and within sheep hydatid cyst fluid. These antigens appear to be precursors of A, B, H, and Le substances or degradation products thereof.

Table 11-4 : Genetic Scheme for the Explanation of Rh Isoantigen Inheritance and Regulation

Chromosomal Loci	Antigenic Determinant	Rh Phenotype
D	D	
C	C	Rh^+
E	E	
D	D	
C	C	Rh^+
e	e	
d	None	
c	c	Rh^-
e	e	

Rh System

Rh red cell isoantigens are medically important in transfusions and to some extent in tissue transplantation. Rh isoantigens have been demonstrated only in the erythrocytes of man and monkey (the term Rh is derived from the *Rhesus* monkey). The phenotypes and genotypes of the Rh isoantigens are summarized in Table 11-4. Rh isoantigens have no reciprocal natural antibodies but are so highly immunogenic that improper transfusion from an Rh-positive (Rh^+) to an Rh-negative (Rh^-) individual results in anti-Rh^+ antibody production in the Rh^- recipient. Similarly, transmission of red cells during parturition from an Rh^+ infant to an RH^- mother (across the placental barrier, for example) can stimulate anti-Rh^+ antibodies in the parent. An Rh^+ fetus conceived in a subsequent pregnancy can be seriously affected by the anti-Rh^+ IgG1 antibodies carried by the mother, since these are able to cross the placenta and enter the fetal circulation. This disorder is known as *Erythroblastosis fetalis* or hemolytic disease of the newborn. Severe destruction of fetal erythrocyte occurs, with release of excessive bilirubin, which causes jaundice and brain tissue damage. Lack of glucuronyl transferase in the infant's immature liver contributes to this phenomenon (Figure 11-2).

Isoantigens of the Rh system are genetically complex. Two acceptable genetic schemes have been suggested as explanations of the expression of the Rh antigens on the erythrocyte surfaces. These are the *Fisher-Race* and *Wiener* theories of Rh isoantigen inheritance. The Fisher-Race theory suggests the presence of five distinct determinants, designated D, C, E, c, and e, which are

288

Fig. 11-2 : Mechanism of jaundice formation in hemolytic disease of the newborn. Jaundice does not occur before delivery, because the bilirubin produced by the breakdown of RBC by the fetal spleen passes via the placenta to the maternal circulation. The fetal bilirubin is transported by the albumin to maternal liver, where glucuronyl transferase (G-T) converts bilirubin to excretable direct bilirubin. B. The liver of a newborn does not produce G-T and thus is unable to convert bilirubin to the excretable form. The consequence of bilirubin accumulation is jaundice and brain tissue damage.

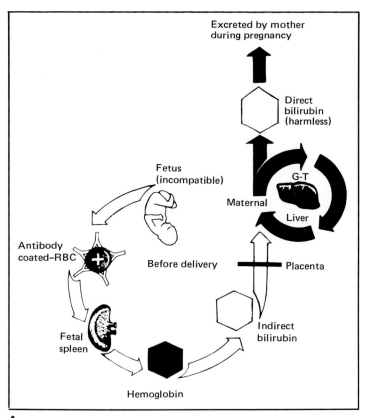

A

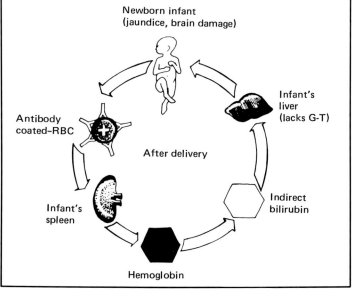

B

Table 11-5 : Wiener's Genetic Scheme for the Explanation of Rh Isoantigen Inheritance and Regulation*

Chromosomal Loci	Antigenic Determinant	Rh Phenotype
R^1	Rh_o	
	rh$'$	Rh^+
	rh$''$	
r$'$	hr$'$	
		Rh^-
	hr$''$	

*In the Wiener scheme, R^0, R^1, R^2, and R^z relate to Rh^+ isoantigen and r, r$'$, r$''$, and r^y represent Rh^-. This is seen in Table 11-6.

products of genes situated at three distinct but closely linked chromosomal loci. Crossing over is infrequent due to the close proximity of the genes to each other. It is thought that one set of three alleles is inherited from each parent. This is similar to the concept of one cistron regulating the product of one antigenic determinant, the Rh phenotype, and is summarized in Table 11-4. *Cistron* refers to a segment of DNA which specifies a single functional unit, such as a protein or enzyme, and within which 2 heterozygous and closely linked recessive mutations are expressed in the phenotype when the cistron is located on two separate homologous chromosomes, but isn't when located on the same chromosome. The gene regulating D is significant, since it expresses the Rh^+ isoantigen important in clinical medicine. This isoantigen is responsible for *Erythroblastosis fetalis* in newborns. It accounts for nearly all (90 percent) of the hemolytic diseases of the newborn resulting from maternal isoimmunization. The alternative allele, small d, is hypothetical. It represents the *absence* of D isoantigen, since the presence of a d isoantigen has not been shown to date.

The second theory (multiple allele), that of Wiener, suggests that one chromosomal locus is responsible for the regulation of several antigenic determinants (multiple allele). This is shown in Table 11-5. Table 11-6 is a detailed summary of the known Rh blood group antigens, their frequency in the caucasoid ethnic group, and the designations of the Wiener and Fisher-Race schemes.

Other Blood Groups   There are approximately twelve other blood group isoantigens of the human erythrocytes. They have been useful primarily in

Table 11-6 : Rh Blood Group: Rh-Hr Phenotypes, Genotypes, and Frequencies in Caucasoid Population

Rh Positive = 83.2%

Reactions with anti-						Designation		Genotypes		Frequencies Caucasoid (%)	Totals
Rh_0 D	rh' C	rh" E	hr' c	hr" e	hr f	Wiener	Fisher-Race	Wiener	Fisher-Race		
+	−	−	+	+	+	Rh_0rh	cDe/c-e	R^0r R^0R^0	cDe/cde	1.9950	
									cDe/cDe	0.0659	2.1
+	+	−	+	+	+	Rh_1rh	CDe/c-e	R^1r, R^1R^0, R^0r'	CDe/cde	32.6808	
									CDe/cDe	2.1585	35.0
+		−	−	+	−	Rh_1Rh_1	CDe/C-e	R^1R^1, R^1R'	CDe/Cde	0.0505	
									CDe/CDe	17.6803	
									CDe/Cde	0.8270	18.5
+	−	+	+	+	+	Rh_2rh	cDe/c-e	R^2r, R^2R^0, R^0r''	cDE/cde	10.9657	
									cDE/cDe	0.7243	
									cDe/cdE	0.0610	11.8
+	−	+	+	−	−	Rh_2Rh_2	cDE/c-E	R^2R^2, R^2r''	cDE/cDE	1.9906	
									cDE/cdE	0.3353	2.3
+				+	−	Rh_1Rh_2	CDe/c-E	$R^1R^2R^1r''$, R^2r'	CDE/CDE	11.8648	
									CDe/cdE	0.9992	
									cDE/Cde	0.2775	13.1
+	+	+	+	+	+	Rh_zrh	CDE/c-e	R^zr, $R^zR^zR^0$, R^0r^y	CDE/cde	0.1893	
									CDE/cDe	0.0125	
									cDe/CdE	0.0003	0.2
+			−	+	−	Rh_zRh_1	CDE/C-e	R^zR^1, R^zr', R^1r^y	CDE/CDE	0.2048	
									CDE/Cde	0.0048	
									CDe/CdE	0.0042	0.21
+	+		−	−	−	Rh_zRh_2	CDE/c-E	R^zR^2, R^zr', R^1r^y	CDE/cDE	0.0687	
									CDE/cdE	0.0059	
									cDE/CdE	0.0014	0.07
+			−	−	−	Rh_zRh_z	CDE/C-E	R^zR^z, R^zr^y	CDE/CDE	0.0006	
									CDE/CdE	0.00001	0.0006

Table 11-6 (continued)

Rh Negative = 16.8%

Reactions with anti-						Designation		Genotypes		Frequencies Caucasoid (%)	Totals
Rho D	rh′ C	rh″ E	hr′ c	hr″ e	hr f	Wiener	Fisher-Race	Wiener	Fisher-Race		
−	−	−	+	+	+	rh	cde/cde	rr	cde/cde	15.102	15.102
−	+	−	+	+	−	rh′rh	Cde/cde	r′r	Cde/cde	0.7664	
			−	+	−	rh′rh′	Cde/Cde	r′r′	Cde/Cde	0.0097	
+	−	+	+	+	+	rh″rh	cdE/cde	r″r	cdE/cde	0.9235	
			+	−	−	rh″rh″	cdE/cdE	r″r″	cdE/cdE	0.0414	
−	+	+	+	+	−	rh′rh″	Cde/cdE	r′r″	Cde/cdE	0.234	
			+	+	+	rh_yrh	CdE/cde	r_yr	CdE/cde	0.0039	
			−	+	−	rh_yrh′	CdE/Cde	r_yr′	CdE/Cde	0.0001	
			+	−	−	rh_yrh″	CdE/cdE	r_yr″	CdE/cdE	0.0001	
			−	−	−	$rh_y rh_y$	CdE/CdE	$r_y r_y$	CdE/CdE	0.000001	

medicolegal and anthropological problems. With the exception of rare transfusion difficulties, the contribution of these groups to diseases has not been ascertained.

Neutrophil- and Platelet-Specific Antigens

There are several unique neutrophil isoantigens, which are specified by two gene loci, NA and NB. The NA gene consists of NA1 and NA2 alleles, while the NB locus is presently composed of one allele, NB1. In addition to these specific isoantigens, neutrophils also have HLA antigens specified by the loci A, B, and C.

The major isoantigens of platelets involved in transplantation are those specified by the HLA system, which includes loci A, B, and C. HLA antigens of the D locus are not found in platelets. Nonetheless, isoantigens specific to platelets alone have been defined. These isoantigens have been implicated in a number of clinical conditions, including sensitization to allografts, thrombocytopenia purpura, and problems of autoimmunization via drugs, particularly in secondary effects on "self" constituents of platelets. The specific platelet isoantigens that have been defined, each having two allelomorphs are KO^a and KO^b; $P1^{E1}$ and $P1^{E2}$; and ZW^a ($P1^{A1}$) and ZW^b. These isoantigens are related to three loci that specify the alleles. Allele is a short form of allelomorph and refers to one of two genes present at a locus, that control a particular characteristic. The frequencies (%) of KO^a and KO^b are 7.4 and 92.6 respectively, while those for ZW^a and ZW^b are 84.5 and 15.5 respectively. These antigens are not found on red cells or leukocytes and are inherited as codominant factors. They are not linked to sex nor to the genes of red blood cells.

Hemolytic Disease of the Newborn Due to Rh Incompatibility

In a first pregnancy, the separation of the placenta following delivery results in the rupture of the placental vessels (villi) and connective tissue, allowing escape of the fetal erythrocytes. Prior to the complete constriction of the open end of the maternal blood vessels, some fetal blood may enter the maternal circulation. The Rh antigen in the fetal erythrocytes if incompatible evokes immune responses, initiating antibody production. In a subsequent pregnancy residual antibodies (IgG) from the response to red cells of the previous incompatible fetus (or also donor) of an incompatible can pass through the placental barrier. These antibodies attach to the specific red cell antigen sites of the fetus (if Rh-incompatible) of the second pregnancy. The life span of the sensitized fetal red cells is shortened, and these cells are readily destroyed in the fetal spleen. The infant will suffer from anemia and its consequences. Jaundice does not occur in the infant before delivery, because the bilirubin produced passes via the placenta to the maternal circulation. Maternal serum albumin transports the fetal bilirubin to the maternal liver, where an enzyme (glucuronyl transferase) converts it to excretable direct bilirubin. The liver of the neonate does not produce glucuronyl transferase and thus is unable to convert bilirubin to an excretable form. Consequently bilirubin accumulates in fetal tissues, causing jaundice and brain tissue damage. Figure 11-2 shows hemolytic disease of the newborn attributed to Rh erythrocyte incompatibility.

Rh isoimmunization can be prevented following the initial and subsequent pregnancies in an Rh-negative mother (with an Rh^+ fetus) by passive immunization with high-titered human anti-Rh_o(D) immunoglobulin (RhoGAM). An intravascular injection of 200 to 300 μg of Rh_o immune globulin to the mother within 72 hours of delivery has proved highly effective in preventing Rh isoimmunization, provided the mother is not already isoimmunized by the time the injection is given and the dose of antigen (from fetus) to which she is exposed is not too great. This preventive procedure must be repeated after each pregnancy. Passive immunization during the third trimester appears not to affect the fetus.

The mode of prevention by passive anti-Rh_o(D) immunization may be as follows: (1) Rh_o isoantigenic red cells are sequestered and destroyed before stimulation of the immune response of the mother can occur through macrophage processing of sensitized fetal red cells; this processing may differ from processing of foreign nonsensitized fetal red cells; and (2) through negative feedback mechanisms, the excessively added IgG immune globulin suppresses antibody synthesis.

The incidence of hemolytic disease in the newborn due to ABO incompatibility is 0.5 to 3.0 percent of pregnancies. Only one out of 300 newborn infants, however, requires treatment for hemolysis due to ABO incompatibility. The ABO hemolytic disease arises when the mother has anti-A or anti-B of the IgG class and the fetus inherits an A_1 or B phenotype from the father. Invariably the mothers are of the group O blood type. Unlike Rh hemolytic disease, the clinical manifestation may occur in the first pregnancy.

Blood Transfusion Reactions

Adverse blood transfusion reactions may result from immunological and nonimmunological factors. Nonhemolytic reactions account for about 95 percent of transfusion reactions.

The immunological factors manifested in transfusion reactions can be attributed to (1) plasma proteins, which generally involve an allergic type reaction resembling that of serum sickness;

Table 11-7 : Nonimmunological Causes of Blood Transfusion Reactions

Air or fat embolism

Circulating overload

Febrile reactions due to pyrogenic factors (endotoxins)

Hypotension and hypothermia due to cold blood

Transmission of infectious disease

Metabolic abnormalities due to acid-citrate-dextrose (ACD) anticoagulant

Thrombophlebitis at site of administration of blood

Hemosiderosis due to hemolytic RBC

(2) erythrocytes, which cause the hemolytic transfusion reactions associated with mediation of the complement system; (3) leukocytes, which cause the transfusion reactions seen especially in multiparous females and in individuals who have received multiple whole blood transfusions: these individuals have anti-leukocyte antibodies, some of which may be to the HLA antigens; and (4) platelets, which, like leukocytes, give rise to transfusion difficulties in multiparous women (age >40) and in individuals receiving multiple whole blood transfusions. Patients generally develop posttransfusion purpura, characterized by petechiae, hemorrhage, and ecchymoses. The nonimmunological manifestations, which occur more commonly than the immunological ones in transfusions, are listed in Table 11-7. In addition to blood transfusion, the blood group isoantigens have been used for paternity testing.

Summary

1. The blood group isoantigens of human erythrocytes are classified into 15 groups on the basis of their distinctive antigenic specificities and structural similarities.
2. The major groups, on which many studies have been done, are the ABO, Lewis, and Rh systems. The isoantigens of these groups are constituents of the structural portion of the erythrocyte membrane.
3. Reciprocal antibody, generally of the IgM class, is normally present, e.g., a B individual has an anti-A antibody in the plasma.
4. The ABO and Lewis group specificities reside in the carbohydrate residues attached via the amino acids threonine or serine to proteins. These isoantigens are important in blood transfusion and in tissue transplantation.
5. The ABO and Lewis isoantigens are expressions of different alleles that occur at a single genetic locus in different individuals of an interbreeding population (genetic polymorphism).

6. The ABO, Hh, Le and Se gene systems determine the synthesis and specificities of the five blood group isoantigens, A, B, H, Le[a], and Le[b].

7. The antigenic specificity of the A, B, H, and Le isoantigens is determined by four sugar residues, D-galactose, L-fucose, N-acetyl-D-galactosamine, and N-acetylglucosamine, linked to two types of backbone precursors, designated 1 and 2.

8. Ii isoantigens are similar to the ABO group isoantigens. Adult erythrocytes have mostly I, while newborn red cells have mostly i.

9. Rh isoantigens have been demonstrated only in the erythrocytes of man and monkey. No reciprocal antibodies are present. Therefore an Rh[-] individual can be sensitized following exposure to Rh[+] erythrocytes.

10. The disorder known as erythroblastosis fetalis (hemolytic disorder of the newborn) is commonly triggered by an Rh[+] fetus of an Rh[-] mother. Severity increases with subsequent pregnancies if not prevented by RhoGAM treatment (anti-Rh[+] antiserum) after the birth of the first child.

11. Rh antigens are modulated by a complex array of genes, either at a single locus (Wiener theory) or at three loci (Fisher-Race theory) on a chromosome. Genetic polymorphism is suggested.

12. Neutrophils and platelets have HLA antigens in addition to their own specific isoantigens.

13. Blood transfusion reactions are mostly nonimmunological (95 percent). The immunological reactions (5 percent) include (1) allergic type reactions; (2) hemolytic reactions involving complement action; (3) antileukocyte-leukocyte reactions; and (4) antiplatelet-platelet reactions.

Bibliography and Selected Reading

General

Hokama, Y. Immunochemistry. In N. V. Bhagavan (Ed.), *Biochemistry* (2nd ed.). Philadelphia: Lippincott, 1978. P. 1075.

Race, R. R., and Sanger, R. (Ed.). *Blood Groups in Man*. Philadelphia: Davis, 1968.

Slomiany, A., Slomiany, B. L., and Glass, G. B. The nature of the ABH blood group antigens in human gastric secretion. *Biochem. Biophys. Acta* 540:278, 1978.

Watanabe, K., Powell, M., and Hakamori, S. Isolation and characterization of a novel fucoganglioside of human erythrocyte membrane. *J. Biol. Chem.* 253:8962, 1978.

Weismann, G., and Clairborne, R. (Eds.). *Cell Membrane, Biochemistry, Cell Biology, and Pathology*. New York: H. P. Publishing, 1975.

Whittmore, M. B., and Shuster, J. Immunohematology. In S. O. Freedman and P. Gold (Eds.), *Clinical Immunology* (2nd ed.). Hagerstown, Md.: Harper and Row, 1976. P. 318.

Wood, C., Kabat, E. A., Ebisu, E., and Goldstein, I. J. An immunological study of the combining sites of the second lectin isolated from *Bandeirraea simplicifolia* (BS II). *Ann. Immunol.* (Paris) 129:143,1978.

Young, E., and Roth, F. J. Immunological cross-reactivity between glycoprotein isolated from *Trichophyton mentagrophytes* and human isoantigen A. *J. Invest. Dermatol.* 92:46, 1979.

Blood Group Isoantigens

Abramson, N., and Schur, P. H. The IgG subclasses of red cell antibodies and relationship to monocyte binding. *Blood* 40:500, 1972.

Morley, G. A study of different rhesus phenotypes and their binding characteristics. *Vox Sang.* 35:382, 1978.

Nagai, N., and Yoshida, A. Possible existence of hybrid glycosyltransferase in heterozygous blood group AB subjects. *Vox Sang.* 35:378, 1978.

Schenkel-Brunner, H., Catron, J. P., and Doinel, C. Localization of blood-group A and I antigenic sites on inside-out and rightside out human erythrocyte membrane vehicle. *Immunology* 36:33, 1979.

Walborg, E. F., Jr. Current Concepts of Glycoprotein Structure. In R. F. Gould (Ed.), *Glycoproteins and Glycolipids in Disease Processes*. Washington, D.C.: ACS Symposium Series 80, 1978. Pp. 1–20.

Watkins, W. M. Blood group substances. *Science* 152:172, 1966.

Zdebska, E., and Koscielak, J. Studies on the structure and I blood-group activity of poly (glycosyl) ceramides. *Eur. J. Biochem.* 91:517, 1978.

Hemolytic Diseases and Transfusion Reactions

Dixon, R., Rosse, W., and Ebbert, L. Quantitative determination of antibody in idiopathic thrombocytopenic purpura. Correlation of serum and platelet bound antibody with clinical response. *N. Engl. J. Med.* 292: 230, 1975.

Eklund, J. Production of plasma with high anti-D concentration in Rh-negative. *Vox Sang.* 35:387, 1978.

Freda, V. J., Gorman, J. G., Pollack, W., and Bowe, E. Prevention of Rh hemolytic disease: Ten years clinical experience with Rh immune globulin. *N. Engl. J. Med.* 292:1014, 1975.

Siskind, G. W. Immunologic suppression of primary Rh antibody formation. *Transfusion* 8:127, 1968.

12 : The Major Histocompatibility Complex and Transplantation Immunology

The biological significance of the chromosomal region, defined as the major histocompatibility complex (MHC), that determines the strong transplantation antigens, is not restricted to allograft survival only, but is involved also in a large array of other biological phenomena, such as the immune responses and susceptibility to disease.

With the advent of tissue transplantation, the histocompatibility lymphocyte isoantigens have become tremendously important to clinical medicine. These isoantigens designated HLA (most of the terminology used in this chapter has been defined in Chapter 10) are found on the surfaces of white blood cells, particularly lymphocytes, and also in platelets, serum body fluids, and all the nucleated fixed tissues of the body. Few or no HLA antigens have been found, however, in human erythrocytes although significant levels have been found in rodent (mouse and rat) red blood cells. These HLA antigens, especially on lymphocyte surfaces, have been the basis for donor selection in organ transplantation.

Major Histocompatibility Complex (MHC) of Man: Histocompatibility Leukocyte Antigens (HLA)

The major histocompatibility complex antigens are recognized or analyzed by (1) the serological technique using lymphocytotoxic antibodies, obtained from multiparous females or from recipients of multiple transfusions, in the presence of complement; and (2) the mixed lymphocyte culture (MLC) assay. The latter uses cell-cell interaction (responding + target cells) and the incorporation or ^{3}H-thymidine following blastogenesis by the responding cell. The serological technique is called the SD or S-determinant method, while the MLC assay is designated as LD or L-determinant. The LD antigens are defined by and are particularly effective in activating the T helper cells (Th), whereas the SD antigens activate Th cells poorly or not at all. The SD antigens are not clearly defined as targets for cytotoxic-mediated lympholysis (CML). Thus cytotoxic determinants (CD) have been established as target antigens for the cytotoxic lymphocytes. Other systems used in defining MHC antigens are the homozygous typing cell (HTC) and the primed LD typing (PLT) assay systems.

Unlike studies with mice, which have employed inbred and congenic recombinant strains, the study of the human MHC has

297

Fig. 12-1 : A, B. Structure of the HLA antigen. C. After detergent solubilization, cleavage with papain occurs at sites 1 and 2, giving fragments F$_H$ and F$_M$. When papain is used directly, cleavage is at 2 (F$_H$ fragment) only.

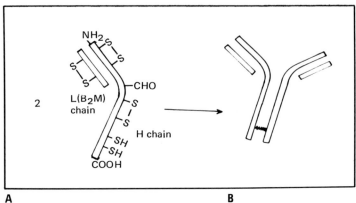

A   B

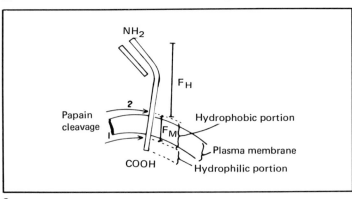

C

relied primarily on population and family studies. The serologically defined and MLR procedures have delineated our present knowledge of the MHC complex in man, which is discussed in this section.

Chemistry of the HLA Antigens

It has been demonstrated that the HLA antigens consist of two chains, linked noncovalently: a β_2-microglobulin, 12,000 (P12)-dalton light chain, and a glycoprotein heavy chain of 44,000 (P44) daltons. The glycoprotein chain, at its carboxyl end, spans the bimolecular layer of the cell membrane and is anchored by the hydrophobic region of the bimolecular cell membrane (Figure 12-1). The β_2-microglobulin (β_2M) light chain has structural homology with the constant region of the γ-chain of IgG. Papain hydrolysis yields F$_M$ and F$_H$ fragments, as depicted in Figure 12-1C. Solubilization of the HLA molecules yields a covalent bond between the two heavy chains of the HLA molecules to give a tetrapeptide structure (Figure 12-1B). β_2-microglobulin has no carbohydrate residues and has no antigenic specificity regarding H-2 or HLA types. On the other hand, the heavy chain is variable and carries the HLA specificity. β_2M is produced by various cells of the body. It was first isolated from the urine of man and is presently used clinically for detection of certain types of kidney disease. The gene that regulates or specifies β_2M is found on chromosome 15.

HLA antigens are shed into body fluids. They develop early in fetal life, at approximately 6 weeks of development, and persist throughout life. HLA antigens are present in all nucleated cells (thus low or absent on human red cells) and constitute about 1 to 2 percent of the membrane proteins of the cells. (See Figure 12–3 for other properties of the HLA antigens.)

HLA Antigens

The genetic control of HLA is maintained by a complex of linked genes at five chromosomal loci. These genes are termed *segregants* or *subloci.* The HLA system is similar to the Rh system in that the linked genes are transmitted in a group (haplotype) from one generation to the next.

The group of allelic genes (pair of HLA allelic determinants) contributed by each parent is referred to as the *haplotype.* Schematically these are shown as segregated, linked genes following mendelian principles of genetics (Figure 12–2). These genes have many alleles within the population and are therefore polymorphic. There are approximately 77 known HLA antigens. Phenotypically, from what is known presently, no individual can have more than one haplotype from each parent. The segregant series of HLA antigens summarized in 1980 (see Terasaki) are shown in Table 12–1. Table 12–1 summarized the serologically defined (SD) and MLC-defined (LD) major human histocompatibility (HLA) loci and the antigens they specify. An increase in numbers of HLA in series A and B has resulted from the further subdivision of some of the originally recognized HLA. For example, HLA-A9 has been subdivided into HLA-Aw23 and HLA-Aw24. It is anticipated that further studies will reveal more new antigens. In Table 12–2 the frequency of HLA antigens in some ethnic groups and chimpanzees is compiled.

The HLA-A, -B, and -C loci have been established through the use of antibodies (antileukocyte) from multiparous women and from recipients of multiple blood transfusions. These antibodies detect the defined cell surface antigens of lymphocytes (the SD approach). The locus HLA-D has been defined via the mixed lymphocyte culture procedure (MLC), in which cell surface differences are examined by the proliferative response of peripheral lymphocytes in vitro (the LD approach). These approaches define the differences in the biological role of, and in the antigenic determinants of, the MHC.

SD ANTIGENS. The HLA complex of man contains four distinct loci, three of which (A, B, and C) are defined by serological means (SD) using anti-HLA antibodies and complement in the

**Table 12-1 : Major Human Histocompatibility Loci
and the HLA Antigens Specified**

	Serologically Defined (SD)	
HLA-A (20)	HLA-B (42)	HLA-C (8)
HLA-A1	HLA-Bw4	HLA-Cw1
HLA-A2		HLA-Cw2
HLA-A3	HLA-B5	HLA-Cw3
	HLA-Bw6	HLA-Cw4
HLA-A9	HLA-B7	HLA-Cw5
	HLA-B8	HLA-Cw6
		HLA-Cw7
HLA-A10	HLA-B12	HLA-Cw8
	HLA-B13	
HLA-A11	HLA-B14	
	HLA-B15	
	HLA-Bw16	
HLA-Aw19		
	HLA-B17	
	HLA-B18	
HLA-Aw23 (9)		
HLA-Aw24 (9)	HLA-Bw21	
HLA-A25 (10)		HLA-Bw49 (w21)
HLA-A26 (10)	HLA-Bw22	HLA-Bw50 (w21)
HLA-A28	HLA-B27	HLA-Bw51 (5)
HLA-A29	HLA-Bw35	HLA-Bw52 (5)
HLA-Aw30	HLA-B37	HLA-Bw53
HLA-Aw31	HLA-Bw38 (w16)	HLA-Bw54 (w22)
HLA-Aw32	HLA-Bw39 (w16)	HLA-Bw55 (w22)
HLA-Aw33	HLA-B40	HLA-Bw56 (w22)
HLA-Aw34	HLA-Bw41	HLA-Bw57 (17)
HLA-Aw36	HLA-Bw42	HLA-Bw58 (17)
HLA-Aw43	HLA-Bw44 (12)	HLA-Bw59
	HLA-Bw45 (12)	HLA-Bw60 (40)
	HLA-Bw46	HLA-Bw61 (40)
	HLA-Bw47	HLA-Bw62 (15)
	HLA-Bw48	HLA-Bw63 (15)

Table 12-1 (Continued)

Lymphocyte Response, Defined (LD)	
HLA-D (12)	HLA-DR (10)
HLA-Dw1	HLA-DR1
HLA-Dw2	HLA-DR2
HLA-Dw3	HLA-DR3
HLA-Dw4	HLA-DR4
HLA-Dw5	HLA-DR5
HLA-Dw5	HLA-DRw6
HLA-Dw6	HLA-DR7
HLA-Dw7	
HLA-Dw8	HLA-DRw8
HLA-Dw9	HLA-DRw9
HLA-Dw10	HLA-DRw10
HLA-Dw11	
HLA-Dw12	

Source: Nomenclature for Factors of the HLA System 1980. In P. I. Terasaki(Ed.), *Histocompatibility Testing,* 1980. UCLA Tissue Typing Laboratory, Los Angeles, California, 1980. Pp. 18–21.
The number in parentheses refers to the original HLA specificity from which the new HLA was derived. For example, HLA-Aw23 and -Aw24 were derived from HLA-A9. The implication is that cytotoxic anti-A9 antibody was not immunospecific. These newly defined HLA specificities are referred to as splits (HLA-Aw23 is a split of HLA-A9).

microcytotoxicity test. These three loci are closely linked (see Figures 12-3 and 12-5), and the region on chromosome 6, group C of man, containing them is approximately 0.8 centiMorgan (cM) or map units. The process of defining these alleles in man has been one of continuous subdivision as more monospecific antiserum has become available. Even today, it is still not possible to establish with complete assurance that each monospecific antibody detects only a single antigen coded by a single distinct allele at each locus. It is clear, however, that a modest number of antisera are capable of defining most individuals within a large population. For the present, assuming that each antigenic specificity represents the product of a different allele, the number of alleles determining these antigens are listed in Table 12-1 for the three SD loci. There are 20 antigenic specificities at the A locus, 42 at the B locus, and 8 at the C locus. Some alleles have the unofficial designation w (workshop), and others have not been defined (blanks represent a homozygote in a haplotype (see p. 300) or missing numbers in Table 12-1.) Table 12-2

Table 12-2 : Ethnic and Chimpanzee Distribution of HLA Antigens in Loci A, B, and C

Loci		Caucasian 629	Negro 317	Mexican 225	Oriental 71	Chimpanzee ?
HLA-A	A1	29	8	12	6	13
	A2	48	34	54	45	0
	A3	23	20	10	1	0
	A9	19	27	30	52	0
	A10	15	6	8	14	0
	A11	12	2	8	28	16
	Aw23	4	20	4	0	ND
	Aw24	15	6	26	52	ND
	A25	4	0	3	0	ND
	A26	11	5	7	14	ND
	A28	10	19	16	0	1
	A29	6	8	10	3	ND
	Aw30	5	23	12	1	ND
	Aw31	4	3	10	11	ND
	Aw32	7	3	6	1	ND
	Aw33	4	19	5	21	ND
HLA-B	B5	10	5	10	8	0
	B7	25	19	15	15	0
	B8	22	7	7	4	0
	B12	25	24	20	11	ND
	B13	5	1	4	11	0
	B14	9	5	12	1	0
	Bw15	10	3	4	14	0
	Bw16	11	7	19	14	1
	Bw17	8	23	2	10	5
	Bw18	10	7	6	0	0
	Bw21	5	8	8	10	0
	Bw22	6	4	1	15	24
	B27	8	3	4	1	2
	Bw35	16	30	33	14	0
	Bw37	4	2	1	1	0
	B38	7	1	8	4	0
	B39	4	6	10	10	0
	Bw40	12	6	12	17	0
HLA-C	Cw1	5	2	6	32	N
	Cw2	5	10	4	0	N
	Cw3	17	13	20	32	N
	Cw4	13	26	29	3	N
	Cw5	5	2	0	1	N

ND = no data; N = not available for chimpanzee.

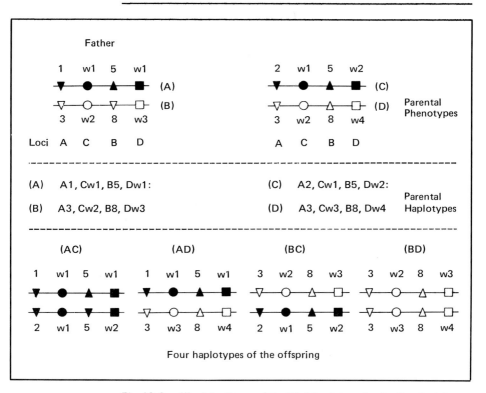

Fig. 12-2 : The inheritance of the HLA haplotype for the four loci A, B, C, and D. It is common practice to label the paternal haplotypes A and B, and the maternal, C and D. Since there can be only two paternal and two maternal haplotypes, there are four possible combinations in the offspring, as indicated in this figure. Thus, in a large family of siblings, it follows that there is a 25 percent chance that two siblings will be HLA-identical, that is, will share two haplotypes. An additional 50 percent will share one haplotype, and the remaining 25 percent will share no haplotypes. Parents share one haplotype with all children and almost always differ for the other.

shows the frequency of HLA antigens in loci A, B, and C in certain ethnic groups and in chimpanzees. The relationships of HLA-A, -B, and -C to transplantation and to disease will be presented later.

LD ANTIGENS. The fourth locus, HLA-D, is determined by the mixed lymphocyte reaction (LD) and represents the genes controlling the strong D locus products of the alleles. Only recently defined and found to consist of eleven alleles, the D locus is closely linked to the B locus as observed in linked disequilibrium findings. Examination for the D locus and its antigenic product is determined by use of panels of different homozygous HLA-D typing cells classified into clusters that share MLR identity. Complex MLR typing results are common and represent genetic complexities not yet delineated. This is to be expected since MLR defined haplotypes may contain two or more antigenic determinants that are in strong linkage disequilibrium. Thus, the degree of genetic polymorphism at the HLA-D locus is still not clear, but the eleven alleles have been used to identify a large number of individuals in select populations. A potentially large number of undetected (blank) alleles may be present in man, and genetic polymorphism similar to HLA-A, HLA-B, and HLA-C loci is anticipated as research continues in this area.

One other locus in the MHC of man, in the vicinity of the HLA-A locus, is suggested by weak mixed lymphocyte reactions. This has been designated LD_2 in Figure 12–3. Figure 12–4 indicates the products of the genes of the four traditional HLA loci as expressed on the lymphocyte membrane.

The association of many diseases with the HLA-B locus (discussed later in this chapter) and the strong linkage disequilibrium of HLA-D with HLA-B suggest that the D locus may play a significant role in disease also. The MLR (hence HLA-D) locus, in transplantation reactions at least, appears to play a significant role with HLA-B.

DR ANTIGENS. The HLA-DR locus refers to *D-locus related* (DR) alleles specifying antigenic determinants primarily related to B lymphocytes. Seven such alleles have been recognized by utilization of the homozygous typing cell method (HTC) in the MLR procedure. Some studies have suggested that HLA-DR locus alleles may be similar to those of HLA-D, since in data collected thus far on families with recombinant HLA genes, D and DR genes have always segregated together. Further, the detection of HLA-D determinant by HTC is associated with detection of the corresponding DR determinant in cytotoxicity typing of B lymphocytes. Additional study shows that antisera to B lymphocytes block the MLR by reacting with the stimulator B lymphocyte (mytomycin-treated). Nonetheless, HTC typing suggests a distinct difference in the HLA-D and HLA-DR loci gene products. Thus the listing of the DR locus and alleles in Table 12–1.

The B lymphocyte antisera is obtained from human alloantibodies and from immunization of animals with B cells. The anti-B alloantibodies appear to be restrictive in that they will react with some B lymphocytes but not all (at least not to self–B cell antigens that are from the same individual the anti-B cell serum is obtained from), whereas the heterologous antibody will react with all B lymphocytes. These antisera can be made

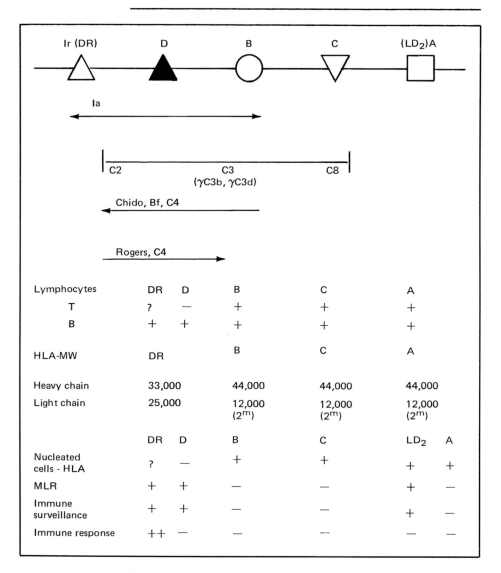

Fig. 12-3 : The HLA gene complex of man and the properties and functions of the genes. The plus (+), and minus (−) refer to the present or absence of the properties specified by the loci indicated.

specific to B lymphocytes by absorption with T cells, HLA-A, HLA-B and HLA-C determinants and by use of platelets, which lack B cell antigens. Nonetheless, these antisera appear to react with monocyte and endothelial cells.

Ia ANTIGENS. Human Ia antigens are analogous to the murine Ia antigens and appear to be similar to the antigens specified by the HLA-DR locus.

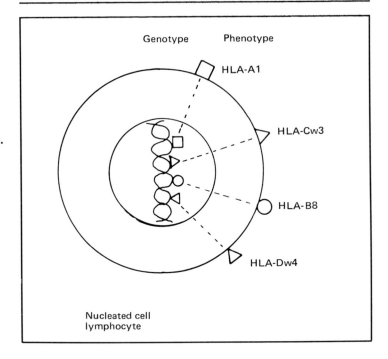

Fig. 12-4 : The products of the genes of the four loci, HLA-A, HLA-B, HLA-C, and HLA-D, as expressed diagrammatically on a lymphocyte surface.

Linkage Disequilibrium

When two alleles appear in a haplotype significantly more often than the randomly assorted expected frequency, this is referred to as *linkage disequilibrium.* For example, the frequency of HLA-A11 in one Caucasian population is 0.12% and the frequency for HLA-B5 is 0.10. If they assorted randomly, the expected frequency would be 0.12 X 0.10 or 0.012. The calculated haplotype for A11, B5 is greater than 0.012. Thus, A11 and B5 appear in the same haplotype significantly more often than would be expected. Examples of linkage disequilibrium are shown in Table 12-3 for HLA loci A : B, B : C, and B : D.

Genetic Linkage

The HLA region on chromosome 6 of humans was recognized through its linkage to phosphoglucomutase-3 (PGM 3), an erythrocyte enzyme. Fusion studies with hamster cells (interspecies hybridomas) showed that the gene for PGM 3 was on chromosome 6. Earlier, PGM 3 was found to be linked to the HLA supergene. Further evidence has been obtained from family studies with visible abnormal chromosomes (pericentric inversion of chromosome 6). A specific HLA haplotype was found in each person with the inversion. A map of chromosome 6, which is being slowly developed, is illustrated in Figure 12-5. Further subdivisions of the HLA complex of man and its antigenic products and associated functions are presented in Figures 12-3 and 12-5. Included in these figures are the genes for complement and erythrocyte, which are specified within the MHC. Map distances have

Table 12-3 : Examples of Linkage Disequilibrium for HLA-A, HLA-B, HLA-C, and HLA-D Loci

	Loci A : B	Loci B : C	Loci B : D
Haplotypes	A1, B8	B5, Cw1	Bw35, Dw1
	A3, B7	Bw22, Cw1	B7, Dw2
	A2, B12	B27, Cw1	B8, Dw3
	A3, B7	Bw40, Cw2	Bw15, Dw4
	A10, Bw16	B27, Cw2	Bw16, Dw5
	A11, B5	Bw40, Cw3	
	A29, B12	Bw15, Cw3	
	Aw30, B13	Bw22, Cw3	
	Aw33, B14	Bw35, Cw4	
		B12, Cw5	

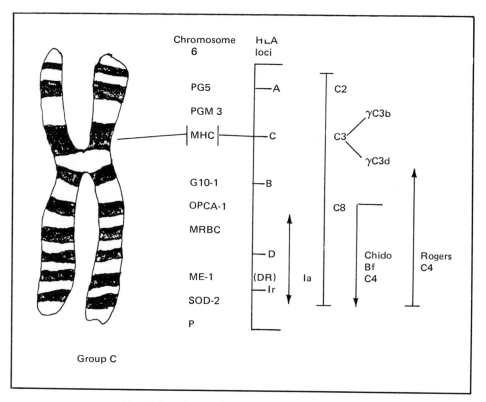

Fig. 12-5 : A map of chromosome 6, group C, of man, specifying gene loci of various enzymes and antigens. PG5 = pepsinogen 5; GI0-1 = glyoxalase-1; PGM3 = phosphoglucomutase-3; OPCA-1 = olivopontocere-bellar atrophy I; MRBC = B cell receptor for monkey cells; ME-1 = malic enzyme 1; SOD-2 = superoxide dismutase 2; P = P blood group; C2, C3, C4, and C8 = complement components; Bf = properdin factor (factor B); Chido and Rogers = erythrocyte antigens; γC3b and γC3d = receptors for C3b and C3d (C3 fragments).

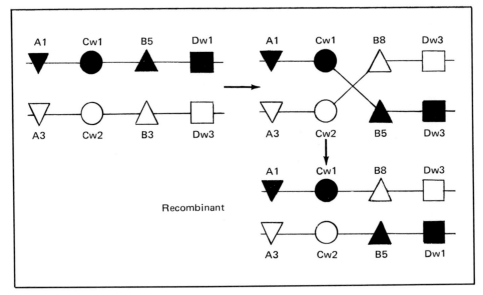

Fig. 12-6 : Hypothetical cross-over in the HLA region between HLA-C and HLA-B loci, during meiosis, resulting in a recombinant.

been established by the crossing over and the frequency of the cross-over of the HLA-ABCD genes. As more cross-over families are typed for all these gene products, the precise location of each gene will be elucidated.

A cross-over is illustrated in Figure 12–6. A hypothetical situation is shown whereby cross-over occurs during meiosis between the HLA-C and HLA-B loci to give recombinant haplotypes. Cross-over between the HLA-A and HLA-C loci has been demonstrated in family studies, with the recombinant haplotype demonstrated in the siblings. Recombinants occur about 1 percent of the time. This type of study, that is, the formation of recombinants, is useful in deducing the position of loci in the HLA system. The more commonly occurring HLA genes in various ethnic groups are listed in Table 12–4.

The MHC of the mouse is discussed in detail in Chapter 10, primarily with emphasis on the association of the H-2 complex of the mouse with the immune response gene (Ir). Comparison of Figure 10–2 for the H-2 complex of the mouse and Figure 12–3 for the MHC of humans reveals similarities in many areas with respect to the genes and the functional expressed products (phenotypes). However, the H-2 complex of mouse is found in chromosome 17. Great insight has been gained into the relationship between immune responses and genetics through the study of mouse and guinea pig Ir genes (see Chapter 10).

Table 12-4 : The Common Occurring HLA Genes in Various Ethnic Groups

HLA Genes	Ethnic Groups — Frequency (%)		
	Caucasian	Negro	Oriental
HLA-A1	23	17	rare
HLA-A3	23	—	rare
HLA-A23	—	common	rare
HLA-A24	15	—	52
HLA-B18	10	7	rare
HLA-Cw2	5	10	rare
HLA-Bw17	7	26	—
HLA-Bw21	4	10	—
HLA-Bw35	17	32	—

Blank spaces = no information available

Table 12-5 : Worldwide Summary of Organ Transplantation

Organ Transplanted	Year					
	1972	1973	1974	1975	1976	1977
Kidney	5418	6207	6477	7546	7320	6030
Liver	—	29	34	19	43	21
Heart	—	28	21	30	26	42
Bone Marrow	—	125	260	263	267	275

Source: Data compiled by National Institute of Allergy and Infectious Diseases and the American Cancer Society.

Transplantation Immunology

Transplantation of organs and tissues, especially of the kidney, is now a common practice in medicine, although still an imperfect therapeutic procedure. Table 12-5 summarizes worldwide statistics of kidney, liver, heart and bone marrow transplants from 1972 to 1977. The major source of organs, especially of heart and liver, has been from cadavers. A high percentage of unsuccessful transplantation of the heart and liver has been due primarily to unrelated donors. Although the technical aspect of surgery in transplantation has advanced tremendously, unfortunately other problems relating to human allografts have not kept pace. These include techniques for tissue preservation of organs and the moral and legal aspects of organ procurement.

Table 12-6 : Transplantation Immunology: Terminology

Nature of Graft	Tissue	Definition
Autograft	Autologous	Graft from one part of the body to another in the same individual
Isograft	Isologous	Graft from genetically identical individuals (identical twins, inbred strains of animals)
Allograft	Homologous	Graft from a genetically dissimilar donor of the same species
Xenograft	Heterologous	Graft from a donor of another species (heterograft); often referring to more distantly related species (xenograft)

Table 12-7 : Terminology of Genetics of Transplantation

Term	Definition
Allele	Genetic determinant that specifies a product (Ag marker)
Locus (sublocus)	Genetic location on chromosome
Haplotype	Genetic information on one chromosome (2 haplotypes—one from each parent = genotype)
Genotype	Genetic information on one pair of chromosomes
Phenotype	Expressed specified products (antigens) of a genotype, detectable or measurable
First-set phenomenon	Temporal sequence and events leading to graft rejection following initial exposure of a recipient to the tissue of a donor
Second-set phenomenon	Temporal sequence and events leading to graft rejection following subsequent exposure of the recipient to tissues of the same donor

This section of the chapter will be confined to an immunological discussion of allograft rejections and their associated problems.

Organs and tissues that have been used in transplantation include kidney, heart, liver, pancreas, lung, intestines, cornea and sclera, bone and cartilage, skin, hair, and bone marrow.

The terms used in transplantation immunology to define the nature of the graft and tissues are summarized in Table 12-6. The terminology used in the discussion of the genetics of transplantation is included in Table 12-7.

*Typing for
Transplantation*

The HLA-A, -B, and -C loci are determined with allogeneic lymphocytotoxic antibodies in the presence of rabbit serum as a complement source. The injured membrane is revealed in a variety of ways: (1) staining of dead cells by trypan blue; (2) separation of living and dead cells with eosin by the phase contrast method; (3) loss of fluorescent label (retained by living cells); and (4) leakage of ^{51}Cr from labeled injured cells. The endpoint method, phase contrast microscopy with eosin, is used routinely in most laboratories typing for HLA in microcytotoxicity testing (Figure 12-7).

Since there are only two paternal and two maternal haplotypes within a family, the offspring can exhibit only four possible combinations. Two siblings have a 25 percent chance of having the same HLA types (identical), a 50 percent chance of sharing one haplotype, and a 25 percent chance of differing for both haplotypes. Since the frequency of cross-over in the HLA region is relatively rare (1 percent), if two siblings share the same haplotypes at the HLA-A and HLA-B loci, the implication is that the HLA-C and HLA-D loci and other genes within the same regions are identical. This is fortunate, since in most laboratories HLA-A and HLA-B loci can be typed readily. In some cases of HLA typing within a family, fewer than two antigens may be detected at any one locus (a "blank"). This represents homozygosity at a locus (example, HLA-D) for the one antigen detected or else indicates the presence of an antigen that cannot yet be identified. The frequency of blank genes in ethnic groups other than caucasians is large. For the caucasians the frequency of blank genes at HLA-A is 5 percent and at HLA-B is 10 percent.

Two or more human gene loci are present on the same chromosome (syngenic) when they are present or absent *simultaneously* in the hybrid cell population following somatic cell hybridization. Hybrids are referred to as *hybridomas* in some systems. Thus PGM 3 and HLA loci have been shown to be in *syngeny*. In these studies the usual markers are enzymes and antigens.

The lymphocytotoxic antibodies are obtained from the sera of multiparous women and individuals who have received multiple transfusions. No natural reciprocal cytotoxic antibodies are found in normal serum the way they are for the ABO blood group. These antibodies are usually of the IgG class and may be cytotoxic (activate complement) or agglutinating and are most frequently multispecific; that is, sensitized individuals generally produce more than one specific HLA antibody. Occasionally, however, monospecific antibody is induced.

The original method in HLA detection was based on the agglutination technique employing mixed leukocytes from peripheral

Fig. 12-7 :
A. Microlymphocytoxicity plate containing cytotoxic antibody and lymphocytes along with rabbit C. Used in the eosin exclusion endpoint assay. Schematic representation of the cytotoxic antibody and rabbit C on the lymphocyte.

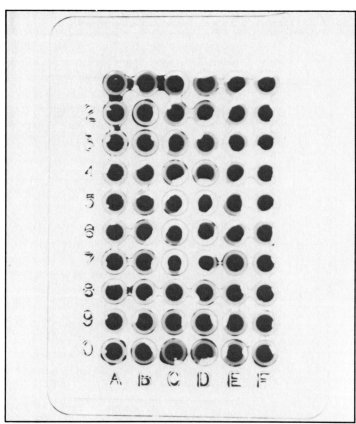

A

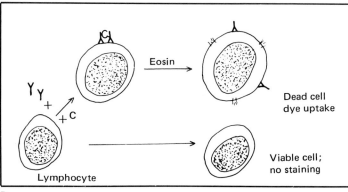

B

blood as target cells. Under these conditions granulocytes were the only cells reacting. This procedure was abandoned for the following reasons: (1) It requires freshly collected target cells; (2) these cells must be ABO-group compatible; and (3) the procedure gave many false-positive reactions. The complement-fixation test using platelets as target cells has been employed for HLA detection, but this technique appeared to be insensitive and lacked a sufficient battery of typing antisera.

The presently accepted method is the *microlymphocytotoxicity* technique. The lymphocytes to be assessed are obtained from donor and recipient and separated by placing the diluted whole blood or mixture of the buffy layer of leukocytes in diluted plasma on Hypaque-Ficoll (Lymphoprep) of an appropriate specific gravity and centrifuged. The mononuclear layer between the Lymphoprep and the aqueous or diluted plasma is removed and washed and used in the lymphocytotoxicity procedure. Both the donor and the recipient cells are tested against a panel of standard cytotoxic antibodies in the microplate (Figure 12-7A). The advantages of this procedure are that (1) lymphocytes need not be ABO-compatible; (2) reactions are reproducible; and (3) lymphocytes maintain valid reactivity better than granulocytes. Lymphocytes can be typed after shipment of cells in culture medium without refrigeration for long distances and can be stored with dimethyl sulfoxide and liquid nitrogen for a long time. Rabbit complement must be used for the lymphocytotoxicity testing because of its sublytic antihuman antibody levels. Thus HLA-A, -B, and -C are defined by the use of antibodies, the serological approach (SD).

The HLA-D gene products were initially recognized by mixing of allogeneic lymphocytes obtained from Lymphopreps. One individual's lymphocytes are treated with x-irradiation or with mitomycin C to inhibit DNA synthesis (these become the *stimulator cells*). These cells are then cultured with the other person's untreated lymphocytes (responder cells) for 5 days, after which time ^{3}H-thymidine is added; and, following a shorter incubation period, the cells are harvested, washed, and the incorporated radioactivity counted in a beta-counter. This test (Figure 12-8A) is referred to as the mixed lymphocyte reaction (MLR). Both the donor and recipient lymphocytes are tested in MLR, that is as stimulator and responder. A similar type of procedure using ^{51}Cr target lymphocytes and measurement of the escaping ^{51}Cr from the target cells is called *cell-mediated lymphocytoxicity* (CML) (Figure 12-8B). The target antigen on the stimulator cells in the MLR specifies the gene products of the D locus of HLA. In MLR the responder cells presumably have had no previous exposure to the HLA-D in the stimulator cells. In the

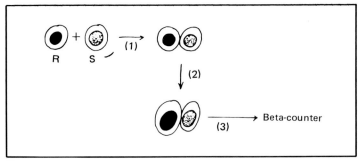

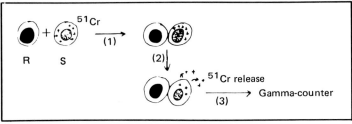

Fig. 12-8 : A. One-way mixed lymphocyte reaction (MLR) and analysis of DNA synthesis in the responder cell (R) against the target lymphocyte (S) (in S, DNA synthesis has been stopped by radiation or mitomycin C treatment) as measured by ^{3}H-thymidine assay. B. Cell-mediated lymphocytotoxicity (CML) using ^{51}Cr-labeled lymphocytes. In this procedure, the ^{51}Cr release following lysis of target lymphocyte is assayed in the gamma counter.

MLR the incorporation of ^{3}H-thymidine by the responder cell occurs following the stimulation by the differences in HLA-D antigens (between the two individuals being examined) in the transformation of the responder lymphocytes to lymphoblasts during active DNA synthesis. If no increase in ^{3}H-thymidine incorporation is shown, and if the amount incorporated is similar to the amount incorporated by the control, then compatibility of the two individuals at the HLA-D locus may exist. In this procedure a known standard panel of donors (stimulator cells) of HLA-D gene products must be available. Few laboratories are equipped to type for HLA-D determinants. Many laboratories, however, can perform the MLR between donor (stimulator)-recipient (responder) and recipient (stimulator)-donor (respondent) cross-match. This test will define the extent to which cells react to the HLA-D locus differences without defining the specific D determinant.

Stimulator cells homozygous for the HLA-D locus are referred to as *homozygous typing cells* (HTC). These HTC are obtained

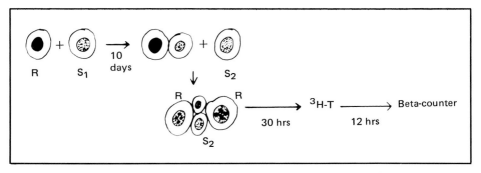

Fig. 12-9 : Primed lymphocyte typing (PLT) assay. Responder (R) lymphocyte is mixed with S_1 (stimulator) cells for 10 days; ^{3}H-thymidine incorporation will occur in R cell (DNA synthesis) if R and S_1 are incompatible; R + S_1 are mixed with S_2 (stimulator) and incubated for 30 hours; results: (a) enhanced DNA synthesis by R + S_1 + S_2 could indicate that $S_1 = S_2$; (b) no increase in DNA synthesis by R + S_2 would indicate that essentially R = S_2 and S_1 is not equal to S_2.

from individuals in family studies. When HTC cells are used as stimulator cells, any responder cells that show little or no increase in ^{3}H-thymidine uptake in the MLR are considered to share similar HLA-D determinants. On the other hand, all responder cells lacking the HLA-D locus genes would be expected to react strongly with HTC in the MLR with increased ^{3}H-thymidine incorporation. This, however, is not the case in practice. Intermediary reactions have been demonstrated. It has been suggested that genes other than those in the HLA-D locus may be present in the region between HLA-A and HLA-B. Furthermore, the accuracy of HLA-D typing using HTC is not always certain. Other problems include difficulties in assessing homozygous HLA-D cells and the instability of the HLA-D gene products.

Other methods have been sought to type the HLA-D locus. *Primed lymphocyte typing* (PLT) is one (Figure 12-9). The initial steps are similar to those of the MLR, with incubation of the activated responder (R) and treated stimulator cells (S_1), but the mixed cells are incubated for a longer period (10 days). This stops the incorporation of ^{3}H-thymidine. At this stage, if additional original stimulator cells (S_1-S_2) are added, there is a marked increase of ^{3}H-thymidine uptake when the ^{3}H-thymidine is added 30 hours after the second stimulation (addition of more S_1 or the related S_2 cells). The ^{3}H-thymidine incorporation is determined 12 to 16 hours after the addition of ^{3}H-thymidine. If the second addition of unrelated stimulator cells is done 30 hours prior to ^{3}H-thymidine addition, and if there is a burst of ^{3}H-thymidine incorporation, this is interpreted to mean that the second stimulator cells have HLA-D deter-

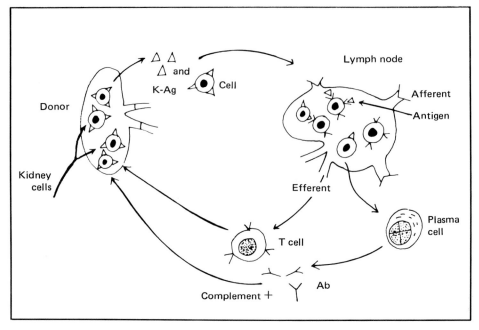

Fig. 12-10 : Sensitization of recipient to donor's kidney antigens in transplantation.

minants similar to those of the first stimulator cells. The MLR using HTC and the MLR-PLT have a significant correlation. Nevertheless, discrepancies arise; the differences, however, appear to be due to the reaction of PLT to the target cell surface, not related to HTC antigen.

The PLT procedure has the following advantages: (1) PLT cells kept frozen can be used to type unknown cells within 24 hours; (2) the method does not require HTC; and (3) PLT cells can be prepared from families with well-defined HLA genes.

Factors Affecting the Outcome of the Allograft

The rejection phenomenon involves both humoral and cell-mediated responses. Preexisting antibodies (in the serum of recipients) to donor cells can trigger the hyperacute response, which is irreversible by immunosuppressive therapy. The resulting immediate or accelerated graft rejection is accompanied by platelet aggregation and fibrin deposition in the graft vessels and subsequent invasion of the neighboring tissues by the granulocytes. A delayed and slowly progressive rejection is accompanied by mononuclear cellular infiltration of the graft tissue. The immediate and primary types of histological tissue rejection patterns are illustrated in Figure 12-11. The mechanism of humoral (hyperacute) and cellular sensitization is shown in Figure 12-10.

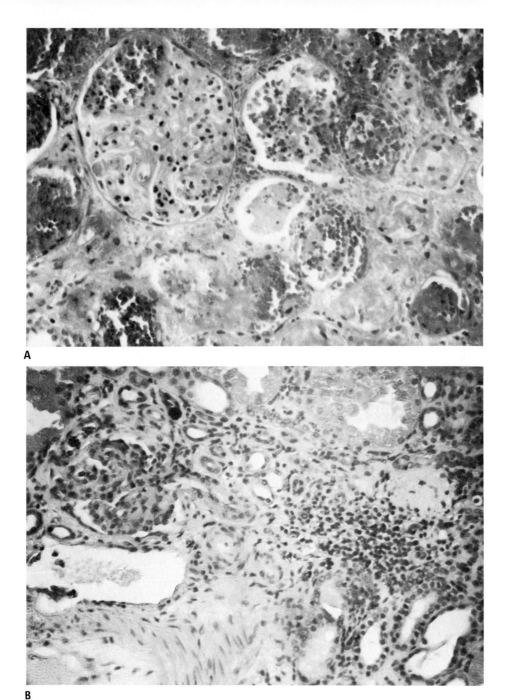

A

B

Fig. 12-11 : A. Hyperacute type of kidney rejection. Fibrin deposition
and infiltration of polymorphonuclear cells are common in this type of
reaction (characteristic of a humoral-mediated rejection). B. Primary acute
rejection in the kidney, mediated by mononuclear cells. This appears to be
a cell-mediated type of rejection. Infiltration of mononuclear cells (lymphocytes and monocytes) predominates in this type of rejection. (H & E,
X 400)

The presently recognized major antigens involved in allograft rejection can be attributed to the ABO group antigens and the HLA-A, -B, -C, and -D gene products. The ABO and the HLA-A, HLA-B, and HLA-C antigens are associated with the humoral cytotoxic or blocking antibodies, while the HLA-D locus antigens are related to the lymphocytotoxic cells. Since it has been demonstrated that 50 percent of kidney grafts with ABO incompatibility never functioned following transplantation, ABO compatibility is of great importance. The A_1 antigen in the ABO group appears to be a major factor (strong antigen).

The major antigens involved in transplantation immunology are the HLA antigens. Appropriate matching by tissue typing, which defines the gene products of the HLA-A, HLA-B, HLA-C and HLA-D, is of importance to the longer survival of kidney or other organ transplants. Table 12–8 summarizes various possible degrees of compatibility of HLA-A and HLA-B loci (match types) as assessed by the lymphocytotoxicity test. In addition to SD testing for compatibility, a cross-match utilizing the MLR test system is employed to assess compatibility between donor and recipient HLA and other, as yet unrecognized, antigens.

Kidney Allograft Rejection

The acute or primary rejection is generally associated with the first-set phenomenon, involving stimulation of the cell-mediated system. Either soluble histocompatibility antigens released by the donor's cell or the same antigens in the donor cell surface trigger the recipient's T lymphocytes to blast cell transformation (6 to 7 days) and subsequent proliferation of sensitized lymphocytes. These T-effector cytotoxic cells attack the donor cells, contributing to the acute or primary rejection of the donor allograft. The sensitization process is illustrated in Figure 12–10. The B cell system is also stimulated, with subsequent antibody formation. The acute primary rejection is associated with the CMI system, however. The graft is usually rejected 10 to 14 days after transplant. If recognized early, this type of rejection can be reversed with immunosuppressive therapy. Following the initial rejection, the second kidney transplant can be rejected in an accelerated manner if a high level and diverse kinds of antibodies are prevalent against the second donor's tissue. The histological pattern of hyperacute rejection has been discussed and is shown in Figure 12–11. In some cases, however, blocking antibodies may prevail, in which case the graft survival is prolonged. These phenomena are similar to those of tumor immunology (Chapter 16).

It is difficult to judge which major immune system is involved in chronic rejection of a kidney graft—that is, the humoral or the cellular system. Grafts of this nature survive for months or

Table 12-8 : Tissue Typing on the Basis of the Major HLA Antigens

Match Type	Hypothetical Recipient Genotype	Hypothetical Donor Genotype	Remarks
A	A2, B5 : A3, B8	A2, B5 : A3, B8	Identical HLAs in both donor and recipient (e.g., identical twins or inbred strains—isologous)
B	A2, B5 : A3, B8	A2, B5 : A3, B5	No group mismatches but donor is missing one antigen found in the recipient
C	A2, B5 : A3, B8	A2, B5 : A3, B7	One group mismatch; donor has one antigen that recipient does not have (i.e., one unrelated antigen)
D	A2, B5 : A3, B8	A10, B12 : A3, B8	Two group mismatches, both on the same chromosome (i.e., one haplotype is completely different between donor and recipient)
E	A2, B5 : A3, B8	A2, B12 : A3, B7	Two or more group mismatches involving both chromosomes (i.e., both donor haplotypes are at least partially different from recipient haplotypes)
F	—	—	Match is classified as type F if the recipient has an antibody to one of donor's HLA antigens. This can occur even in identical twins if one of them has an autoimmunity to one of his own HLA antigens.

years. The immunopathological picture is associated with changes in the vessels and glomeruli and the presence of deposits of C3, C4, and immunoglobulins. The pattern appears to be one of recurrence of the original disease. This is very plausible, since it must be remembered that organ replacement does not eliminate the etiology of the original disease. Thus, even transplants of isografts or kidney between identical twins ultimately succumb to the original disease after many years. In chronic rejection, the immunological mechanism probably involves both the low affinity antibodies and the sensitized effector cells, or possibly cells such as the ADCC cells. Table 12-9 summarizes the immune mechanisms involved in transplantation rejection. Table 12-10 summarizes the differences and similarities of some of the important features of the ABO and Rh blood groups and the HLA complex.

Bone Marrow Transplants

The salient features of bone marrow transplantation are as follows: (1) the marrow cells consist of immunocompetent lymphoid cells capable of mounting an immunological response, both humoral and cell-mediated, against host tissue (graft-versus-host reaction or GVHR); (2) the donor lymphoid cells contain strong HLA antigens, thus if undetectable incompatibility

Table 12-9 : In Vitro Correlation of Systems Involved in Graft Destruction

System	Target Antigens	Target Antigen Destroyed by
Cytotoxic antibody (IgG) + complement	HLA, A, B, C ABO group (Others?)	Antibody + complement
T effector cells (specific)	HLA-D products	T lymphocytes
K cell	HLA, A, B, C	Cytotoxic cells armed with antibody
ADCC (nonsensitized) (Null cells)	ABO group (Others?)	

Table 12-10 : Comparison of ABO, Rh, and HLa Isoantigens

Characteristics	Blood Group System		
	ABO	Rh	HLA
Clinical significance	Transfusion reaction Hemolytic disease of the newborn	Erythroblastosis fetalis	Transplantation and transfusion reactions
Techniques for the immunosuppression of the humoral and cell-mediated responses	None	Specific anti-Rh antibody given to Rh⁻ mother just prior to Rh exposure	Steroids; anti-lymphocyte serum (ALS)
Genetic polymorphism	Moderate	Extensive	Extensive
Chromosome loci	Single	Complex	Complex
Chromosome number	9 (short arm)	1	6 (short arm)

exists (MLR test–negative), these donor cells are readily rejected; and (3) successful transplantation of bone marrow is restricted to acute aplastic anemia, acute leukemias, and congenital combined immunodeficiency disease (CID). Reasonable clinical success has been achieved in acute aplastic anemia and CID (50 percent), and 20 percent success in acute leukemias. In 70 percent of patients receiving bone marrow transplant, GVH reactions occur, and 20 percent of these are irreversible. In acute aplastic anemia good clinical results are achieved if the transplantation is performed prior to blood transfusion (prior to sensitization).

One of the major concerns in the bone marrow transplantation has been the graft-versus-host response (GVHR) phenomenon. Since the recipient's immune system is completely obliterated by drugs and x-irradiation prior to bone marrow transplant, the donor's competent immune cells will (if any incompatibility exists) mount an immune response against the recipient's tissue. Nevertheless, bone marrow transplant has promising clinical value in aplastic anemias and certain types of leukemia. Great care must be taken, however, to ascertain maximum compatibility matching between donor and recipient.

Paternity and Anthropological Testing

The frequency of certain HLA genes is markedly different in various ethnic groups. These HLA genes are shown in Table 12-5 for caucasians, blacks, and orientals. Some not listed include HLA-Bw46 and HLA-Bw54, which appear to be unique to the Chinese and Japanese, respectively. Thus, HLA typing utilizing the 77 allele markers provides another practical means of obtaining data about the interrelationships of population previously documented by other genetic markers (ABO system, etc.).

The polymorphism of the five HLA-linked loci with the present 92 allelic markers also provides a means of assessing paternity. The usefulness of HLA for paternity testing has been recognized by the American Medical Association and the American Bar Association. HLA has been recommended as the next step if red cell testing provides insufficient information.

The frequency of most of the HLA antigens is low, that is, in most cases it is highly probable that HLA typing will exclude a male wrongfully accused. The putative father can also be included—along with any other male within an ethnic group—as the possible biological father by HLA testing. This is done by calculating the probability of the putative father's contributing the required genes to the offspring, and comparing this with the probability of any random male of the appropriate ethnic group's contributing those particular genes. The courts, however, do not as yet require the admittance of evidence on the probability of a defendant's being the biological father. This is in contrast to the evidence ruling out the possibility (of paternity).

HLA and Disease

The relationship of gene product expression—such as the ABO group antigens—to disease conditions has been examined extensively. With very few exceptions, these studies have shown no clear correlation between disease and antigenic markers. Such studies are presently being carried out in an attempt to relate HLA antigens to disease states. These studies appear to show a promise of helping in the diagnosis of, and in revealing high risk individuals' susceptibility to, certain illnesses, especially the autoimmune type of disease. Autoimmune diseases involving the immune response appear to show a significant relationship to HLA genes.

Table 12-11 : HLA and Disease Association

Disease	Racial Group	HLA Type	Antigen Frequency Patient	Antigen Frequency Control	RR	
Joint diseases						
Ankylosing spondylitis	Haida Indians	B27	100	50	34	
	Pima Indians	B27	36	18	3	
	Japanese	B27	68	0	306	
	Caucasian	B27	90	8	88	
Reiter's disease	Caucasian	B27	78	8	36	
Juvenile rheumatoid arthritis	Caucasian	B27	26	9	5	
Rheumatoid arthritis	Caucasian	Dw4	42	16	3	
	"	Dw3	30	17	3	
Sjögren's syndrome	Caucasian	B8	51	24	3.2	
	"	Dw3	53	17	5.2	
Gastrointestinal tract						
Chronic acute hepatitis	Caucasian	A1	42	28	2	
	"	B8	41	20	3	
	"	Dw3	60	22	7	
			25	22	1	(NS)
Ulcerative colitis	Japanese	B5	81	41	9	
	Caucasian	B5	14			(NS)
Celiac disease	Caucasian	A1	64	30	4	
	"	B8	71	23	9	
	"	Dw3	98	15	278	
Skin						
Psoriasis	Caucasian	B13	20	5	5	
	"	Bw17	26	8	5	
	"	Bw37	8	1	5	
Behçet's disease	Japanese	B5	75	31	7	
	Caucasian	B5	35	11	4	
Herpes lobialis	Caucasian	A1	56	21	4	
	"	B8	33	17	3	
Others						
Hodgkin's disease	Caucasian	A1	31	39	1.4	
	"	B5	11	16	1.6	
	"	B8	24	29	1.3	
	"	Bw18	7	13	1.9	
Acute lymphocytic leukemia	Caucasian	A2	60	54	1.3	
	"	B8	29	24	1.3	
	"	Bw18	29	25	1.3	
Sarcoidosis	Black	B7	46	16	6.0	
Anterior uveitis	Caucasian	B27	57	8	15.4	
Takayasu disease	Japanese	Bw52	44	13	5.5	
Endocrine glands						
Thyroid; Graves's disease	Caucasian	B8	37	22	2	
	"	Dw3	50	22	4	
	Japanese	Bw35	57	21	5	
Adrenal; Addison's disease	Caucasian	B8	50	23	4	
	"	Dw3	70	22	11	

Table 12-11 (Continued)

Disease	Racial Group	HLA Type	Antigen Frequency Patient	Antigen Frequency Control	RR
Pancreas; diabetes	Caucasian	B8	37	22	2
Pancreas; juvenile diabetes	Caucasian	Bw15	23	15	2
	''	Dw3	50	5	5
Neurological disease					
Multiple sclerosis	Caucasian	A3	(27) 36	(30) 26	2 (NS)
	''	B7	(45) 34	(27) 24	2.2
	''	Dw2	(54) 60	(21) 15	(5) 9
	Black	A3	16	14	0 (NS)
	''	B7	35	16	2
	''	Dw2	34	0	—
Myasthenia gravis	Caucasian	A1	45	26	3
	''	B8	58	23	4
	''	Dw3	48	17	4
Schizophrenia	Caucasian	A28	19	5	5

RR = relative risk (see text); NS = not significant

There are two major approaches to the study of a genetic system, in this case HLA, and its relationship to a disease or to an unusual condition. One is the population studies approach, in which the frequency of the HLA genotypes in a group of unrelated patients is compared with the corresponding (age, sex, and ethnic background) frequency in a group of healthy individuals (control). The second approach is to study families in order to see if affected relatives show similar haplotypes more often than shown by the accepted genetic frequency of the general population. The population studies give only information about the association between HLA markers and the disease examined, whereas family studies can reveal genetic linkage between the HLA marker locus and a major disease-controlling gene. *Association* and *linkage* have different connotations in these studies. Association between two characteristics can occur without linkage between the corresponding loci, and linkage between two loci does not imply association between corresponding characteristics. In the HLA system, however, association may be found between some alleles at two closely linked loci.

Population studies are easier to perform but have the major drawback that the HLA genes under study may not include the particular ones responsible for the disease susceptibility. Difficulties of family studies are related to biased sampling of patients and hampered by incomplete penetrance and varying ages of disease onset.

Basically, in population studies, the HLA phenotypes in a group of unrelated patients and in a group of unrelated individuals (controls) of the same homogeneous ethnic origin are analyzed. From the data obtained it can be determined whether there is a statistically significant deviation in the frequency of the HLA genes in patients and in controls. A general statistical analysis using the classic Chi-square test may be employed.

The statistical significance can be distinguished from the relative risk (RR). The *relative risk* is the risk of developing a disease when an HLA antigen is present in an individual relative to the risk of developing the disease when the antigen is lacking. Thus, the strength of the association is determined by:

$$\text{Relative risk (RR)} = \frac{\text{Patient } (+) \times \text{Control } (-)}{\text{Control } (+) \times \text{Patient } (-)}$$

The *relative risk* is estimated as being the cross-product ratio (RR) of positive patients $\times$ negative controls to positive controls $\times$ negative patients. The relative risk is higher than one (1+) when an antigen is found more frequently in the patient than in the controls. A relative risk of less than 1 ($-$1) (negative association) reflects a decreased frequency of antigen in the patient. The statistical significance and RR may not be parallel in some cases; thus both values need to be found. Relative risk may be considered a measure of biological significance.

Table 12-11 lists examples of various diseases in different ethnic groups, their statistical significance, and the relative risks. Of interest is the striking HLA-B27 antigen frequency found in ankylosing spondylitis for various ethnic groups (90 percent), which has led to typing for HLA-B27 in the diagnosis of suspected cases of this disease.

Summary

1. The major histocompatibility complex (MHC) of man resides in chromosome 6. The MHC includes HLA, which consists of the four loci designated A, B, C, and D and the lesser understood Ir (DR) and LD_2 loci; the alleles for the complement components, C2, C3, C4, and C8; the red cell antigens, (Chido and Rogers); and the properdin factor Bf.
2. MHC has been demonstrated in ten other species of animals. These include the chimpanzee, rhesus monkey, dog, pig, rabbit, guinea pig, rat, chicken, mouse, and *Xenopus laevis* (amphibian).
3. The HLA antigens consist of two chains, the β_2-macroglobulin (MW 12,000) and the heavy chain glycoprotein (MW 44,000). The latter chain designates the specificity of the HLA.

4. HLA antigens are present in all membranes of nucleated cells and in tissue fluid at low levels. They are essentially absent in erythrocytes. HLA appears early in fetal life (at 6 weeks of development) and persists for life.

5. The genetic control of HLA is accomplished by a complex of linked genes at five subloci on chromosome 6 (man). There are presently 92 known HLA antigens. This number will continue to expand.

6. The HLA antigens are determined by serological means, using specific cytotoxic antibodies and complement for their detection (serologically defined, or SD). They are also determined by the MLC reaction. This is referred to as lymphocyte-defined (LD) determination. Loci A, B, and C are determined by SD while locus D by the LD determination. The locus DR is also defined by LD determination of B cell antigens (Ia).

7. The MHC plays a significant role in transplantation immunology. Long-term allograft survival requires good HLA matching. This is especially critical in bone marrow transplantation.

8. Recently there has been great interest in the use of HLA typing in association with disease. In some diseases a significant association has been demonstrated between HLA antigens and the disease. For example, individuals with HLA-B27 are at high risk for ankylosing spondylitis (see Table 12-11). Patients with this disease have a 67 to 100 percent probability of having the HLA-B27 antigen, depending on their ethnicity.

9. HLA analysis is also used in paternity and anthropological assessment.

Bibliography and Selected Reading

General

Announcement. WHO-IUIS Terminology Committee: Nomenclature for factors of the HLA systems. *Cell. Immunol.* 21:382, 1976.

Bach, F. H., and Van Rood, J. J. The major histocompatibility complex—genetics and biology. Part 1. *N. Engl. J. Med.* 295:806, 1976.

Bach, F. H., and Van Rood. J. J. The major histocompatibility complex—genetics and biology. Part 2. *N. Engl. J. Med.* 295:872, 1976.

Bach, F. H., and Van Rood, J. J. The major histocompatibility complex—genetics and biology. Part 3. *N. Engl. J. Med.* 295:927, 1976.

Bodmer, W. B. Jr., Bodmer, J. G., Festenstin, H., and Morris, P. J. (Eds.). *Histocompatibility Testing.* Copenhagen: Munksgaard 1977.

Gill, J. J., Cramer, D. V., and Kunz, H. W. The major histocompatibility complex—comparison in the mouse, man and the rat. *Am. J. Pathol.* 90:735, 1978.

Perkins, H. A. The Human Major Histocompatibility Complex (MHC). In H. H. Fudenberg, D. P. Stiles, J. L. Caldwell, and J. V. Wells (Eds.), *Basic and Clinical Immunology*. Los Altos, Calif.: Lange, 1978. P. 165.

Van der Weerdt, Ch. M. The Platelet Agglutination Test in Platelet Grouping. In H. Balner, S. J. Cleton and J. G. Ernesse (eds.), *Histocompatibility Testing*. Baltimore: Williams & Wilkins, 1965. P. 11.

Major Histocompatibility Complex

Dorval, G., Welsh, K. I., Nilsson, K., and Wigzell, H. Quantitation of β_2 microglobulin and HLA on the surface of human cells. I. T and B lymphocytes and lymphoblasts. *Scand. J. Immunol.* 6:255, 1977.

Lamm, L. U., Kissmeyer-Neilson, F., and Henningsen, K. Linkage and association studies of two phosphoglucomutase loci (PGM 1 and PGM 3) to eighteen other markers. *Hum. Hered.* 20:305, 1970.

Lamm, L. U., Friedrich, V., Peterson, G. B., Jorgensen, J., Nielsen, J., Therkelsen, A. J., and Kissmeyer-Nielsen, F. Assignment of the major histocompatibility complex to chromosome number 6 in a family with a pericentric inversion. *Hum. Hered.* 24:273, 1974.

Meo, T., Atkinson, J. P., Bernoco, M., Bernoco, D., and Ceppelini, R. Structural heterogeneity of C_2 complement protein and its genetic variants in man: A new polymorphism of the HLA region. *Proc. Natl. Acad. Sci. USA* 74:1672, 1977.

Sheehy, M. J., Sondel, P. M., Bach, M. L., Wank, R., and Bach, F. H. HLA LD (lymphocyte defined) typing: A rapid assay with primed lymphocytes. *Science* 188:1308, 1975.

Snary, D., Barnstable, C., Bodiner, W. F., Goodfellow, P., and Crumpton, M. J. Human Ia antigens, purification and molecular structure. *Origins of Lymphocyte Diversity,* Cold Spring Harbor Symposia on Quantitative Biology, XLI. Cold Spring Harbor Laboratory of Quantitative Biology, Cold Spring Harbor, L. I., New York, 1977. Pp. 379–386.

Springer, T. A., and Strominger, J. L. Detergent-soluble products of the HLA region. *Transplant. Proc.* IX (suppl.) 1:21, 1977.

Strominger, J. L., Mann, D. L., Parham, P., Robb, R., Springer, T., and Terhost, C. Structures of HLA-A and HLA-B antigens isolated from cultured human lymphocytes. Cold Spring Harbor Symposia on Quantitative Biology, XLI, Cold Spring Harbor Laboratory of Quantitative Biology, Cold Spring Harbor, L. I., New York, 1977. Pp. 323–329.

Terasaki, P. I. (Ed.). *Histocompatibility Testing 1980.* Nomenclature for Factors of the HLA System 1980. Los Angeles: UCLA Tissue Typing Laboratory, 1980. Pp. 18-21.

Van Camp, B. G. K., Cole, J., and Peetermans, M. E. HLA antigens and homogeneous immunoglobulins. *Clin. Immunol. Immunopathol.* 7:315, 1977.

Van Someren, H., Westerveld, A., Hagemeiyer, A., Mess, J. R., Meera Khan, P., and Zoalberg, O. B. Human antigen and enzyme markers in man—Chinese hamster somatic hybrids. Evidence for synteny between the HLA, PGM 3, ME_1, and IPO-B loci. *Proc. Natl. Acad. Sci. USA* 71:962, 1974.

Welsh, K. I., Dorval, G., Nilsson, K., Clements, G. B., and Wigzell, H. Quantitation of β_2-*microglobulin* and HLA on the surface of human cells. II. In vitro cell lines and their hybrids. *Scand. J. Immunol.* 6:265, 1977.

Transplantation Immunology

Carpenter, C. B. (Ed.). *Clinical Histocompatibility Testing.* A transplantation proceeding reprint, Vol. 2. New York: Grune & Stratton, 1977.

Cline, M. J., Gale, R. P., Stiehm, E. R., Opelz, G., Young, S. H., Geig, S. A., and Fahey, J. L. Bone marrow transplantation in man. *Ann. Intern. Med.* 83:691, 1975.

Gale, R. P., and Opelz, G. (Eds.). *Immunobiology of Bone Marrow Transplantation.* A transplantation proceeding reprint, Vol. 2. New York: Grune & Stratton, 1978.

Goldfinger, D. Acute hemolytic transfusion reactions: A fresh look at pathogenesis and considerations regarding therapy. *Transfusion* 17:85, 1977.

Skamene, E., and Gold, P. Organ Transplantation. In S. D. Freedman and P. Gold (Eds.), *Clinical Immunology* (2nd ed.). Hagerstown, Md.: Harper and Row, 1976. P. 449.

Thomas, E. D., Buckner, C. D., Banaji, M., Clift, R. A., Fefer, A., Fluornoy, N., Goodell, B. W., Hickman, R. O., Lesner, K. G., Neiman, P. E., Sale, G. E., Sander, J. E., Singer, J., Stevens, M., Storb, R., and Weider, P. L. One hundred patients with acute leukemia treated by chemotherapy, total body irradiation, and allogeneic marrow transplantation. *Blood* 49:511, 1977.

Thomas, E. D., Storb, R., and Buckner, C. D. Total body irradiation in preparation for marrow engraftment. *Transplant. Proc.* 8:591, 1976.

Thomas, J., Thomas, F., Mendez-Picon, G., and Lee, H. Immunological monitoring of long-surviving renal transplant recipient. *Surgery* 81:125, 1977.

Tsoi, M. S., Storb, R., Weiden, P. L., and Thomas, E. D. Studies on cellular inhibition and serum-blocking factors in 28 human patients given marrow grafts from identical siblings. *J. Immunol.* 118:1799, 1977.

HLA and Association with Disease

Bergman, L., Lindlom, J. B., Safvenberg, J., and Krause, U. HLA frequencies in Crohn's disease and ulcerative colitis. *Tissue Antigens* 7:145, 1976.

Buckley, R. H., MacQueen, J. M., and Ward, F. E. HLA antigen in primary immunodeficiency disease. *Clin. Immunol. Immunopathol.* 7:305, 1977.

Dausset, J., and Svejgard, A. (Eds.). *HLA and Disease.* Copenhagen. Munksgaard, 1977.

Dupont, B., Lisak, R. P., Jersild, C., Hansen, J. A., Silberberg, D. H., Whitsett, C., Zweiman, B., and Ciongoli, K. HLA antigens in black American patients with multiple sclerosis. *Transplant Proc.* (Suppl.) 9:181, 1977.

Fu, S. M., Stern, R., Kimbel, H. G., Dupont, B., Hansen, J. A., Day, M. K., Good, R. A., Jersild, C., and Fotino, M. Mixed lymphocyte culture determinants and C_2 deficiency: LD-7a associated with C_2 deficiency in four families. *J. Exp. Med.* 142:495, 1975.

Grosse-Wilde, H., Bertrams, J., Schuppien, W., Netzel, B., Ruppelt, W., and Kurvert, E. K. HLA-D typing in 111 multiple sclerosis patients: Distribution of four HLA-D alleles. *Immunogenetics* 4:481, 1977.

Hoshino, K., Inouye, A., Unokudu, T., Ito, M., and Tsuji, K. HLA disease in Japanese. *Tissue Antigens* 10:45, 1977.

Isohisa, I., Numano, F., Maezawa, H., and Sasazuki, T. HLA-Bw52 in Takayasu disease. *Tissue Antigens* 12:246, 1978.

McIntyre, J. A., McKee, K. T., Loadholt, C. B., Mereuno, S., and Lin, I. Increased HLA-b7 antigen frequency in South Carolina blacks in association with sarcoidosis. *Transplant. Proc.* (Suppl.) 9:1973, 1977.

McMichael, A., and McDevitt, H. The association between HLA system and disease. *Prog. Med. Genet.* 2:39, 1977.

Payne, R. The HLA complex: Genetics and Implications in the Immune Response. In J. Dausset and A. Svejgard (Eds.), *HLA and Diseases.* Copenhagen: Munksgaard, 1977. P. 20.

Tanimoto, K., Horiuchi, Y., Tsuji, T., Yamamoto, K., Kodama, J., Murata, S., Funahashi, S., and Nagaki, K. HLA types in two families with hereditary angioneurotic edema. *Clin. Immunol. Immunopathol.* 7:336, 1977.

13 : Mechanisms of Immunological Injury, Hypersensitivity, and Cellular Cytotoxicity

The term *hypersensitivity* implies an overreaction of the immune system (hyperimmune reactivity) to the extent that the immune process becomes deleterious to *self*. The majority of the hypersensitivity reactions to be discussed in this chapter are triggered by exogenous antigens and in this respect differ from some specific autologous autoimmune diseases (see Chapter 14). Nevertheless, some of the basic features in the mechanism of the immune processes initiating tissue damage are indistinguishable. Hypersensitivities can be separated into two major categories, depending on the antigens involved in the induction of the immune response: *immediate* (humoral) and *delayed* (cell-mediated). Immediate hypersensitivity is manifested by tissue reactions occurring within minutes after the antigen combines with its appropriate antibody. In contrast, delayed hypersensitivity is associated with tissue reactions occurring usually more than 24 hours later, after the antigen interacts with the appropriate sensitized T lymphocyte. This phenomenon has been described in Chapter 3.

Anaphylaxis (anti-phylaxis) is a term sometimes used synonymously with immediate hypersensitivity. It is the antithesis of prophylaxis (prevention against deleterious organisms by active or passive immunization). At the turn of the last century, it was demonstrated that animals can be protected from exotoxins (tetanus and diphtheria toxins) by repeated inoculations of nonlethal doses of the exotoxins. The antitoxins (antibodies) produced neutralize the exotoxins and thus prevent their reaching the specific receptor sites on the target organs (central nervous system). This early discovery of the prophylactic approach in immunology is the forerunner of immunization against toxins of microbial origin.

This chapter encompasses the defined immunological mechanisms by which tissue injury is induced in experimental animals, and which occur spontaneously in humans. Gell and Coombs have classified these reactions into four major types, designated I, II, III, and IV. Types I, II, and III are associated with the B cell or humoral system and the amplification and ancillary systems discussed in Chapters 8 and 9. Type IV is synonymous with the T cell or CMI cytotoxicity system and includes the participation of the amplification and ancillary systems.

Immediate
Hypersensitivity
(Humoral System)

Anaphylaxis

Anaphylaxis, the antithesis of prophylaxis, is manifested in immediate tissue reactions, which occur within minutes of the interaction between a specific antigen and its homologous antibody. Anaphylaxis can be considered as (1) *generalized* or *systemic,* a shock-like syndrome occurring minutes after administration of a specific antigen to a sensitized individual possessing the corresponding antibody; or (2) *localized,* a reaction that may occur rapidly but in a specific target organ or tissue such as the liver, gastrointestinal tract, skin, or nasal mucosa.

Antibodies

Anaphylaxis can be mediated by IgE (type I) or IgG (types II and III) and occasionally by IgA and IgM. Thus the antibodies involved can be categorized as *homocytotropic* or *heterocytotropic.* The homocytotropic antibody is restrictive, and passively transmitted responses occur only within the same species (allogeneic). This is characteristic of IgE antibodies in man and dogs and of the IgG or IgGa (electrophoretic mobility) in guinea pigs and rats. Passively sensitized recipient animals can be challenged cutaneously with the specific antigen within 6 hours of the intravenous administration of IgE, with the maximum cutaneous reaction occurring 48 to 72 hours after IgE antibody injection. The reaction designated as *passive cutaneous anaphylaxis* (PCA) occurs immediately after challenge with the antigen (allergen). The administered IgE can persist for as long as 6 weeks if attached to mast cells in tissue. On the other hand, the heterocytotropic antibodies (IgG, IgA, IgM) also involved in the PCA reactions (immediate reaction) remain in the subcutaneous and skin tissue areas for a shorter period of time. These antibodies detach themselves from the tissue in 12 to 24 hours. The challenge with the specific antigen can be evoked immediately. The optimum response is usually manifested 3 to 6 hours after the intravenous administration of the heterocytotropic antibody. Thus, the optimum time of the appearance of the immediate response following passive antibody transfer is dependent on the concentration of antibody administered according to the following equation: $C = 1/t^2$. An inverse squared relationship exists between the local IgG antibody concentration (C) and the time (t) of the latent period. The latent period can be reduced to near zero time if a high concentration of antibody is passively administered. Heterocytotropic antibody, for example, is demonstrated in rabbits, which can passively sensitize guinea pig skin tissue. Apparently the guinea pig skin tissues have rabbit IgG Fc receptors. In contrast, immunoglobulins of sheep, horse, and goat are not active when passively transferred to guinea pigs.

Homocytotropic antibody such as IgE can be induced in animals in less than 10 days, whereas heterocytotropic antibody is detectable in the peripheral blood 10 to 14 days after active immunization.

Assay for
Anaphylaxis

Anaphylaxis can be examined by several in vitro techniques using smooth muscle tissues from sensitized animals or by passively sensitizing smooth muscle tissues with serum antibodies from hypersensitive animals. When actively or passively sensitized uterus, ileum, tracheal rings, or cardiac tissues are suspended in physiological buffered solution to which are added the homologous antigens, the result is the immediate contraction of the muscles which can be recorded or registered on the physiograph (bioassay). This can be attributed to the various mediators released by the antigen-antibody reaction. Another procedure uses sensitized chopped lung or skin tissues suspended in physiological buffered solution. The addition of the specific antigen evokes the release of mediators, such as histamine or slow-reacting substance of anaphylaxis (SRS-A), which can be measured biochemically or by bioassays. Antigens capable of eliciting anaphylaxis are generally soluble. Such antigens are proteins, chemical haptens conjugated to carriers, carbohydrates, and, on occasion, nucleic acids. Cellular antigens such as erythrocytes or bacteria induce little or weak anaphylactic responses, perhaps because of the solubilized determinants of the complex antigens of the cell membranes. Nevertheless, the fungal antigens, such as those from *Aspergillus,* can contribute readily to immediate hypersensitivity (anaphylaxis) and have caused numerous allergic clinical problems in man.

Classification
of Immediate
Hypersensitivity

TYPE I REACTION IN IMMUNOLOGICAL INJURY. Type I hypersensitivity is mediated by the immunoglobulin IgE. The physicochemical characterization and biological function of IgE have been described in Chapter 2. This section will discuss its role as the antibody associated with type I immediate hypersensitivity.

IgE-Mediated Atopy. IgE-mediated hypersensitivity was earlier referred to as *atopy* (*atopos* = uncommon (Greek)), an abnormal state of hypersensitivity. The humoral factor responsible for this reaction was designated *reaginic* or skin-sensitizing *antibody.* The term *allergy allos,* (other + *ergon, work,* Greek) refers to an

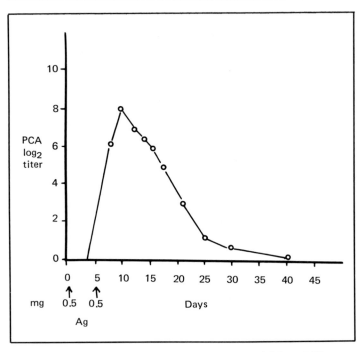

Fig. 13-1 : Primary IgE synthesis in a rat administered 0.5 mg DNP-Ascaris antigen on days 1 and 5 with 1.0 mg B. pertussis as adjuvant. PCA assay was used to quantitate the IgE levels. (Modified from T. Tada and K. Okumura, Collaboration between carrier-specific helper (T) cells and hapten-specific precursors (B cells) is required for maximal anti-hapten IgE antibody response. J. Immunol. 107:137, 1971).

immune deviation from the original state or a "changed reactivity" of an individual. Thus an individual deviating from the expected normal immunological response is one who is allergic. Atopy was first thought to be restricted to humans, but the condition can be demonstrated in dogs and rats and appears to be mediated through the analogous IgE homocytotropic antibody. In rats given two doses of DNP-As (DNP-Ascaris antigen) at day 0 (0.5 mg DNP-As + 1.0 mg Bordetella pertussis vaccine and at day 5 (0.5 mg DNP-As), there is a rapid synthesis of IgE antibody with a maximum titer, as measured by passive cutaneous anaphylaxis (PCA), on the seventh day, followed by a rapid decline with undetectable IgE after the thirtieth day following the initial injection. This is shown in Figure 13-1. As indicated in Chapter 2, the $T_{1/2}$ of IgE is 1.5 days. Figure 13-2 diagrams the interaction between T and B cells in the synthesis of IgE.

Atopic reactions occur in genetically susceptible individuals and may affect one or more primary target organ systems. In man the shock organs are the skin, respiratory, gastro-urinary, and vascular systems. Atopy in the respiratory system is associated

Fig. 13-2 : The T-B cell relationship in the immune response of B cell to IgE synthesis.

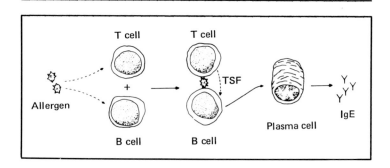

with hay fever, asthma, and serous otitis, affecting the nasal mucosa, bronchioles, and aural mucosa. Urticaria, atopic dermatitis (eczema), and angioneurotic edema are observed when the skin is the reactive, or shock, organ.

When the intestinal and urinary tracts are shock organs the associated hypersensitivity causes vomiting, abdominal pain, diarrhea, and frequency of urination with pain. The vascular involvement in atopy associated with the capillary vessels of the central nervous systems is manifested by headaches, personality changes, and other nervous system alterations.

Genetics of Atopy. Three aspects of the genetics of atopy can be considered: (1) overall susceptibility to allergy; (2) identification of the immunoglobulin IgE (reaginic antibody) in the pathogenesis of atopy; and (3) knowledge of the genetics of the immune response.

That there is a general familial predisposition toward allergic rhinitis, atopic eczema, and asthma has been known for many years. It has been demonstrated that one out of two allergic patients has positive familial history of allergy. In contrast, only one out of seven allergic patients shows a nonallergic family history. Moreover, if both parents have atopic allergy, the offspring have a 75 percent chance of developing an allergy; whereas if only one parent has atopic allergy, the offspring have a 50 percent chance of developing an allergy. It has also been shown that individuals manifest symptoms of atopic allergy in early childhood when both parents have a history of allergy, whereas those with only one parent suffering from allergy often develop symptoms around puberty. Allergic individuals from nonallergic families develop symptoms much later in adulthood.

Individuals do not inherit the disease itself but inherit a general *predisposition* to develop hypersensitivities to a variety of allergens. This is borne out by the fact that children may develop atopic hypersensitivity to different allergens from their parents and that manifestations of the symptoms may vary. In any case it is well established that familial and genetic factors are important in the development of allergic diseases. Nevertheless, the mode of transmission of the hereditary genes of atopic diseases remains controversial. The following have been suggested: (1) a single dominant gene with partial penetrance; (2) a single recessive gene with partial penetrance; and (3) multigenic heredity.

The recognition of IgE immunoglobulin as the major antibody involved in atopic allergy has contributed to our understanding of the immunological basis of this type of hypersensitivity. Recently, methods using radioimmunoassay for detection of the concentration of IgE and for specific recognition of the homologous allergen have contributed to our understanding of the atopic allergy. In general it has been shown that individuals with atopic allergy have higher levels of IgE, although there are overlapping concentrations of IgE levels within normal range.

Although IgE synthesis is regulated by T cell–B cell interaction, which is gene-regulated, gene control of IgE synthesis has not been conclusively established. Experiments with rats suggest that the genetic control of reaginic antibody synthesis is an autosomal trait in which nonresponsiveness is dominant. Furthermore, inbred mice studies suggest that the synthesis of mouse IgE-like antibodies is controlled by many genes (polygenic) rather than a single gene (monogenic).

In immune responses in mice, IgE-like and IgG immunoglobulins were induced against a variety of allergens. The following summation can be made from these studies regarding the distinct types of genetic control of IgE responsiveness in experimental animals: (1) Ir genes possibly linked to the major histocompatibility complex (MHC) have specific control of antigen receptors on lymphocytes; and (2) the ability to synthesize IgE of any specificity is controlled by genes.

In Chapters 10 and 12, the genes associated with the immune response and their association with the MHC were discussed in detail. A general discussion of antigens was presented in Chapter 4. Nevertheless, a brief discussion of the antigens associated with elicitation of atopic hypersensitivity is appropriate at this time.

Allergens. Allergen is a complete antigen that evokes the formation of IgE in susceptible individuals and gives rise to the atopic manifestation. The natural allergens, including enzymes of insects, have distinct physicochemical properties (summarized in Table 13–1). Literally thousands of crude extracts of allergens are available commercially and are prepared from plants, several varieties of mites, and animals, including pets and humans. All these products are crude extracts and consist of mixtures. Investigations of the significant part of these extracts have been made

Table 13-1 : Major Characteristics of Allergens

Properties

1. Molecular weight	1.5 to 4.0×10^6
2. Concentration for sensitization	ng–μg
3. Chemistry	Numerous SH groups, suggesting cross-linkages
4. Color	Brownish—enolyzed sugar-lysine residue (not characteristic of cell allergens)
5. Antigenicity ("allergoids")	Glutaraldehyde treatment: decreases IgE synthesis, no effect on IgG formation

just recently. Table 13-2 lists some of the partially purified allergens from ragweed, fungus, and some insects, especially bee venom.

Type I Reaction. Type I, immediate hypersensitivity, is mediated by IgE in association with mast cells (fixed cells) and basophils (peripheral blood) and the subsequent release of active pharmacological mediators. The physicochemical properties of these mediators are summarized in Table 13-3. Figures 13-3 and 13-4 illustrate diagrammatically the mode by which the mediators are released from the granules. All the details of the sequential mechanism involved in the ultimate release of the active mediators are not clearly understood.

Mechanisms. The sequence of events appears to be as follows: immunoglobulin E (reaginic antibody) attaches through its Fc portion to an IgE Fc receptor on a basophil or mast cell membrane. As indicated earlier, IgE antibodies have great binding affinity to mast cells. This binding can be blocked with the Fc fragment of the specific IgE molecule or an IgG antibody to the Fc receptor on the mast cell membrane. This binding of IgE to mast cells in subcutaneous tissues has been shown to persist for several weeks (up to 6 weeks in humans). The allergen reacts with the Fab portion of the IgE molecule, and the formation of cross-linkages (bridges) between the IgE's through the allergen triggers the release of granules and the subsequent elaboration of the active mediators (Figure 13-3). The postulated sequence of biochemical events occurring within the mast cell is shown in Figure 13-4. Several steps are involved in the process, with varying energy requirements for each step. Following the interaction of the allergen with IgE and the subsequent binding, the sequence is as follows: (1) Activation of proesterase to esterase, which requires Ca^{++}, thus an increase in intracellular Ca^{++} due to the antigen-antibody complexing at the membrane surface.

Table 13-2 : Characteristics of Some Fractionally Isolated Allergens of Ragweed, Honey Bee Venom, and Aspergillus Involved in Hypersensitivity

Allergens: Fractions	Characteristics
Ragweed	
a. Acidic proteins	
E, most active	Allergen E: MW 3.8×10^4, consists of 2 polypeptides (2.18×10^4 and 1.57×10^4 daltons) bound by noncovalent forces, dissociated by urea, guanidine, HCL, sodium dodecylsulfate, $<0.5\%$ carbohydrates.
K, second most active	Allergen K: MW 3.8×10^4 daltons.
b. Basic proteins	RA-3, 1.5×10^4 daltons; RA-5, 5.0×10^3 daltons; BPA-R, 2.8×10^4 daltons; all three are weak allergens that may contain the active antigenic components, but in lesser amounts.
Honey bee venom	
a. Gel filtration (SG75) fractions	
Fraction 1	MW $> 7.5 \times 10^4$, 3 subfractions; most active allergen in RAST for IgE.
Fraction 2	Hyaluronidase: $5.5-6.1 \times 10^4$ daltons, second most active allergen; glycoprotein containing mannose and glucosamine; enzyme that hydrolyzes endo-*N*-acetyl-hexosaminic bonds of hyaluronic acid and chondroitin-sulfuric acids A and C to tetrasaccharide residues. Stabilized by NaCl, inhibited by Fe^{++}, Mn^{++}, and Ca^{++}. Acts as an allergen.
Fraction 3 Phospholipase A (phosphatide 2-acyl hydrolase)	A protein: may consist of isomers ($A\alpha$ & $A\beta$), enzyme; hydrolyzes the fatty acyl ester at the 2-position of phospholipids—releases fatty acid and lysophosphatide; inhibited by Zn^{++}, and Ba^{++}, and Mn^{++}; activated by Ca^{++}; stability $90^{\circ}C$ and pH 3.0 for ~ 5 minutes. Secondary allergen as far as IgE RAST is concerned.
Fraction 4 Melittin	26-amino acid peptide, ruptured mast cell with histamine release, strong hemolytic activity, constitutes $\geqslant 50\%$ of honey bee venom.
Fractions 5, 6, and 7	Apamin, neurotoxin, complex mixtures of lower MW materials with pharmacological activity.
Aspergillus	
a. Trichloracetic acid supernatant fraction (TCA-Fum)	Preparation from sonicated mycelial culture of *A. fumigatis* reacts with IgE and also IgE and IgM; soluble in 10% TCA and 50% $(NH_4)_2SO_4$, anionic mucopolysaccharide, insensitive to DNAse and RNAse.

Table 13-3 : The Active Mediators Released by Mast Cells in Type I Hypersensitivity

Compounds	MW	Properties and Activity
Histamine	111	Vasoactive amine; increases capillary permeability; secondary to partial interruption of vascular endothelium; causes smooth muscle constriction (increases respiratory and air way resistance); erythema and angioedema; histidine (precursor); affected by antihistamines (receptor-dependent).
SRS-A	400-500	Slow reacting substance of anaphylaxis; increases capillary permeability; contraction of smooth muscle (reverse with epinephrine), not affected by antihistamines, acidic lipid not preformed in granules; involved in the prolonged bronchospasm in asthma; antagonists, diethylcarbamazine; arylsulfatase from eosinophil splits SRS-A into 2 fragments, also suppresses SRS-A formation.
ECF-A	500-600	Eosinophil-chemotactic factor; acid peptide—preformed state in granules of mast cells.
Serotonin	176	5-hydroxytryptamine; occurs in mast cells and human platelets; preformed in granules; antagonist-lysergic acid, increase permeability and capillary dilation; constriction of smooth muscle (some species) not as important in type I hypersensitivity in man unless platelets are activated and granules are released.
PAF	450-550	Platelet activation factor; induces platelet aggregation; releases serotonin and histamine (rabbit); contains phosphoryl choline and related to lecithin.
Bradykinin	1060	Formed by action of kallikrein on kininogen (α_2-globulin in serum); consists of 9 amino acids, non-apeptide. Chemotaxis; smooth muscle constriction; dilation of peripheral arterioles (increases capillary permeability), increases mucous secretion of bronchus. Stimulates pain fibers; induces symptoms of hay fever, angioedema (associated with painful swelling), asthma.
Heparin		Acidic mucopolysaccharide; contributes to the metachromatic staining of mast cell granules (bind basic dyes); contributes to anaphylaxis in dogs, but not in humans; transient anticoagulation in humans.
Prostaglandins	400-500	Fatty acid derivatives; increase permeability and dilation of capillary, contraction of smooth muscle and bronchial constriction; causes alteration in pain threshold; E_1 and E_2 feedback control for synthesis. E_1 and E_2 stimulate c-AMP via receptor other than β-adenyl cyclase, role in asthma, effect cyclic nucleotide synthesis in target cells.
HETE (12, L-hydroxy-5.8. 10.14-eicosatetraenoic acid)		Product of arachidonic acid and formed by lipooxygenase; chemotaxis.

This step can be inhibited by diisopropyl fluorophosphate (DFP) and is associated with the microfilaments. (2) Further autoactivation of proesterase (broken lines in Figure 13-4). (3) Microfilaments move the granules alongside the microtubules or plasma membrane. This step requires energy and is inhibited by deprivation of glucose. (4) A further step (block with deoxyglucose) involving Ca^{++} and c-AMP, which enhances the release of granules

Fig. 13-3 : Activation and release of mast cell mediators through the reaction of sensitized IgE antibody to its corresponding allergen (type I reaction).

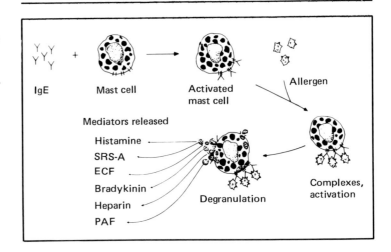

Fig. 13-4 : The postulated biochemical sequence of the release of granules and the elaboration of the active mediators by target mast cells in type I hypersensitivity.

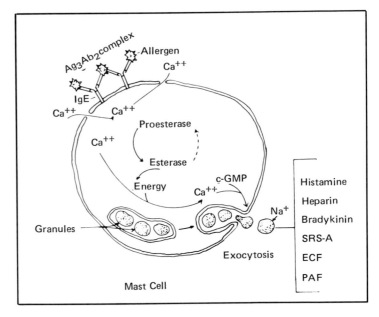

and elaboration of the vasoactive amine and other mediators from the granules. The release from granules requires possible exchange with Na^+.

The step involving Ca^{++} can be inhibited by ethylenediaminetetraacetic acid (EDTA), and the sequence involving the release of the active mediators by an increase in c-AMP. The postulated role for the cyclic nucleotides in type I hypersensitivity will be discussed in detail later in the paragraphs to follow.

The active mediators elaborated from the granules, which contribute to the clinical symptoms seen in type I hypersensitivity, have been summarized in Table 13-3.

Clinical Features. Type I hypersensitivity can be artificially separated into generalized and localized anaphylaxis. The generalized reaction is manifested by widespread dissemination of the antigen with systemic symptoms of edema, urticaria, and bronchial constriction. The localized reaction is primarily a result of diagnostic skin testing. The administration of large concentrations of allergen during skin tests can result in a systemic or generalized allergic reaction. Type I reactions are associated with the following recognized clinical hypersensitivites: (1) allergic rhinitis (hay fever), allergen-induced (pollens, fungal spores, dust (mites), and animal danders) atopic hypersensitivity; (2) atopic dermatitis, associated with allergic rhinitis and asthma (atopic and nonatopic forms); (3) anaphylaxis, usually caused by drugs, insect venom, or food hypersensitivity: IgE is the major immunoglobulin involved, but it may be evoked by IgA and IgM through activation of the complement system and formation of anaphylatoxins or generations of kinins (Chapter 9); (4) urticaria and angioedema, cutaneous forms of anaphylaxis. The acute form is usually caused by food or drugs, nonimmunological forms are associated with chronic urticaria; (5) a rare form of hereditary angioedema due to autosomal mendelian dominant deficiency of C1 inactivator (C1 esterase inhibitor), repeated episodes of urticaria and angioedema; (6) drug hypersensitivity, which can occur also in the other three types (II, III and IV) of hypersensitivity, depending on the immunogenicity of the drug; and (7) food allergy associated with systemic anaphylaxis, urticaria, and recurrences of atopic allergy, a sensitivity induced via the gastrointestinal system and thus dependent on maturation of the GI tract, hence more common in newborn and youngsters.

Asthma. Asthma is a chronic disease characterized by hyperirritability of the bronchial mucosa with eosinophils. It occurs at any age and is manifested by wheezing and dyspnea, which can range from mild discomfort to life-threatening respiratory failure. Patients with asthma can be free of symptoms between episodes of attack or can have chronic obstruction of the air passage. Asthma can be separated into two aspects: (1) extrinsic (allergic, atopic, or immunological asthma); and (2) intrinsic (nonallergic, nonatopic, idiopathic asthma). Extrinsic asthma is mediated by IgE and can be associated with allergic rhinitis and urticaria. All the symptoms associated with atopy and reaginic antibody are manifested. Skin tests are positive to specific allergens, and the levels of IgE are generally elevated. It is common in early infancy and childhood, and about 50 percent of asthmatics have evidence of atopic allergy. On the other hand, intrinsic or nonatopic asthma occurs primarily in adults and usually after an infectious respiratory ailment. Intrinsic asthma pursues a more chronic and recurrent course, with bronchial obstructions unrelated

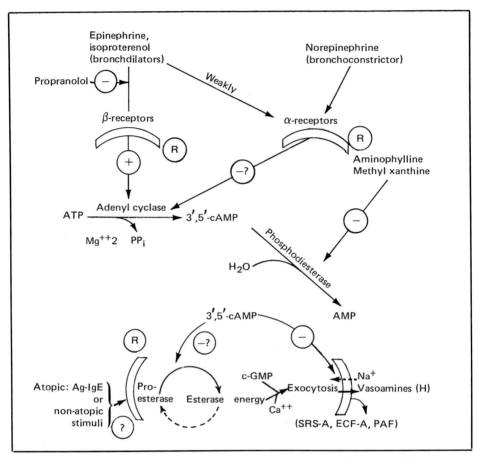

Fig. 13-5 : Postulated mechanism for the allergic release of histamine and slow-reacting substance of anaphylaxis (SRS-A), showing the influence of the catecholamines epinephrine and norephinephrine. Norepinephrine is known to have an effect opposite to that of epinephrine, but it remains to be shown (indicated by -?) that it acts directly on adenyl cyclase. Cyclic AMP inhibits the release of vasoamines (histamine H), slow-reacting substance of anaphylaxis (SRS-A), eosinophilic chemotactic factor (ECF-A), and platelet-activating factor (PAF). Decrease in c-AMP results in an increase in c-GMP, which results in increased release of H, ECF-A, SRS-A, and PAF. Stimulators of α-receptors will also tend to stimulate c-GMP levels. − = inhibitory (suppresive) effect on the indicated process; + = stimulatory effect on the indicated process; and R = receptors (IgE-Ag = Fc receptor).

to seasonal allergens or exposure to allergens. Skin tests are negative to the atopic allergens, and serum IgE level is generally normal. Family histories are negative for atopic disease. Yet the general clinical manifestations are similar to those of allergic asthma. Thus it has been suggested that the mechanisms that induce the clinical picture are similar. To explain this similarity the adrenergic theory was proposed (Figure 13-5).

The sympathetic system mediates the release of catecholamines, which include epinephrine, norepinephrine, and dopamine. A synthetic compound, isoproterenol, acts similarly to epinephrine and is an agonist. The parasympathetic (craniosacral outflow) system mediates the release of acetylcholine (ACh) and is synonymous with the cholinergic system. Through their mediators or neurotransmitters these two systems maintain the homeostasis of bronchial smooth muscle tonicity by alternately relaxing (epinephrine or norepinephrine acts as a hormone) and constricting (Ach) in the normal physiological state. Thus presumably in both atopic and nonatopic asthma the end result or clinical manifestations are similar, since the terminal mechanisms on the effect on bronchial smooth muscles are similar, although the initiating agents, immunological or infections, etc., are dissimilar.

Adrenergic Concept. The bronchial system is affected by the catecholamines. Those affecting the α-receptor, such as norepinephrine, induce bronchoconstriction, and those affecting the β-receptor (e.g., epinephrine) induce bronchial relaxation. Under normal circumstances, homeostasis exists between these two influences. The β-receptor is linked to adenyl cyclase, an enzyme that catalyzes synthesis of cyclic $3', 5'$-c-AMP (c-AMP) from ATP in the presence of Mg^{++} ions. It has been postulated that patients with bronchial asthma, eczema, rhinitis, etc., have a deficiency in β-adenyl cyclase in the cells of the affected tissues, since the key to suppression or release of histamine and SRS-A is the cyclic nucleotides c-AMP (suppresses) and c-GMP (stimulates). Diminished levels of c-AMP, due to insufficient synthesis via β-adenyl cyclase or hyperactive degradation (to AMP) via the enzyme phosphodiesterase, would increase the amount of histamine (H), eosinophilic chemotactic factor (ECF-A), platelet-activating factor (PAF), and SRS-A released in response to the presence of IgE-Ab complexes, infections, or other agents.

Experimentally, suppression of adenyl cyclase by *propranolol* (a β-adrenergic blocking agent; antagonizes the action of epinephrine), along with an increase in α-receptor stimulation, will suppress c-AMP production and cause an increase in c-GMP production, leading to increased histamine and SRS-A release following either atopic or nonatopic stimulation. *Isoproterenol,* which stimulates β-receptors, together with aminophylline or methylxanthine (which inhibits phosphodiesterase), would increase the levels of c-AMP and thus cause suppression of histamine and SRS-A release; the level of c-GMP would be diminished.

Immunotherapy. Hyposensitization or desensitization in type I immunological injury mediated by IgE has been one of the procedures for treatment of atopic allergy caused by known allergens.

Fig. 13-6 :
A. Probable mechanism of allergen blockage by IgG in hyposensitization therapy. B. Probable blocking mechanism, by pentapeptide fragment from the Fc of IgE, of the Fc IgE receptor sites on a mast cell.

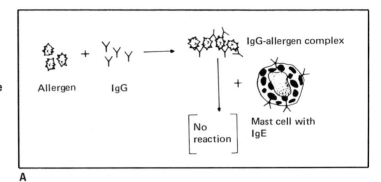

A

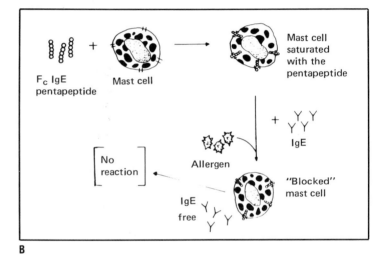

B

Generally the allergenic extracts used have been crude preparations. Immunotherapy by administration of extracts of the allergen has been effective in reducing symptoms in atopic allergies (hay fever), especially those in patients with seasonal pollen hypersensitivity. This type of treatment also may be effective in desensitization with molds and house dust (mites) allergens. A complete state of desensitization is not achieved, however. The mechanisms associated with successful hyposensitization have been explained as follows: (1) Hyposensitization with allergens is associated with the production of specific blocking IgG antibodies against the allergen. The IgG antibody formed is not involved in type I hypersensitivity but appears to bind circulating allergens and thus interferes with the interaction of IgE on mast cells. This blocking by IgG is illustrated in Figure 13-6A. It has also been suggested that IgG synthesis against the allergen induces a feedback mechanism for suppression of synthesis of IgE by B cells. (2) An increase in suppressor T cells, regulators of IgE synthesis by B cells, also may play a role during hyposensitization with allergen. (3) Allergenic extracts contain monomeric or tolerogenic polypeptides, which are incomplete and which bind to T or B cells, thus preventing interaction between T and B cells for synthesis of IgE (haptenic capacity but no carrier effect). Thus there is an incomplete transmission of any message or sufficient signal for active transformation of B cell to synthesize IgE (see Chapter 10). This induction of tolerance and subsequent inability of the T and B cells to react with the polymeric or aggregated immunogenic antigens can result in suppression of IgE synthesis.

A novel method of inhibiting the symptoms of atopic allergenic patients is the use of a synthetic pentapeptide consisting of Asp-Ser-Asp-Pro-Arg, a component of the H-chain homology of the amino acid sequence numbers 320 through 324 of IgE. This pentapeptide inhibited 60 to 89 percent of the Prausnitz-Küstner (P-K) reaction under examination. This approach assumes that the pentapeptide structural unit of IgE will localize in, or displace, the IgE Fc on the mast cell or basophil, and thus prevent the attachment of the sensitized complete IgE molecule. This is shown in Figure 13-6B. A drawback to such interference by the pentapeptide may be that the peptide may bind all mast cells and basophils if excessive amounts are given and thus interfere with normal functions of these cells.

TYPE II REACTION IN IMMUNOLOGICAL INJURY. The type II reaction encompasses all immunopathological mechanisms in which lesions are produced by cytotoxic antibodies reacting with accessible antigens on cells, or on the tissue membrane of cells. The antigen may be a natural constituent of the membrane or may be an antigen adsorbed to the membrane of the cell or tissue. In the majority of these reactions, complement is implicated in the cell or tissue destruction, and the formation and release of C mediators is involved in the inflammatory condition. In addition to complement action, tissue destruction can occur through the mononuclear cell intervention. The nature of these cells is discussed in detail later in the chapter. These cells have been designated *antibody-dependent cytotoxic cells* (ADCC) and are neither T nor B cells nor macrophages but are part of the null cell population of the peripheral blood. Thus these killer cells (K cells) possess Fc receptors but no surface Ig nor T cell markers such as HTLA, HTL or T antigens (see Chapter 3). The mechanism by which K cells destroy target cells is unknown at present. It has been suggested, however, that channels are formed (by enzymatic action?) in the bimolecular layers of the membrane, initiating electrolyte loss or changes between the cytoplasm and the external microenvironment of the target cell. This leads to the demise of the cell.

Antibodies. All antibodies reacting with membrane antigens are not necessarily cytotoxic. For example, antibodies to thyroid tissue have been shown to stimulate formation of the thyroid hormone. This phenomenon has been described and noted as *long-acting thyroid stimulator* (LATS) and has been attributed to a specific antibody to thyroid-producing cells. Other examples of nondestructive antibodies, sometimes referred to as *enhancing* or *blocking* antibodies, have been demonstrated in the sera of experimental animals and humans with cancer. These antibodies tend to protect the target organ or disrupt the normal expected antigen reactions with the cell or cytotoxic antibody. Thus, the IgG antibody that reacts with an allergen and masks the antigenic determinant sites will prevent the allergen from binding with the IgE immunoglobulin and prevent the sequence of events leading to the release of vasoactive amines from mast cells (Figure 13-6A). Blocking antibodies have been demonstrated in transplantation studies in which histocompatibility antigens have been masked by the antibody and hence have permitted the transplant to escape rejection by the sensitized T cell. Similar observations of a masking effect by antibody have been demonstrated for the maintenance of tumors in man and animals (see Chapter 16).

Mechanisms. Figure 13-7 summarizes in diagrammatic form the type II reactions that lead to destruction of the target cells. Figures 13-6A and 13-7B also illustrate the masking effect. Figure 13-7B, up to antigen coated target cell, represents the masking effect.

Some authors have suggested the addition of types V (13-7B) and VI classifications (13-7B when C is activated and lysis of cell occurs) for the masking or enhancing antibody and the K cell (ADCC) reactions, respectively. Until these are better understood, the present types I to IV appear to be satisfactory in the explanation of the basic mechanisms involved in immunological injury.

Type II Disorders. Some immunological diseases associated with type II mechanisms mediated via complement action are summarized in Table 13-4. The most commonly recognized autoimmune diseases of type II immunological injury appear to be those associated with destruction of red blood cells. These are the immune hemolytic anemias, in which the erythrocytes are readily destroyed by autoantibodies and complement action. Two types of antibodies based on reactions at different temperatures have been recognized in autoimmune hemolytic anemia: (1) warm antibody and (2) cold antibody. The former consists of IgG antibodies (rarely, IgA or IgM) generally directed to antigens of the Rh system (see Chapter 11) and reacting best at 37°C or 20°C. Cold antibody consists of IgM (rarely, IgA) and reacts best at 4°C as cold agglutinins but can react up to 32°C.

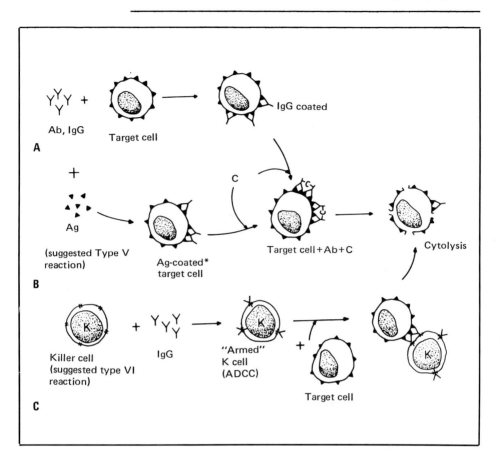

Fig. 13-7 : Type II immunological injuries initiated by an IgG antibody.
A. Antibody (IgG) reacts with Ag on target cell plus complement results in
lysis of cells. B. Antigen coats target cell plus antibody (*) to this step
masking phenomenon if C not activated, if C activated and lysis of target
cell (B suggested type V reaction). C. Killer cell armed with antibody via
Fc receptor and attached to target cell and cytolysis (suggested type VI
reaction). B and C reactions have been designed types V and VI, respectively, by some workers.

A rare form of autoimmune hemolytic anemia, paroxysmal cold
hemoglobinuria, is mediated by IgG antibody and complement.
Sensitization of the erythrocyte by antibody and binding of C
occurs at 15°C, and the heavily sensitized cells are hemolyzed
at 37°C. The antibody has been designated Donath-Landsteiner,
and is responsible for a classic biphasic temperature phenomenon.
Antigen of the erythrocytes involved in the cold agglutinin
syndrome is of the I blood group; while for the classic biphasic
Donath-Landsteiner antibody, the target antigen appears to be
of the P blood group.

Table 13-4 : Immunological Injury or Disease Due to Type II Mechanisms and Complement Action

Disease	Target Tissue
Autoimmune hemolytic anemias	Erythrocytes
Drug-induced immune hemolytic anemias	''
Alloantibody-induced hemolytic anemias	''
Idiopathic (autoimmune) thrombocytopenic purpura (ITP)	Platelets
Secondary autoimmune thrombocytopenia	''
Drug-induced immune thrombocytopenia	''
Posttransfusion purpura	''
Neonatal immune purpura	''
Alloantibodies, destruction of transfused platelets	''
Goodpasture's disease	Kidney and lung basement membrane
Autoimmune neutropenia	Neutrophil
Drug-induced autoimmune neutropenia	''

Alloantibody-induced hemolytic anemia is associated with the various antigenic systems of erythrocytes—ABO, Kell, Lewis, etc.—and is particularly observed in blood transfusion anemias. Hemolytic disease of the newborn can be placed in this category (see Chapter 11). A diagrammatic scheme of lysis of the red blood cells is shown in Figure 13-8 for autoimmune and drug-induced hemolysis. The mechanism for the alloantibody-induced sequence should be similar to that shown for autoimmune hemolytic anemia (Figure 13-8A).

Thrombocytopenia may be due to a variety of factors: (1) increased platelet destruction, (2) decreased platelet production or (3) abnormal platelet distribution—pooling to the spleen, for example. Autoimmune thrombocytopenia is associated with an increase in platelet removal and destruction through enhanced opsonization by macrophages. This leads to generalized bleeding and purpura. The major clinical features associated with idiopathic thrombocytopenia purpura (ITP) are: (1) demonstrable antiplatelet antibody, (2) shortened half-life, (3) usually, preceding viral infections, and (4) commonly, CMI to platelets. Presumably autoantibodies are formed to viral antigens bound to platelets and to platelet antigens in the region of the bound viral antigens. The drug-induced antibodies to platelets are formed similarly to drug-platelet complexes, with the drug acting as hapten and the platelet representing the carrier moiety. The

Fig. 13-8 :
A. Autoimmune
hemolytic anemia.
Lysis of target
erythrocyte with
warm (IgG) or
cold (IgM) anti-
bodies and comple-
ment. B. Drug-
induced hemo-
lytic anemia.

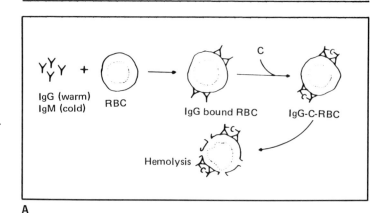

A

B

drugs most commonly used in therapy, such as sulfonamides, chlorothiazide derivatives, chlorpropamide, quinidine, and aspirin, have been implicated in drug-induced thrombocytopenia. The mechanisms shown in Figure 13-8 for red blood cells might be involved similarly in the processes leading to thrombocyto-penia, except that macrophage opsonization (through its Fc receptors), rather than the complement system, may be more commonly involved in the destruction of platelets. The drugs involved in induction of autoimmunity in hemolytic anemia and thrombocytopenia are listed in Table 13-5.

Thrombocytopenia mediated through immunological means has been demonstrated in blood transfusions and in newborns. In such cases it is due to alloantibodies (transfusion and maternal sensitization) and autoantibodies (ITP).

The autoimmune destruction of neutrophils contributes to leukopenia. Leukopenia is the reduction of the number of

Table 13-5 : Some of the Drugs Implicated in the Induction of Immune Hemolytic Anemia and Thrombocytopenia

Drugs	Target Cell
Acetoazolamide	P
Allymid	P
Aminosalicylic acid (PAS)	P&E
Aspirin	P
Antihistamines	P&E
Carbamazepine	P
Cephalothin	P&E
Chlorothiazide	P&E
Chlorpropamide	E
Digitoxin	P
Isoniazid	E
Meprobamate	P
Levadopa	E
Methyldopa	P
Quinidine	P&E
Quinine	P&E
Rifampicin	P&E
Stibophen	P&E
Sulfonamides	E
Thioguanine	P
Tetracyclines	E

P = platelet; E = erythrocyte.

circulating leukocytes to below 3,500 to 4,000 cells/μ1. A decrease in granulocytes (granulocytopenia) occurs more commonly than in lymphocytes (lymphocytopenia). This decrease in granulocytes may be due to (1) decreased production of granulocytes in the bone marrow, (2) increased utilization of granulocytes (abnormal distribution), and (3) increased destruction through utilization (short half-life, see Chapter 8). Decreased production of granulocytes has been demonstrated in aplastic anemia, leukemia, and other diseases involving the bone marrow. Increased destruction or utilization of granulocytes occurs in autoimmune neutropenia and some forms of drug-induced leukopenia. Autoimmune neutropenia appears to be mediated through antineutrophils and complement. Recent studies suggest that lymphocytotoxic K cell through the ADCC mechanism may be the major mode of action.

Drug-induce neutropenia is commonly mediated through the direct effect of the drug on bone marrow. Nevertheless, a mechanism similar to that acting in the drug-induced hemolytic anemias (anti-red cells + C) and in thrombocytopenia (antiplatelets + macrophages or C) may play a part in drug-induced destruction of granulocytes through immunological reactions.

Another example of the type II reaction of immunological injury is glomerulonephritis associated with specific autoantibodies to the glomerular-basement membrane (GBM) of the kidney. This is demonstrated clinically by *Goodpasture's syndrome* and experimentally by studies with rabbit antirat kidney basement membrane antibody (as antibody injected into rats will induce *Masugi glomerulonephritis,* which resembles Goodpasture's disease (see Chapter 14 for the autoimmune mechanism in kidney diseases). Complement and the leukocytes (neutrophils) contribute greatly to the tissue injury area through the C-activated components and the enzymes of the leukocytes (see Chapter 8).

Allogenic cytotoxic antibodies to lymphocytes are readily demonstrated in postpartum multigravidae or in individuals who have undergone a series of whole blood transfusions. These sources of sera have been used in the development of the HLA serological detection methods (see Chapter 12). These antibody-lymphocyte reactions bind complement, with the subsequent destruction of the lymphocyte. In some diseases, such as systemic lupus erythematosus (SLE), autoantibodies to T cells have been found that specifically lyse these cells. These same antibodies appear to bind to brain cells of individuals with SLE and thus may be the significant factors in the cerebral manifestations. The existence of cross-reacting antigens between T cells and brain cells of mice has been established experimentally.

Type II reactions associated with deposition of antibodies (IgG, IgA, IgM, and IgD) and C components of the classic and alternative pathways along the basement membrane of the dermal-epidermal junction of the skin can be demonstrated in pemphigoid disorders.

The etiological basis for the immune responses that evoke the antibodies to "self" antigens remains undiscovered in many diseases, although the pathogenetic results of the antibody-antigen reaction leading to activation of C, K cells, T and B cells, and macrophages have been documented both clinically and, in particular, experimentally. Transfusion reactions and the ensuing hemolytic diseases (hemolytic anemia, leukopenia, and thrombocytopenia), as well as erythroblastosis fetalis of the newborn, can be attributed to isosensitization or allosensitization from imcompatible blood transfusions or pregnancy. In addition, individuals can produce an antibody to an exogenous product, such as the lipopolysaccharides of gram-negative organisms, which

Fig. 13-9 : Type III, immune complex-mediated immunological injury. There is activation of complement by Ag-Ab complexes in extravascular reactions and attraction of PMNs.

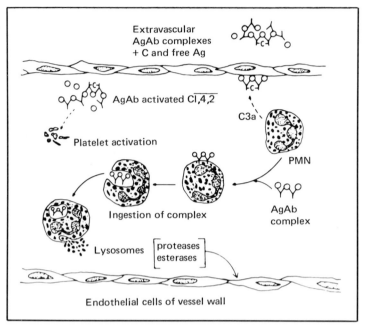

Extravascular AgAb complexes + C and free Ag

AgAb activated C1̄,4,2̄

Platelet activation

C3a

PMN

Ingestion of complex

AgAb complex

Lysosomes [proteases esterases]

Endothelial cells of vessel wall

may cross-react with common antigens found on target cells or react directly with cells to which LPS may be bound. This is probably common in areas of inflammation (especially chronic). Induction of autoantibodies will be considered further in Chapter 14.

TYPE III REACTION IN IMMUNOLOGICAL INJURY. Injury initiated by interaction of specific antibody (IgG or IgM) with freely dispersed (soluble or suspension) antigenic molecules constitutes the type III reaction. This reaction is characterized by deposition and localization of antigen-antibody complexes in tissues. Inflammation is the cardinal feature, with activation of the classic complement system. The active fragments of the complement components are formed through the classic pathway of activation (see Chapter 9). The subsequent physiologically activated components (C3a and C5a) attract the polymorphonuclear (PMN) cells to the active site. The PMNs then phagocytize the excessive complexes and other products with consequent exocytosis of lysosomal enzymes (hydrolases), including the proteases, glycosidases, and esterases, which exacerbate the inflammatory lesion. The homologous formation of complexes between IgG antibody and soluble antigen and the initial binding of C to the Fc portion of the antibody-antigen complexes are depicted in Figure 13-9.

Mechanisms. The pathogenesis of the immune complex diseases and the initial inflammatory lesion that is characteristic of the

Type III reaction can be summarized as follows: (1) antigen-antibody complexes, generally with excess antigen, form intravascularly or near the surface of the endothelial cells of the capillary; (2) complement is fixed by the complexes through the Fc portion of the antibody (two antibody molecules are required for IgG and one for IgM); (3) formation through appropriate cleavage of C components by the classic pathway results in formation of the chemotactic factors (C3a, C5a, or C$\overline{567}$); (4) damage or activation of platelets initiates release of vasoactive amines and prostaglandins, which results in increased vascular permeability; (5) Ag-Ab complexes localize simultaneously in vessel walls and in extracellular tissues; (6) further fixation of complement and release of active fragments such as the chemotactic factors (C3a, C5a, and C$\overline{567}$) occur; (7) PMNs are attracted to the area of the complexes and inflammatory lesion with subsequent ingestion of the immune complexes by the neutrophils; (8) the release of lysosomal enzymes, such as proteases, glycosidases, and esterases, initiates damage to adjacent cells and tissues; (9) the activation of fibrinogen (Chapter 9) ensues, with deposition of fibrin; (10) either the lesions heal and regress after a single exposure of excessive antigen, or inflammation and tissue injury are maintained, with persistent formation of immune complexes. Two major classic immune reactions of type III have been demonstrated in experimental animals: (1) the Arthus reaction and (2) serum sickness. The sequence of events described in the preceding paragraphs occurs in both types and also in the clinically observed immune complex diseases, some of which are listed in Table 13-6.

Arthus Reaction. In the Arthus reaction, the sensitized individual has high antibody levels (detectable) in the circulatory plasma, which interact with an equally high level of the homologous antigen in subcutaneous tissues and in blood vessel walls (through injections). Massive precipitation of the complexes triggers the focal inflammatory conditions previously described (thrombus formation, aggregation of platelets, infarction, hemorrhage, and tissue necrosis). A pattern of acute vasculitis can be demonstrated in histological sections. Intradermal injection of antigen in the sensitized host (experimental animal) results in local swelling at the site of antigen deposition in 1 to 2 hours. This reaction increases to a maximum at 3 to 6 hours after antigen injection and disappears in 10 to 12 hours. Temporal examination of the lesion shows neutrophil infiltration followed by macrophages (monocytes and eosinophils) and resultant phagocytosis of complexes and reduction of the inflammatory condition. The Arthus reaction can be demonstrated passively by administration of antibody subcutaneously, followed by administration of the homologous antigen in the same region of the skin.

Table 13-6 : Some Examples of Human Diseases Associated with Immune Complexes Detectable in Serum and in Target Organs

Autoimmune disorders	Hashimoto's thyroiditis; rheumatoid arthritis; systemic lupus erythematosus
Disseminated malignancy	Carcinoma: breast, colon, lung; leukemia: acute lymphoblastic, chronic lymphoblastic; Hodgkin's disease; malignant melanoma
Drug reactions	Serum sickness; penicillamine nephropathy
Microbial infections	Bacterial: acute streptococcal glomerulonephritis, lepromatous leprosy, mycoplasmal pneumonia, shunt nephritis (staphylococcal), subacute bacterial endocarditis, syphilis; viral: acute viral hepatitis, viral hepatitis B infection, Guillain-Barré syndrome, HBsAg in polyarteritis nodosa, infectious mononucleosis, glomerulonephritis, dengue, hemorrhagic fever, cytomegalovirus in respiratory diseases; fungal: allergic bronchopulmonary aspergillosis, extrinsic allergic alveolitis
Parasitic infections	Leishmaniasis, malarial nephrotic syndrome, schistosomiasis, tropical splenomegaly, trypanosomiasis syndrome
Others	Celiac disease, Crohn's disease, dermatitis herpetiformis, essential mixed cryoglobulinemia, Henoch-Schönlein nephritis, hepatic cirrhosis, pemphigoid, postpericardiotomy syndrome, sickle cell anemia

The immunological diseases that may be due to the Arthus-type reaction can be seen clinically in various examples of hypersensitivity pneumonitis and extrinsic allergic interstitial alveolitis (caused by breathing dust containing fungal microflora, mites, and heterologous proteins such as danders of animals or avian proteins). For example, in extrinsic allergic interstitial alveolitis, circulating antibody can encounter a large concentration of molecularly dispersed antigen absorbed from the alveolar sacs and react with the precipitating antibody in the pulmonary capillaries. The precipitating complexes initiate the characteristic clinical manifestations of allergic interstitial alveolitis. The disease may be acute or chronic, depending on the persistence of antibody and exposure to the causative antigen. Fungi generally involved are thermophilic *Actinomyces, Aspergillus,* and *Micropolyspora faeni.* The mites in house dust have been attributed to the *Dermatophagoides* species.

Serum Sickness. Classic serum sickness caused by the injection of serum into human subjects for antitoxin or antibacterial therapy is less common than it was two to three decades ago. The widespread immunization program and the advent of potent antibiotic agents and increasing use of purified human antibodies, for example, RhoGAM for erythroblastosis fetalis and antihepatitis-A γ-globulin all have contributed to the declining incidence of serum sickness. Nevertheless, serum sickness-like reactions due to nonprotein antigens—for example, penicillin—remain a problem. Table 13-7 summarizes some of the causes of serum sickness.

Table 13-7 : Proteins and Nonproteins Implicated as Causes of Serum Sickness

Foreign proteins	1. Horse: antitetanus toxin, antirabies, botulism, and snake venom.
	2. ACTH
	3. Bee venoms
	4. Antithymus cell (heterologous serum)
Nonproteins	1. Penicillin
	2. Sulfonamides
	3. Arsenic compounds
	4. Hydantoin compounds
	5. Piperazine citrate

Administration of a single large dose of antigen such as BSA in 500 to 1,000 mg concentrations intravenously will result in the formation of antibody. The antibody will then react with the residual antigen remaining in circulation, forming complexes that deposit in the capillaries of various target organs (kidney, spleen, lung and/or heart) to initiate vasculitis and the series of events associated with inflammation. This predilection of the antigen-antibody complexes for capillaries of the glomerulus, heart, joint capsules, and lung is still not clearly understood. Recent evidence suggests, for example, the presence of C3 receptors on endothelial membrane surfaces of capillaries of the glomeruli. Whether this is the mode by which complexes of Ag-Ab-C3 attach through known available receptors in certain regions of the blood vessels remains to be explored.

Schwartzman Phenomenon. It was shown in Chapter 9 that complement activation may occur either through the classic pathway or, by activation of C3, through the alternative pathway. It has been suggested that activation of the C system through the alternative pathway in massive amounts would lead to platelet damage and release of platelet factor III, thus initiating intravascular coagulation. This seems to be the necessary component of the Schwartzman phenomenon, wherein hemorrhagic and necrotic lesions occur either at local sites in the skin or in the adrenals and kidney. The Shwartzman reaction involves two steps: (1) an initial *preparatory* phase, with the intradermal injection of a culture filtrate of a gram-negative organism; and (2) an intravenous *provocative* dose of the same culture filtrate 24 hours later. In a few hours a hemorrhagic and necrotic inflammatory lesion appears at the site of the initial preparatory intradermal injection. It has been demonstrated that the antigen given in the preparatory intradermal injection need not be related to that given in the provocative dose. The length of time between the preparatory and provocative doses is important in the development of the lesion, however. The 24-hour period appears to give the maximum response. Although the inflammatory lesion resembles that of the Arthus reaction, the Shwartzman phenomenon has been shown to be nonimmunological although, as already mentioned, it may be triggered by the activation of the alternative complement pathway. In this regard it is interesting to note that the first preparatory antigen tried in the Schwartzman reaction was the lipopolysaccharide or endotoxin of *Salmonella typhi*. Endotoxins of gram-negative organisms have been implicated in the activation of the alternative pathway of C activation (see Chapter 9). The significance of the Shwartzman reaction becomes understandable when the histological lesions and clinical manifestations are seen to resemble immunological injury.

Immune Complex Disorders. The mechanism for the immunological pathogenesis of the immune complex disorders has been presented. These immune complex disorders are modulated by various factors, including the nature of the host, antigen, antibody (IgG, IgM, and occasional IgA especially in rheumatoid arthritis), complexes (ratio of Ag to Ab), complement, blood clotting and fibrinolysis, platelets, and leukocytes.

Host. Experimental animals vary in the degree of intensity to which they develop the lesions of the immune complex disorders. Rabbits have been examined extensively. When given single or multiple injections of large concentrations of purified foreign protein such as BSA, they show a generalized acute and transient vasculitis in various tissues (especially the heart, spleen, lung, and glomerulus). Complement levels measured as CH_{50} units also decrease during the formation of the antigen-antibody complexes in the blood. The rapid removal of the Ag-Ab complexes, with a subsequent increase in free circulating antibody diminishes the inflammatory vasculitis, and the rabbit recovers to its normal state. Similar manifestations have been observed with foreign serum proteins given to guinea pigs. Figure 13–10 shows typical inflammatory changes around blood vessels with cellular infiltrates in the heart, lung, and kidney, including enhanced phagocytosis of autologous RBC in the spleen. The lesions are similar to the histological changes demonstrated in SLE patients.

Other species show chronic immune complex disorders with persistence of virus as the antigen source. These include lymphocytic choriomeningitis in mice, Aleutian mink disease, and possibly SLE-like disease in NZB/W mice. That genetic control plays a significant role in the immune response and in the host susceptibility that leads to immune complex disorders is highly suggestive. Clinical studies with the major histocompatiblity complex (MHC), especially the HLA complex, implicate the sig-

Table 13-8 : Antigens Associated with Type III Immunological Injury

Antigen	Immunological Disease
DNA	Systemic lupus erythematosus
Ig	Rheumatoid arthritis
Streptococcal antigen	Acute streptococcal glomerulonephritis
Viral	Acute viral hepatitis
Penicillin	Serum sickness
Malaria	Malarial nephritic syndrome
Thyroid tissue antigens	Hashimoto's thyroiditis

nificance of genetics in the predilection immune complex disorders.

Antigen. A multitude of antigens are involved in the immune complex disorders. In general, any antigen eliciting IgG or IgM synthesis should be able to initiate an immune complex disorder. Some of the antigens—including bacterial, viral, fungal, and parasitic antigens—and their related diseases are listed in Table 13-8. In cancer patients immune complexes have been found in plasma and deposited in areas of inflammation and lesions. The antigens involved in many of the malignancy diseases, however, have not been identified. Some of the antigens involved in the immune complexes of autoimmune disorders have been characterized, especially those in SLE (DNA, nucleoproteins, glycoproteins, RNA, and various enzymes—DNAse, RNAse, etc.).

The DNA-antibody complex has been suggested as one of the causative factors in the pathogenesis of glomerulonephritis in SLE, although many other autoantibodies have been demonstrated in SLE. A variety of antigens have been demonstrated in thyroiditis (see Chapter 14), and an altered form of IgG has been suggested in rheumatoid arthritis. The etiology of the immune complex disease of the autoimmune disorders is presently unknown.

Antibody. The classes of antibody involved in the type III immune complex disorders are IgG, IgM, and occasionally IgA. There are considerable variations in their affinity and avidity in the formation of complexes. The genetic characteristics of the host and the kind, route, and timing of antigen administered define the nature or affinity of the antibody produced. Both precipitating and nonprecipitating antibodies may be found, and both appear equally capable of eliciting either acute or chronic immune complex disorders.

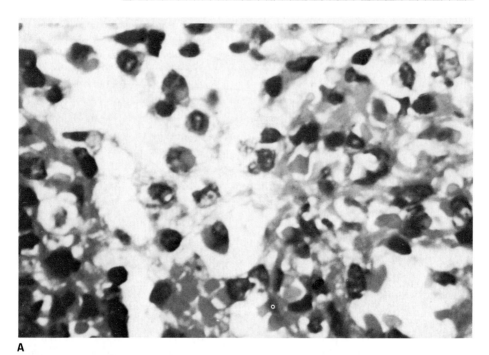

A

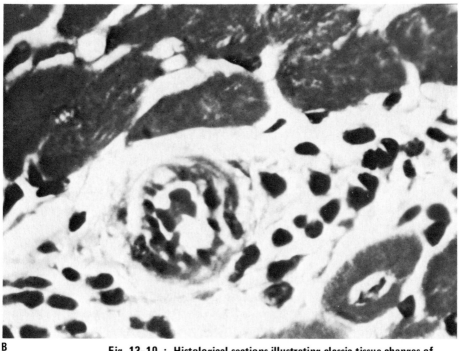

B

Fig. 13-10 : Histological sections illustrating classic tissue changes of serum sickness in a guinea pig given horse serum (H & E stain). A. Spleen, showing active ingestion of autologous erythrocytes by macrophages (erythrophagia) (X 400). B. Vasculitis in the heart of the same animal,

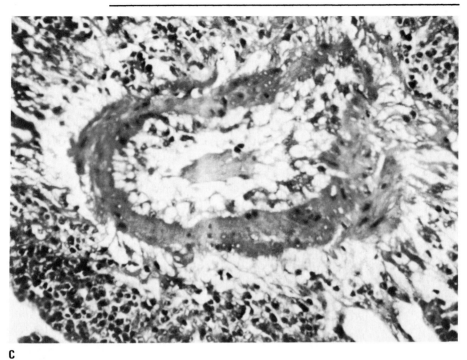

C

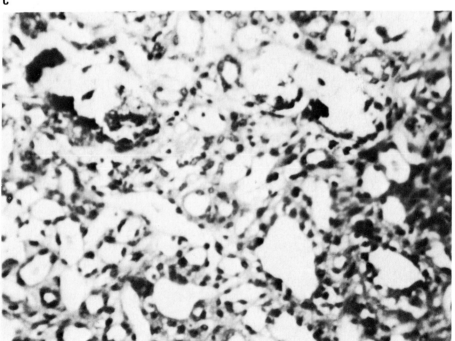

D

with perivascular infiltration of mononuclear cells (X400). C. Lung tissue, with thickening of vessel wall, acute vasculitis, and extravascular infiltration of mononuclear cells (cuffing) (X125). D. Calcification (dark residues) and myeloma-like kidney of the same guinea pig (X125).

Immune Complexes. The formation of immune complexes is dynamic and is governed by a variety of conditions: the levels and kinds of antibody and antigen, and the kinetics of formation in the peripheral plasma or capillary walls in the presence of many other cellular elements and serum proteins. The nature of the complexes, that is, the ratio of antigen to antibody, can be constantly changing, thus the size and accessibility of the regions of the binding sites to the tissue surfaces of the complexes are in a constant variable state. Studies in experimental animals have shown that chronic persistence and size (hence Ag-Ab ratios) play a significant role. Whether complexes persist or clear rapidly is based on their size and can dictate the target vessels in the immune complex disorder. For example, ^{125}I-labeled immune complexes larger than 11S (Ag_2-Ab_2 complexes) are rapidly removed by macrophages, especially those of the liver ($>$than 99 percent). Saturation of the macrophages in the liver results in persistent circulation of the complexes in plasma with subsequent deposition in tissues such as the glomeruli of the kidney. Uptake by liver macrophages and other organs of the reticuloendothelial system of the immune complexes may be mediated via the Fc portion of the antibody in the antigen-antibody complex.

In general, analysis of animal studies would indicate that the persistence of the complexes in circulation and the size of the complexes in the region of antigen excess contribute to the toxicity of the complexes. The ability of the complexes to activate complement is also important in pathogenesis, as is the avidity of the antibody produced and the strength of its binding to antigen to form stable complexes.

Role of Complement. Activation of complement through the classic pathway produces the active components contributing to inflammation, including increased vascular permeability (C3a anaphylotoxin activates the basophils to release histamine, SRS-A, etc.). Immune complexes also attach to lymphocyte (T_γ and T_μ lymphocytes, Fc receptors on T cells for IgG and IgM Fc portions, repsectively) and platelet surfaces. Release of the immune complex from these surfaces is called *complex release activity* (CRA) and the complexes remain as soluble forms in the plasma. This appears to be mediated through the alternative C pathway activation; Mg^{++} is required for the CRA and the lack of which leads to C4 and C5 deficiency. This phenomenon increases with age.

Platelets. The binding of immune complexes to platelet membrane (via the Fc receptor) causes activation of platelets and release of vasoactive amines and increases synthesis of prostaglandins. The prostaglandin synthetic pathway is depicted in Figure 13–11.

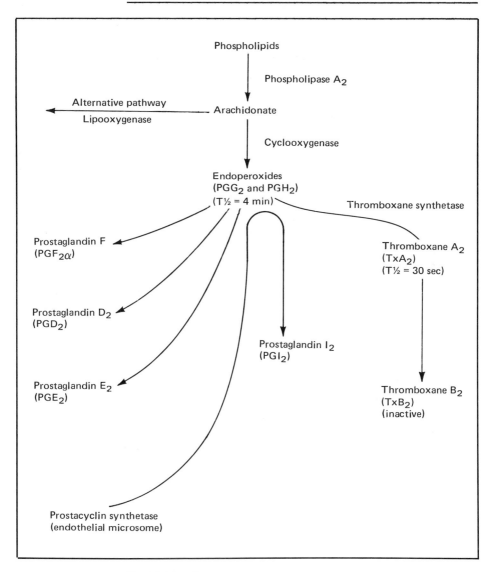

Fig. 13-11 : Prostaglandin and thromboxane synthetic pathway demonstrated in the activation of platelets.

Formation of PGE_2 contributes to an increase in c-AMP production in target cells, such as basophils (mast cells), and thus minimizes further release of granules and vasoactive amines. Release of the vasoactive amines (serotonin by platelets and histamine by basophils) contributes to the vascular permeability of the capillaries. Platelets bind more readily with complexes in the region of antibody excess. Immune complexes found in the antigen excess region frequently do not activate platelets.

Leukocytes (PMN). Activation of complement or release of 12, L-hydroxy-5.8.10.14-eicosatetraenoic acid via lipooxygenase in platelet activation will stimulate chemotaxis of PMNs into the area of immune complex deposition. Phagocytosis of complexes ensues, and the release of granules containing the proteases, glycosidases, esterases, and other hydrolases increases tissue damage. Immune complexes bind to neutrophils through the Fc receptor, thus enhancing opsonization. Since PGE_2 is released by platelets in the same milieu or lesion, the effect of this molecule on the PMNs induces an increase in c-AMP and thus suppresses further release of lysosomal granules, which should ultimately minimize the inflammatory condition. The presence of Ca^{++} is important for the enhanced release of lysosomal enzymes by PMNs. Concentrations greater than 2 mM, however, inhibit release of the lysosomal enzymes.

Detection of Immune Complexes. Tissue-bound immune complexes are readily identified by immunofluorescence or by enzyme-coupled antibody. Since in many cases the antigens are unknown, the specifically isothiocyanate fluorescein-labeled heterologous antibody is directed to the Fc antigenic portion of the antibody or to C1q, C4, and C3 components of the complex. Horseradish peroxidase–labeled antibodies are similarly used. There are advantages and disadvantages to all systems that have been tried, but with experience these procedure have been proved to be extremely valuable and useful in clinical medicine. Soluble complexes to which complement is bound can be examined using Raji cells (B lymphoblasts), which possess C3 receptors, using ^{125}I-labeled Ag-Ab-C complexes as a standard.

Type III Disorders. Some of the diseases in the pathogenesis of which immune complexes play a part are summarized in Table 13-6. Immune complexes have been demonstrated in plasma and at the site of the injured tissues in these disorders (see Figure 13-10).

Cell-Mediated Hypersensitivity

Type IV Reaction in Immunological Injury

Type IV immune reactions are mediated by T cells sensitized to specific antigens and occur without the involvement of antibody and complement. Interactions between a small number of the actively sensitized T cells and specific antigen result in tissue injury through the release of lymphokines, direct T cell cytotoxicity, or, more likely, both phenomena.

DELAYED HYPERSENSITIVITY (T CELL–MEDIATED. The classic lesion of cell-mediated immune reaction is the delayed skin reaction associated with the administration of purified protein

Fig. 13-12 :
Classic delayed
hypersensitivity
(DTH)–CMI reac-
tion (type IV)
against target cells
or soluble antigens
with release of
lymphokines.

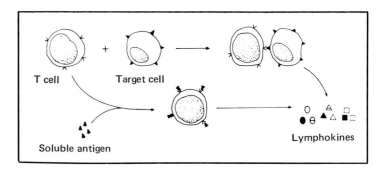

T cell Target cell

Soluble antigen

Lymphokines

derivative (PPD) to a sensitized individual. This reaction develops over a period of 24 to 48 hours with the characteristic mononuclear infiltration. Figure 13-12 depicts a delayed hypersensitivity reaction. The details of CMI reaction and the role of lymphokines have been presented in Chapter 3. Briefly, the lesion is initiated by a small number of sensitized T cells, which react with specific antigen through their receptors (unknown) and undergo transformation and the subsequent release of lymphokines. Lymphokine release results in the movement of a variety of cells, polymorphonuclear leukocytes, monocytes, and lymphocytes (T and B cells) to the site of the lesion. Ultimately, in the later stages, the characteristic histological pattern is that of a predominantly mononuclear infiltration (lymphocytes and macrophages). Part of the increase in sensitized T cells may be through release of transfer factor. Excessive macrophage cellular infiltration can result in release of hydrolases, which can initiate serious tissue injury and lesions. The lesions ultimately resolve through normal repair mechanisms, but in some cases the normal tissue patterns are permanently altered (scar tissue).

The extent and duration of delayed hypersensitivity may be increased by involvement of the amplification and ancillary systems discussed in Chapters 8 and 9. These include the clotting and kinin systems.

TYPE IV DISORDERS. The various delayed hypersensitivity reactions that can be considered as Type IV cell-mediated immunity were summarized in Table 3-3, Chapter 3. Another example is experimental allergic encephalitis, induced by a polypeptide and adjuvant isolated from the myelin of the central nervous system (CNS).

The classification set forth by Gell and Coombs facilitates the understanding of hypersensitivity and the roles of the T and B cell systems. Nevertheless, it is to be expected that reactions of both immediate and delayed hypersensitivity can occur simultaneously or in sequence. These reactions are basically dependent on the nature of the inciting agent. For example, mediators such as those released by mast cells can be demonstrated in the allergic contact dermatitis type of delayed hypersensitivity of skin reactions in humans. This may also be the case in classic delayed hypersensitivity skin reactions. In addition to the mononuclear cell infiltrates of the classic descriptions, the following have been demonstrated for infiltration of basophilic allergic contact dermatitis (dinitrochlorobenzene, DNCB) and classic delayed hypersensitivities: leukocytes and piecemeal degranulation of these cells and fixed mast cells (including replication); increased vascular permeability leading to dermal and epidermal edema; vascular compaction and erythrocyte extravasation; microvascular alterations affecting endothelial cells and pericytes; compromised vessel lumina and basement membrane thickening; and activation of the clotting system with fibrin deposition in a characteristic intervascular pattern in the reticular dermis. There appear to be greater numbers of basophilic infiltration in delayed contact dermatitis with DNCB than in classic delayed hypersensitivity elicited with microbial antigens. The fixed connective tissue mast cell appears to play a greater role in delayed skin reactions in man than in guinea pigs, in which the mobile basophil plays a greater role. The histological pattern exhibited in contact-delayed hypersensitivity with DNCB is associated with mast cells and the clotting system (Jones mote type of delayed hypersensitivity).

Cell-Mediated Cytotoxicity

Cell-mediated cytotoxicity is the direct destruction of target cells or tissue by mononuclear cells. These mononuclear cells include the T cells and their subsets, K cells, NK cells, and macrophages. The cytotoxicity may take the form of cytolysis (lysis of target cell) or cytostasis.

The mode by which T cells kill is not known, but the mechanism attributed to macrophages may be similar to that which has been demonstrated for neutrophils (see Chapter 8). The generation of superoxide (O_2^-) has been implicated in killing by alveolar and peritoneal cavity–activated macrophages. Cytolysis can be measured by the release of chromium 51 (^{51}Cr) from labeled target cells. The important cytotoxicity categories are illustrated in Figure 13-13. The target cells used can be various tumor cells, allogeneic lymphocytes, and red blood cells (chicken, sheep, human), etc. A T cell subset is activated by alloantigen, as can be demonstrated in the mixed lymphocyte cytoxicity test, or induced by an allograft containing the unrelated alloantigen. The interaction between the effector T cell and target cell is specific (Figure 13-13A). A subset T cell or an "armed" macrophage (with antibody to the tumor antigen), with specificity, will react specifically with the homologous target tumor cells containing the inciting tumor membrane antigen (tumor-specific antigen) or nonspecifically with other target cells containing similar membrane antigens (Figure 13-13B). T cells can also be activated or sensitized by soluble antigen specifically or non-specifically (PHA or Con A stimulation) and by cells capable of cytotoxicity nonspecifically against a nonspecific target cell (Figure 13-13C). The mixture of lymphocytes, mitogen (Con A or PHA), and allogeneic or syngeneic cells acts as follows: (1) a continuous culture of mitogens, lymphocytes, and syngeneic target cells results in cytotoxic destruction of the syngeneic target cells (X); and (2) if lymphocytes, mitogen, and allogeneic target cells are mixed and mitogen is subsequently removed, then specific cytotoxicity is demonstrated for the allogeneic target cell (Z) (Figure 13-13C). Removal of mitogen abrogates the cytotoxic effect of the lymphocytes on the syngeneic target cells (nonspecific effect). This latter reaction (shown in Figures 13-13A and 13-13C) is also referred to as *cell-mediated lympho-cytotoxicity* (CML). Antigens can also activate T cells specifically. These sensitized T cells then act on specific target cells (Z, Figure 13-13C), which have the same antigenic determinants on their membranes.

The effector K cells (null cell–derived) and macrophages can be armed by specific antibody via the Fc receptors and the antibody binding sites (variable portions of the Fab) attached to specific antigenic determinants on target cells and in this manner destroy target cells (Figure 13-13D and E). In this case the K cells and macrophages are nonspecific and are armed specifically by the antibody. These cells are referred to as *antibody-dependent cytotoxic cells* (ADCC).

A fifth category of cytotoxic mononuclear cells, which are neither T nor B cells and, like the ADCC K cells, are found in the null cell population of the peripheral blood, "natural" killer cells (NK) (Figure 13-13F). Like the ADCC K cell, the NK cells do have Fc receptors. In addition, the NK cells are directly cytotoxic to the target cell without mitogen or antigen activation. Here the cytotoxicity is achieved through direct effector cell target interaction. The nature of the binding sites involved in the effector and target cells is unknown.

Table 13-9 summarizes the various modes by which humoral and cell-mediated cytotoxicity cells can destroy target cells.

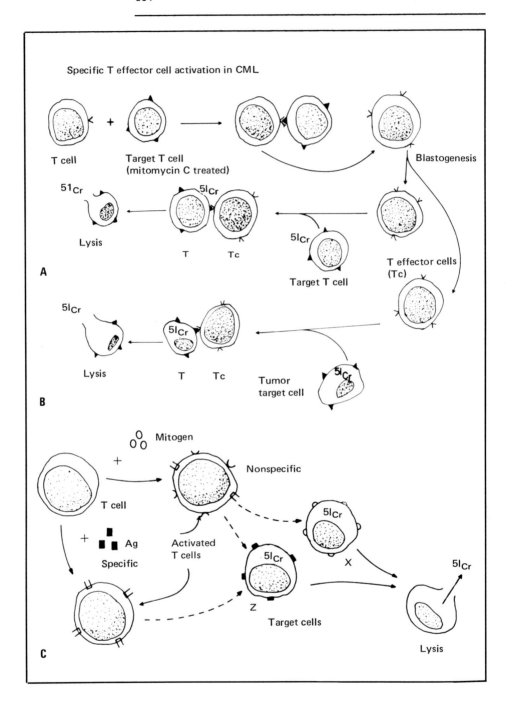

Specific T effector cell activation in CML

T cell + Target T cell (mitomycin C treated) → Blastogenesis

^{51}Cr Lysis ← ^{51}Cr T Tc ← ^{51}Cr Target T cell ← T effector cells (Tc)

A

^{51}Cr Lysis ← ^{51}Cr T Tc Tumor target cell ^{51}Cr

B

Mitogen + T cell → Nonspecific Activated T cells

+ Ag Specific

^{51}Cr ^{51}Cr Z Target cells X ^{51}Cr Lysis

C

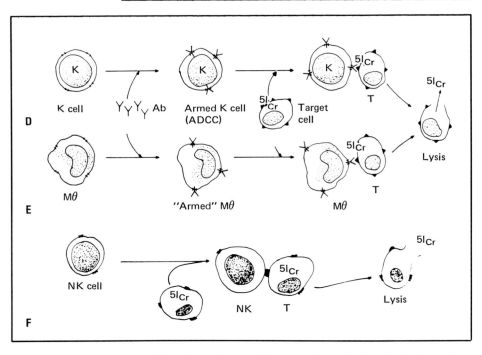

Fig. 13-13 : Various aspects of specific and nonspecific cytotoxic mechanisms in the destruction of target cells (T). A, B. Specific effector T cell (T cytotoxic cell, Tc). C. Activation of T cell nonspecifically with mitogen or specifically with antigen. D, E. Arming of K cell or macrophages with specific antibody to a specific target cell. F. Direct action of natural killer (NK) cell on target (T) cell. (X represents nonspecific target cell, Z is the specific target cell).

Table 13-9 : The Major Effector Cells Involved in Direct Cytotoxicity

Effector Cells	Specificity		Activating Factors	Induced by
	Effector Cells	Target Cells		
T cells	Specific	Specific	Alloantigens	Allograft
T cells and "armed"	Specific	Specific	Tumor antigen-induced	Tumor-specific Ag (TSA)
macrophages	Nonspecific	Nonspecific		Cell membrane Ag (CMA)
T cells	Nonspecific (Ag)	Nonspecific	PHA soluble Ag	Mitogen
K cells and macrophages	Nonspecific	Nonspecific (ADCC)	IgG or IgM (?)	Ab (Ab-dependent)

Summary

1. The mechanisms of immunological injury have been class-ified into four types: three types involve the humoral immune system and are referred to as *immediate hypersensitivity;* the fourth type, the cell-mediated immune system, is referred to as *delayed hypersensitivity.* The term *anaphylaxis* (coined as an antonym of *prophylaxis*) is used to define a thoroughly char-acterized immunological injury of immediate hypersensitivity.

2. Type I immediate hypersensitivity is mediated by IgE and involves the basophils or mast cells, which release mediators from their cytoplasmic granules. These mediators initiate the inflammatory condition and express the clinical manifesta-tions characteristic of type I immunological injury. The mediators include histamine, SRS-A, ECF-A, PAF, heparin, serotonin, and others. Diseases mediated by the type I mech-anism include atopic allergy (hay fever, urticaria, a form of asthma, etc.). Essentially complement is not involved, but platelet may be indirectly involved. Desensitization (hypo-sensitization) is helpful for some forms of type I hypersensi-tivity, especially those involving seasonal allergens.

3. Type II immediate hypersensitivity is mediated by IgG or IgM and involves complement or K cell (ADCC). The target of the antibodies is the antigen on the cell surface or an antigen bound to the cell surface (drugs, for example). The character-istic inflammatory lesions occur through the formation of C-activated fragments and the accumulation of neutrophils. Diseases in which type II mechanism is involved include auto-immune hemolytic anemia, idiopathic thrombocytopenia, leukopenia (neutrophils), Goodpasture's disease, and many others.

4. The type III mechanism involves the interaction of antibody with soluble antigen and the subsequent formation of immune complexes that activate complement. The major antibody in-volved is IgG or IgM, but occasionally IgA may be involved, also.

5. The nature of the host, antibody, antigen, size, and ratio of Ag-Ab complexes is of significance in the pathogenesis of type III immunological injury. Complement, leukocytes, and platelets play a major role in the pathogenesis. Diseases, either primary or secondary, in the immune complex disorders are numerous. They include systemic lupus erythematosus (SLE), serum sickness (primarily drug-induced), Arthus-type disorders (bacterial, viral, and fungal antigens and avian proteins), glomerulonephritis, and vasculitis.

6. Type IV immunological injury is mediated by T lymphocytes and is also referred to as *delayed hypersensitivity.* The inflam-mation and activation of the disease process involves the re-lease of lymphokines following the interaction of the sensi-tized T cells with the antigen (soluble antigen or a target cell).

7. The release of lymphokines initiates the characteristic lesions associated with delayed hypersensitivity (24 to 48 hours after T cell–Ag interaction). Complement is not required. The lymphokines (mediators from T cells) and macrophages—the latter through their enzyme hydrolases—play a major role in the pathogenesis of these lesions.

Bibliography and Selected Reading

General

Coombs, R. R. A Immunopathological mechanisms. *Proc. R. Soc. Med.* 67:525, 1974.

Denvert, G. Thymus-derived killer cells: Specificity of function and antigen recognition. *Transplant. Rev.* 29:59, 1976.

Irvine, W. J. Autoimmune mechanisms in endocrine disease. *Proc. R. Soc. Med.* 67:499, 1974.

Marchalonis, J. J. (Ed.). *The Lymphocyte: Structure and Function,* Part I. New York and Basel: Dekker, 1977.

Sell, S. Teaching monograph: Immunopathology. *Am. J. Pathol.* 90:211, 1978.

Willoughby, D. A. Inflammation. *Endeavour* 2:57, 1978.

Wilson, G. S., and Miles, A. A. (Eds.). *Topley and Wilson's Principles of Bacteriology and Immunity.* Baltimore: Williams & Wilkins, 1975.

Immediate Hypersensitivity (Humoral System)

Bardana, E. J., Jr. Culture and antigen variants of *Aspergillus. J. Allergy Clin. Immunol.* 61:225, 1978.

Beaven, M. A. I Histamine (first of two parts). *N. Engl. J. Med.* 294:30, 1976.

Beaven, M. A. II. Histamine (second of two parts). *N. Engl. J. Med.* 294:320, 1976.

DeWeck, A. L., Blumenthal, M., Yunis, E., and Jeannet, M. HLA and Allergy. In J. Dausset and A. Svejgaard (Eds.), *HLA and Disease.* Baltimore: Williams & Wilkins, 1977. Pp. 196–221.

Frick, O. L. Immediate Hypersensitivity. In H. H. Fudenberg, D. P. Stites, J. L. Caldwell, and J. V. Wells (Eds.), *Basic and Clinical Immunology* (2nd ed.). Los Altos, Calif.: Lange, 1978. Pp. 246–266.

Goetz, E. J., and Austin, K. F. Cellular characteristics of the eosinophil compatible with a dual role in host defense in parasitic infections. *Am. J. Trop. Med. Hyg.* 26:142, 1977.

Gupta, S., Safai, B., and Good, R. A. Subpopulations of human T lymphocytes. IV. Quantitation and distribution in patients with *Mycosis fungoides* and Sezary Syndrome. *Cell. Immunol.* 39:18, 1978.

Hamburger, R. N. Peptide inhibition of the Prusnitz-Küstner reaction. *Science* 189:389, 1975.

Hoffman, D. R., and Shipman, W. H. Allergens in bee venom. 1. Separation and identification of the major allergens. *J. Allergy Clin. Immunol.* 58:551, 1976.

Ishizaka, K., and Dayton, D. H., Jr. (Eds.). *The Biological Role of the Immunoglobulin E System.* Washington, D.C.: DHEW, 1972.

Okudaira, H., and Ishizaka, K. Reaginic antibody in the mouse. III. Collaboration between hapten-specific memory cells and carrier-specific helper cells for secondary anti-hapten antibody formation. *J. Immunol.* 111:1420, 1973.

Parker, C. W. The Role of Prostaglandins in the Immune Response. In P. W. Ramnel and B. B. Phariss (Eds.), *Prostaglandins in Cellular Biology.* New York: Plenum, 1972. Pp. 173–194.

Tada, T., and Okumura, K. Collaboration between carrier-specific helper (T) cells and hapten-specific precursors (B cells) is required for maximal anti-hapten IgE antibody response. *J. Immunol.* 107:137, 1971.

Delayed Hypersensitivity (Cell Mediated Immunity)

Dvorak, H. F., Mihm, M. C., Jr., Dvorak, A. M., Johnson, R. A., Manseau, E. J., Morgan, E., and Colvin, R. B. Morphology of delayed type hypersensitivity reactions in man. *Lab. Invest.* 31:111, 1974.

Eylar, E. H., Salk, J., Beveridge, G. C., and Brown, L. V. Experimental allergic encephalomyelitis, and encephalitogenic basic protein from bovine myelin. *Arch. Biochem. Biophys.* 132:34, 1969.

Thomas, J., Thomas, F., and Lee, M. H. A Search for Mechanisms Facilitating Human Non-Identical Allograft Survival: Some Parameters of Cell-Mediated Immunity in Long-Term Human Renal Transplant Recipients. In M. Welsler, S. D. Litwin, R. R. Riggio, and G. W. Siskind (Eds.), *Immune Effector Mechanisms in Diseases.* New York: Grune & Stratton, 1977. Pp. 77–104.

Wells, J. V. Immune Mechanisms in Tissue Damage. In H. H. Fudenberg, D. P. Stites, J. L. Caldwell, and J. V. Wells (Eds.), *Basic and Clinical Immunology.* Los Altos, Calif.: Lange, 1978. Pp. 267–282.

Cell-Mediated Cytotoxicity

Asjo, B., Kiessling, R., Klein, G., and Povey, S. Genetic variation in antibody response and natural killer cell activity against a Maloney virus-induced lymphoma (YAC). *Eur. J. Immunol.* 8:544, 1977.

Hebeman, R. B. Natural Cell-Mediated Cytotoxicity Against Tumor. In M. E. Weksler, S. D. Litwin, R. R. Riggio, and G. W. Siskind (Eds.). *Immune Effector Mechanisms in Disease.* New York: Grune & Stratton, 1977. Pp. 147–172.

Paul, W. E. Immune Effector Mechanisms: Duality of Recognition Functions. In M. E. Weksler, S. D. Litwin, R. R. Riggio, and G. W. Siskind (Eds.), *Immune Effector Mechanisms in Disease.* New York: Grune & Stratton, 1977. Pp. 129–146.

Quinnan, G. V., Manischewitz, J. E., and Ennis, F. A. Cytotoxic T lymphocyte response to murine cytomegalovirus infection. *Nature* 273:541, 1978.

Strober, W. The Cellular Basis of "Nonspecific" Cytotoxicity Reactions. In M. E. Wekler, S. D. Litwin, R. R. Riggio, and G. W. Siskind (Eds.), *Immune Effector Mechanisms in Disease.* New York: Grune & Stratton, 1977. Pp. 173–194.

14 : Autoimmunity

The body is endowed with mechanisms to distinguish *self* from *nonself*. However, there are many pathways for the breakdown of the central mechanisms underlying self recognition, a breakdown that results in autoimmune responses. Autoimmunity can be defined as *a failure of an organism to recognize self, and this includes any immune response of an individual to antigens normally present in the host's own tissue,* whether this response be humoral (e.g., circulating antibodies) or cellular (e.g., delayed hypersensitivity). There are several mechanisms by which an autoimmune response is initiated. Fundamentally, there is a disruption of the normal pathways of interaction of T and B cells with autoantigens.

Autoimmunity is a concept that helps explain the pathogenesis of a number of clinical diseases. The term *autoimmune disease* generally has been used to describe certain conditions in which the autoimmune response is the primary and major factor in initiating tissue injury and lesions. There are other diseases in which the autoimmune response is secondary to tissue injury resulting from other causes, but in which the autoimmune response may help perpetuate tissue injury. Not surprisingly, in many instances the autoantibodies formed, which are capable of reacting with host tissue antigens, may not cause tissue injury and disease.

Autoimmune disorders are frequently associated with malignancies, immune deficiency syndromes, and aging. A possible autoimmune pathogenesis for a given disease is indicated when one observes (1) the existence of autoantibodies; (2) amyloid deposits of denatured γ-globulin; (3) hypergammaglobulinemia with presence of various immunoglobulins; (4) vasculitis, serositis, and glomerulonephritis (which suggest an immune complex disease); or (5) the existence of other diseases, such as endocrinopathies, known to be associated with autoimmune disorders.

A classic example of a true autoimmune disease is organ-specific autoimmune thyroiditis, in which it has been shown that humoral autoantibody is the major factor in eliciting tissue injury. Another autoimmune disease is experimental allergic encephalitis. In this case the cell-mediated autoimmune response is the major mechanism of tissue injury. In other diseases autoantibodies have been observed but have not been shown to induce tissue lesions. Examples are the antimitochondrial and anti-smooth muscle antibodies present in autoimmune liver disorders.

The term *autoallergic* is often used interchangeably with *autoimmune.* The term *allergy* was used by von Pirquet in 1906 to describe an altered reaction to repeated injections of heterologous gamma globulin to diphtheria toxin. Thus, allergy is often used to mean harmful altered reactions, secondary to immune mechanisms. Today, the term *allergy* is most commonly applied to disease characterized by hypersensitivity reactions, such as hay fever and asthma, which are mediated by cytophilic IgE antibodies. *Hypersensitivity* has been used to describe immune reactions similar to allergy and also to describe nonimmunological reactions such as nonimmune hypersensitivity to drugs.

Autoimmunity, which is observed in clinical and experimental circumstances, can also be defined by an apparent termination of the natural unresponsiveness to self. Immunological tolerance is the result of an active physiological process and is not simply the lack of immune response. There are two types of immunological tolerance. One results in a central unresponsive state characterized by an irreversible loss of competent lymphocytes, while the other is a peripheral inhibition in which competent cells are present but are suppressed. A definition of *unresponsiveness* is inability to make a detectable immune response to an antigenic challenge, as distinguished from so-called *tolerance,* a term commonly used in transplantation immunology to include factors in addition to nonimmunological events, such as the increased resistance to the ill effects of drugs and toxins. However, for the purposes of this chapter, the terms *unresponsiveness* and *tolerance* will be used interchangeably, since the discussion will be confined to immune mechanisms.

Interrelationship of the Unresponsive State (Tolerance) and Autoimmunity

Currently, it is believed that a person becomes tolerant or unresponsive to his own tissue antigens during fetal development and that the natural unresponsive state develops as a result of direct contact between the self constituents and receptor sites on the surface of lymphocytes reactive to these antigens. This is a phenomenon predicted by Burnet, who developed the clonal selection theory, which proposed that the contact of antibody-forming cells with their respective antigens during fetal or early postnatal life leads to destruction or inactivation of the corresponding clones. The maturation of lymphocytes occurs continuously, and the autoantigen must be present to induce tolerance in the newly arising lymphocytes. If the particular autoantigen is not present and in contact with the newly arising

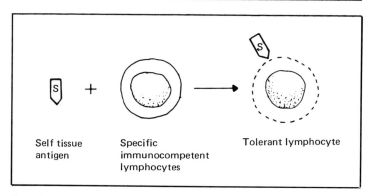

Self tissue antigen + Specific immunocompetent lymphocytes → Tolerant lymphocyte

Fig. 14-1 : Induction of natural unresponsive state. Clones of immuno-competent cells capable of reacting to self antigens during fetal development are either eliminated or made unresponsive by early exposure to self antigen.

lymphocytes, then termination and breakdown of tolerance will occur. This has been demonstrated experimentally: removal of the pituitary gland from a tree frog before metamorphosis results in rejection of the same pituitary when it is reimplanted into the same frog in the adult stage.

In concert with the principles just stated, many investigators have artificially induced an unresponsive state to a wide variety of antigens during the newborn period, when an immature immune system is present.

The mode of induction of the natural unresponsive state probably depends on two mechanisms: (1) clones of immunocompetent cells capable of reacting to self antigens are eliminated by a mechanism of the clonal theory of Burnet; and (2) antigen-producing cells are made unresponsive by early exposure to self antigen (Figure 14-1). The clonal selection theory was not easily reconciled with observations on the experimental induction of autoimmunity. Weigle and co-workers showed that injections of cross-reacting thyroglobulins of other species, in the absence of adjuvant, elicited formation of autoantibodies against thyroglobulin and experimental thyroiditis. It became clear that the T and B cells interact in the production of autoantibodies and that the mechanisms of induction of the unresponsive state at the cellular level differ between T cells and B cells.

On the cellular level, macrophages, B cells, T cells, and antibody-producing B cells from the bone marrow are involved in unresponsiveness. The evidence for direct cooperation between T and B lymphocytes is well confirmed. Specifically reactive T cells and B cells must both interact with specific antigen-sensitive cells for production of antibodies. Although macrophages play

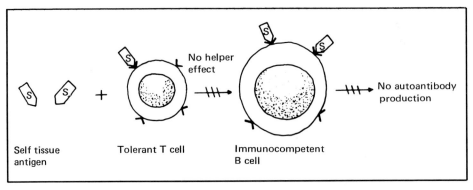

Fig. 14-2 : Natural unresponsive state. Autoantigens, such as the protein hormone thyroglobulin and solubilized membrane antigen, circulate in very low concentration. The natural unresponsive state is developed
and maintained in T cells only. The B cells do not develop tolerance to
these antigens. No autoantibody is produced, however, because of a lack
of T cell helper signal.

a major role in the establishment of unresponsiveness, they
appear to be nonspecific and under genetic control.

Both T and B lymphocytes can become unresponsive or tolerant.
However, the kinetics of tolerance in these two lymphocyte
populations differ greatly. Many autoantigens such as thyroglobulin, protein hormones, and solubilized membrane antigens
circulate in limited concentrations in the body fluid. With limited
concentrations of these self components, the unresponsive state
is maintained only in the T cells and not in the B cells. The
natural unresponsive state is maintained to antigens such as
native thyroglobulin because of the lack of T cell helper signal;
thus autoantibody production is *not* initiated (Figure 14-2).

On the other hand, *high doses of antigen* can induce *unresponsiveness in both T and B lymphocytes.* This was shown experimentally with injection of human γ-globulin in mice. Experiments in mice have shown that thymocytes become tolerant to
human γ-globulin within 24 hours of exposure, and this tolerance
lasts for 100 days. By contrast, B cell tolerance requires an
induction period of 15 to 21 days. The long latent period between exposure and tolerance to human γ-globulin in mice may
indicate that the bone marrow cells are relatively resistant to
tolerance or that thymic cell–bone marrow interaction is required
before tolerance can be induced. Even with high doses of antigen,
the unresponsive state of B lymphocytes is often incomplete,
and some antibody of low affinity can still be formed.

In the case of thyroglobulin and its involvement in thyroiditis,
only the T lymphocytes may be tolerant, leaving B-lymphocytes

able to respond to autoantigens suitably presented to them with T lymphocyte help. Mechanisms allowing the requirement for specific T lymphocytes responding to autoantigens to be by-passed will be discussed. Tolerance of autoantigen on the basis of the selective unresponsiveness of T lymphocytes can be easily bypassed by various viral or microbial infections and other events.

In contrast to their unresponsiveness to thyroglobulin, neither T nor B cells appear to be unresponsive to basic protein, and specific antigen-binding cells to basic protein have been detected to both T and B cell populations. By deleting either the T or B cells it has been demonstrated that T cells and not antibody are responsible for induction of experimental allergic encephalitis.

Recent studies have demonstrated the existence of antireceptor or antiidiotypic antibodies, which may arise as a result of various T cell bypass mechanisms (described later). An idiotype is a unique configuration of the variable portion of a lymphocyte's receptor and can include the actual combining receptor site to the antigen. The idiotype can stimulate specific antibody production. Such antibodies are called *antiidiotypes* and can bind to the specific lymphocyte receptor site.

These antireceptor or antiidiotypic antibodies may block the expression of an immune response and produce a tolerance-like situation to self antigen. When an animal makes an immune response to a given antigen, autoantibodies directed to the antibody, which are made as the result of the antigenic stimulus, may also be produced. The idiotypic determinants characteristic of a given antibody may also be present on lymphocytes with receptor for the antigen. Thus, the autoantibody to the idiotype may block or suppress the immune response to a given antigen.

Genetic and Viral Factors in Autoimmunity

Autoimmune phenomena have been observed with increased incidence in certain families. There is considerable evidence that genes associated with the major histocompatibility locus in man (HLA) are important in immune regulation and in the pathogenesis of autoimmunity. The differences in susceptibility to various viruses and the intensity of the cellular immune response or graft-versus-host (GVH) reaction is also controlled within the cluster of genes located within the major histocompatibility region. Genetically determined cell surface antigens, termed Ia, are important immunological factors in antigen recognition, cellular interaction, and cellular cooperation.

Many of the human autoimmune disorders have been found to be associated with a particular HLA haplotype. The majority of the associations are with the second loci (HLA-B and -D) genes, and this locus may be close to the immune response (Ir) genes in man. The association of HLA antigens is marked in cases of ankylosing spondylitis, in which patients are found to possess HLA-B27 antigens in as many as 90 percent of cases. It should be noted that the association does not imply that the disease is caused by possession of the HLA-B27 antigen. Certain autoimmune diseases, particularly the organ-specific disorders, such as idiopathic Addison's disease, Graves' disease, chronic active hepatitis, and Sjögren's syndrome, occur more frequently in individuals who have HLA-B8. Other diseases, such as multiple sclerosis and rheumatoid arthritis, appear to be associated with lymphocyte-defined genetic loci, whose products on the cell membranes are responsible for mixed lymphocyte reactivity.

Autoimmunity and autoimmune diseases are frequently associated with genetic and viral factors that interact with the immune system and influence regulation. Genetically determined lymphocyte membranes in man determine the magnitude of the response in mixed lymphocyte reactions (MLR), and may be closely associated with the development of autoimmunity. Although the exact mechanisms by which genetic factors and autoimmunity are related are unclear, it is likely that the immune response (Ir) genes, lymphocytic surface antigen, and possible receptors for specific viruses are involved. Viruses and other infectious agents are often associated with autoimmunity. Many virus buds from cell surfaces can incorporate normal membrane constituents as part of their viral envelope. Such a combination of viral and host tissue antigens may become immunogenic and give rise to autoimmune responses.

General Mechanisms of Autoimmunity

Autoimmunity arises when there is an abnormal interaction of T and B cells with autoantigen. The immunological imbalance may arise from a disturbance of the suppressor and helper activities of regulatory T cells. Either an excess of T cell helper activity or a deficiency of suppressor activity can initiate the autoimmune reaction. The immunological imbalance is probably modulated by various viral, genetic, and environmental factors. The autoimmune state may be induced by any one or more of the following mechanisms:

T Cell Specificity Bypass Mechanism

There may be a bypass either of T cell specificity or of the need for specific T cells in the presence of competent B cells.

In the normal state, there is no T cell response to many autoantigens, such as thyroglobulins, protein hormones, and soluble membrane antigens, which circulate in very low doses. Prolonged exposure to these would produce selective tolerance in T lymphocytes, leaving B lymphocytes able to bind autoantigens and be

Fig. 14-3 : T cell
bypass mechanism.
A. In the normal
state the T cell is
tolerant and the B
cell is competent,
and no autoanti-
body is formed be-
cause of the absence
of T cell helper sig-
nals. B. The T cell
bypass mechanism
may be initiated
when the self anti-
gens from immuno-
genic units initiate
the T cell helper
signal. Allogeneic
cells or adjuvants
that can nonspecif-
ically activate
lymphocytes can
also stimulate the
production of
autoantibodies.

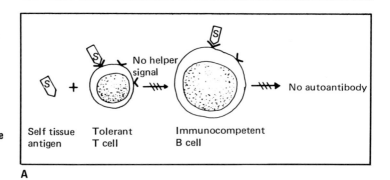

A

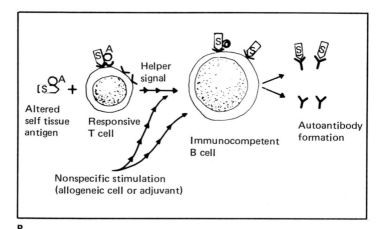

B

stimulated by autoantigens presented to them with appropriate
T lymphocyte help. Under such circumstances, the requirements
for specific T lymphocytes responding to autoantigenic determinants can be bypassed (Figure 14-3).

In the normal state, the T cell is tolerant and the B cell is competent; no autoantibody is formed, because the absence of the T
cell helper signals the presence of the autoantigen. On the other
hand, autoantigens will form immunogenic units with antigens,
which are able to initiate the T cell helper signal, to stimulate
the existing immunocompetent B cell. Among the helper determinants are viruses, or bacteria, and drugs. Any factor that
nonspecifically activates lymphocytes, such as adjuvants or a
GVH reaction with allogeneic cells, can stimulate production of
autoantibodies by the bypass of T cell specificity. The types of
autoimmune reactions that involve bypass of T cell specificity
will be discussed in more detail.

Sequestered Antigen
Release Mechanism

Another mechanism involves the stimulation of competent T
cells and/or B cells by sequestered self antigens.

Fig. 14-4 : Sequestered antigen release mechanism. A. Normally, host T and B cells are responsive or non-tolerant to sequestered antigen. No autoantibody is formed as long as the antigen remains sequestered and is not able to react to the responsive cells. B. When sequestered antigen is released, the competent T and B cells are stimulated, with initiation of both the cell-mediated reaction and auto-antibody formation.

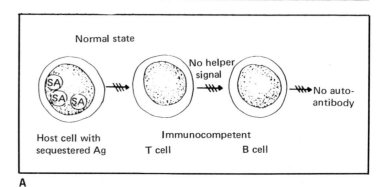

A

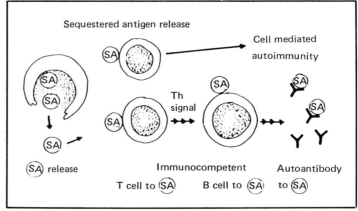

B

A sequestered antigen is an antigen that is not readily available for recognition by the immune system. Its release into the system is often caused by some tissue injury. When the sequestered antigen is released, the host T cells recognize it as foreign, the helper signal is released, and the B cells divide and proliferate, producing autoantibody (Figure 14-4). In contrast to their state of unresponsiveness to thyroglobulin, neither T nor B cells appear to be unresponsive to basic protein, and antigen-binding cells specific to basic protein have been detected in both T and B cell populations. By deleting those cells, T or B, that specifically bound to basic proteins, it was demonstrated that T cells and not antibody were primarily responsible for induction of experimental allergic encephalitis. Thus, the cellular immune mechanism of injury is primarily responsible for the demyelinization and tissue injury found in allergic encephalitis.

Loss of Suppressor Activity

Suppressor cell activity may be lost. Under normal conditions, if self antigen has triggered a T cell helper signal, autoantibody production can be halted by the presence of a suppressor T cell

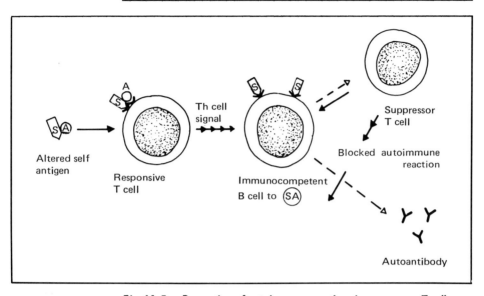

Fig. 14-5 : Prevention of autoimmune reactions by suppressor T cells. Suppressor T cells normally prevent the autoimmune reaction by suppressing B cell proliferation: they halt the response of B cells to the T cell helper effect.

(Fig. 14-5). The suppressor T cells arrest the division and proliferation of the competent B cells. Consequently no autoantibody is formed. With the loss of this population of T lymphocytes, proliferation and division of the competent B cells can occur, and the production of autoantibody is induced.

Depending on the disease, any one or a combination of the above mechanisms may play a role in the induction of the autoimmune state. The autoimmune reactions can be either humoral or cellular or both.

Modes of Reaction Involved in T Cell Specificity Bypass Mechanism of Autoimmunity

The T cell bypass mechanism of autoimmunity is a means by which a nontolerant immunocompetent B cell can be stimulated to produce autoantibody without the need for a specifically immunocompetent T cell. The B cells may be stimulated by two general pathways:

1. The autoantigens may form immunogenic units and initiate T cell helper signals to stimulate the existing nontolerant immunocompetent B cells. Among the helper determinants are drugs, viruses, and bacteria.
2. Substances that nonspecifically stimulate lymphocytes, such as adjuvants or a GVH reaction with allogeneic cells, can bypass T cell specificity and stimulate the immunocompetent B cells to produce autoantibodies.

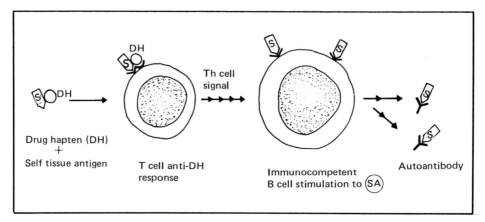

Fig. 14-6 : Autoimmunity following drug administration. The drug (as a drug hapten) can combine with host tissue to form immunogenic units. The anti-drug hapten response of T cells will initiate the T cell helper effect without the intervention of, and eliminate need for, specific T cells. The immunocompetent B cells are activated to produce autoantibodies.

Autoimmunity Following Administration of Drugs

A coupling of the drug or metabolite to an autoantigen may initiate a host T lymphocyte response against the drug. In addition the drug may initiate a T cell helper signal that stimulates immunocompetent B cells reactive to autoantigen, with production of autoantibodies (Figure 14-6).

There are many examples of autoimmune manifestations following drug administration. The production of nuclear antibodies in a syndrome similar to that of systemic lupus erythematosus is relatively common in patients treated with procainamide or hydralazine.

Virus Infections

Virus infections can initiate autoantibody formation by either one of two pathways. First, the viral antigens and self tissue autoantigens may combine to form immunogenic units. Second, certain viruses, such as the Epstein-Barr (EB) virus, may stimulate proliferation of the B lymphocyte cell line directly.

Viral and host antigens can form immunogenic units on the surface of infected host cells. The viral antigens also may form complexes and modify histocompatibility antigens and other membrane constituents. The modified viral-host antigens can stimulate the T cell helper effect and elicit autoantibody production (Figure 14-7).

There are many examples of autoantibodies against nuclei, lymphocytes, platelets, and smoothe muscle infections. In experiments with mice, Zinkernagel et al. have shown that cell-mediated immune damage of cells expressing viral antigens is

Fig. 14-7 : Auto-immunity following viral-host tissue interaction. Viral antigens can combine with a wide variety of host tissue antigens to form immunogenic units that induce autoantibody formation.

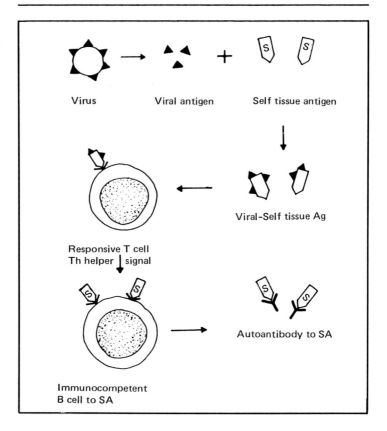

Virus   Viral antigen   Self tissue antigen

Viral-Self tissue Ag

Responsive T cell
Th helper signal

Autoantibody to SA

Immunocompetent
B cell to SA

not against normal self but altered self (self associated with a foreign antigen). They have shown that there is universal H-2 restriction of murine T cell-mediated immune function. The T cell immune reactions compare self with nonself and not with foreign nonself cells. For example, virus-specific cell-mediated cytotoxicity is directed against infected self cells.

Adjuvant Effect and Bacterial Infections

Immunological adjuvants are nonspecific stimulators of lymphocytes and can help initiate autoimmune responses. Lipopolysaccharides or purified protein derivatives of tuberculin are polyclonal B cell activators, and Freund's complete adjuvant is a nonspecific T cell stimulator. The need for a specific T cell is bypassed (Figure 14-8).

Bacterial infections with liberation of products of adjuvant activity, such as *Bordetella pertussis* infection, could produce polyclonal lymphocyte activation and autoimmunity.

Bacteria can provide helper determinants in different ways. In rheumatic fever-associated streptococcal infections, there are cross-reactive determinants of the streptococcal organism and

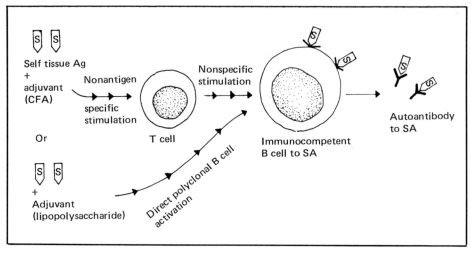

Fig. 14-8 : Nonspecific stimulation by immunological adjuvants in initiation of autoimmune reaction. Adjuvants can help initiate autoimmune reactions by bypassing the need for specific T cells. The adjuvants nonspecifically stimulate T cells to initiate a T cell helper effect. In the case of lipopolysaccharides, direct activation with polyclonal stimulation of B cells can occur, with production of autoantibodies.

host tissues. If the determinants of bacteria form complexes with host tissue, these complexes can activate host T lymphocytes and initiate the T cell helper effect for autoantibody production.

Degradation and Alteration of Autoantigens

Tissue damage with alteration of host antigens may elicit an autoimmune reaction. Partial degradation can expose antigenic determinants that are not available in the native molecules, and these can react with T lymphocytes to induce autoimmunity. Many bacterial, viral, and parasitic infections are associated with transient positive tests for antiglobulin of the rheumatoid factor type, and among the underlying mechanisms is either partial degradation or alteration of host antigens.

Allogeneic Cells

When live allogeneic lymphocytes are injected into a recipient, the primary event is a GVHR reaction. The donor T lymphocytes will respond to the major histocompatibility complex of lymphoid and hernatopoietic cells of the recipient. The stimulation of the lymphoid tissue in the recipient is manifested by profound lymphoreticular hyperplasia, with germinal center enlargement and plasmacytosis. The donor T cell reaction initiates proliferation of the recipient B cells (Figure 14-9.)

In a normal person, autoantibody formation does not occur, because T lymphocytes are unable to react to autoantigens; however, when host B cells are nonspecifically stimulated by the

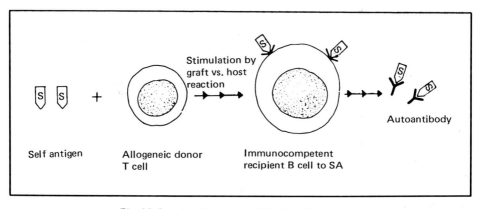

Fig. 14-9 : Autoimmunity following allogeneic cell stimulators. Allogeneic donor T cells will react to the major histocompatibility complex
of the lymphoid cells of the recipient. The donor T cell initiates a signal
and induces proliferation of recipient B cells, with resultant autoantibody
production.

donor T cells, as in the GVH reaction, there is an allogeneic
effect leading to the production of antibodies. By this mechanism, the need for carrier-specific T lymphocytes can be bypassed; hence, the GVH reaction results in the formation of
autoantibodies.

**Organ-Specific
Autoimmune
Diseases and T Cell
Specificity Bypass
Mechanism of
Autoimmunity**

In the various endocrine organs frequently associated with
autoimmune diseases, the self tissue antigens circulate in extremely low concentrations. These low concentrations of self
tissue antigens are sufficient only to induce and maintain tolerance at the level of the T cells; tolerance is not induced in the B
cells.

Various animal and human clinical investigations have demonstrated that thyroglobulin, which previously was thought to be
a sequestered antigen, is actually present in the circulation in
very small amounts after birth and is able to equilibrate between
the intravascular and extravascular fluid compartments. Also, in
animals and man, tolerance to the thyroglobulin antigen was
found at the level of the T cells, but the B cells were found to be
immunocompetent.

In the normal state, tolerance at the T cell level will prevent
formation of autoantibody. This is not a completely healthy
condition, since other factors, such as viral transformation and
genetic mutation, may cause alteration of the host antigen to
form immunogenic units activating responsive T cells. The need
for specific T cells is bypassed with an alternative T cell helper
signal to initiate proliferation of the immunocompetent B cells
with autoantibody production (Figure 14-10).

Fig. 14-10 :
Autoantibody
formation in certain
organ-specific
autoimmune dis-
eases. In most
organ-specific
diseases, such as
thyroiditis, toler-
ance to the self
tissue antigen is
found at the T cell
level and not at the
B cell level. When
the self tissue anti-
gen is altered by
genetic mutation or
viral transforma-
tion, the altered self
tissue antigen ac-
tivates a responsive
T cell to stimulate
immunocompetent
B cells, with re-
sultant autoanti-
body production.

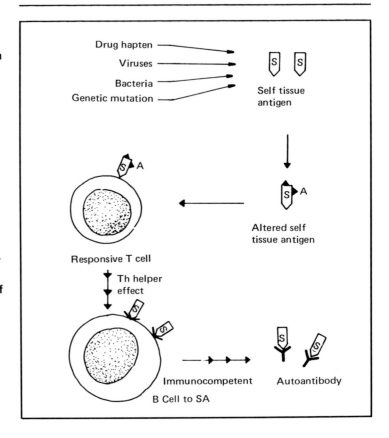

In studies of experimental thyroiditis, as well as human thyroid-itis, there is overwhelming evidence that the major factor in initiating tissue injury is the humoral autoantibody response. The same mechanism involved in thyroiditis may operate in other organ-specific diseases, such as primary adrenal gland atrophy, parathyroid hypoplasia, and primary ovarian atrophy. These organs release extremely small concentrations of self antigens during the development of the natural unresponsive state, and tolerance is developed at the T cell level and not at the B cell level.

Sequestered Antigen
Release Mechanism
and Allergic
Encephalitis

It was formerly believed that many autoantigens are secluded from immunocompetent cells in the body (sequestered); however, many antigens formerly thought to be secluded, such as thyro-globulin protein hormones, are now known to circulate in extremely small amounts. Cell membrane constituents, such as major histocompatibility antigens, are likewise known to circulate in low doses. However, there may well be segregation of some antigens in normal persons.

The basic protein of myelin is effectively secluded from im-munocompetent cells and does not normally elicit immune

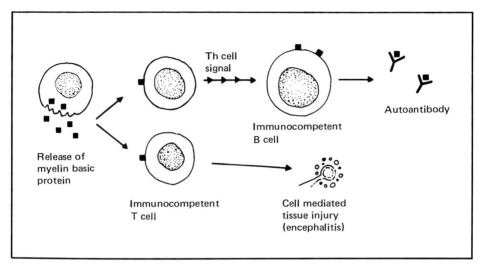

Fig. 14-11 : Sequestered antigen release mechanism of autoimmunity in experimental and postinfectious encephalitis. The sequestered antigen is basic protein, and, when released by various means such as viral inflammation, it will stimulate both immunocompetent T and B cells. The primary mechanism of injury in experimental and postviral encephalitis is a cell-mediated injury.

responses. In normal human adults, neither T nor B cells appear to be tolerant of basic protein, and specific binding cells to basic protein can be detected in both T and B cells. This can explain the observation that T cells and the cellular (delayed sensitivity) mechanism are the primary mechanisms of injury in experimental allergic encephalitis (Figure 14-11). The release of the sequestered basic protein, which in turn initiates a cellular immune response, is believed to play a significant role in post-viral infectious encephalitis. A viral infection, such as mumps, may cause release of myelin basic protein, which in turn triggers the immune system to initiate encephalitis.

Loss of Suppressor Cell Activity in Autoimmunity

Several investigators have hypothesized that T cells act in the control of B cells by suppressing B cell–dependent synthesis of autoantibody. As shown in Figure 14-5, the T lymphocytes can inhibit autoimmune responses and provide a general mechanism for preventing or delaying autoimmune responses. Evidence has accumulated that there is a distinct population of T lymphocytes with suppressor and helper effects. The major evidence for suppressor control is that antibody is made at a fairly steady rate, which is not influenced by injecting more antigen; injection of antilymphocyte serum induces a large temporary rise in the number of autoantibody-secreting cells, and tolerance to many self components may be maintained by active suppressor.

With loss of suppressor cell activity—through aging, immune deficiency syndromes (e.g., thymic hypoplasia), or other disease mechanisms—the self-reactive B cells are permitted to proliferate, with resultant production of autoantibody and autoreactive lymphocytes.

There is experimental evidence to support the concept of loss of suppressor T cell activity in development of autoimmune reactions. Following early thymectomy, a strain of Leghorn chickens developed a more severe form of autoimmune thyroiditis than the thyroiditis that occurs spontaneously. Spleen cells from old New Zealand Black (NZB) mice, transplanted to young NZB mice depleted of T cells by antilymphocyte serum, will induce a persistent Coombs' positive hemolytic anemia.

Classification of Autoimmune Diseases

Human autoimmune diseases can be broadly separated into three main groups: organ-specific diseases, non-organ-specific diseases, and non-organ-specific diseases with lesions in one, or few, organs. There is a high frequency of association of many of the different autoimmune diseases in comparison to the incidence of their association in a random population. The diseases in each group may be related genetically, with an overlap of clinical lesions. The characteristics of each group of autoimmune disease will be discussed here, and a characteristic example given for each disease group.

Organ-Specific Autoimmune Diseases

The organ-specific disorders are characterized by chronic inflammatory changes in a specific organ. The autoantibodies exhibit specificity for antigens of the diseased organ. Examples of this group are (1) autoimmune thyroiditis; (2) primary hypothyroidism; (3) thyrotoxicosis (Graves' disease); (4) chronic atrophic gastritis; (5) primary adrenal atrophy; (6) post-rabies vaccination encephalomyelitis; and (7) myasthenia gravis.

The mere presence of an antibody or sensitized lymphoid cell to an autoantigen does not establish that immune mechanisms are responsible for the pathogenesis of the disease and observed tissue injury. Four conditions should be satisfied before an autoimmune response can be implicated in a given disease:

1. A demonstrable immune response to cellular tissue antigens should be detected at some time during the course of the disease.
2. The specific antigen should be identified, localized, and characterized as to host and origin.
3. An animal model of the particular disease should be established. This model should be characterized by the presence of specific antibodies in actively sensitized animals, associated

with the appearance of tissue lesions similar to those of the human disease.

4. Experimentally the disease should be transferable from a diseased animal to a normal animal by means of serum antibodies or sensitized lymphoid cells.

AUTOIMMUNE THYROIDITIS. Autoimmune thyroiditis has been shown to fulfill the four conditions listed above and can be used to illustrate the mechanism of organ-specific autoimmune disease.

Many autoantigens, such as thyroglobulins, protein hormones, and solubilized membrane antigens, circulate in very low concentrations in the body fluid. In the development of the natural unresponsive state to thyroglobulin and thyroid epithelial antigen the host maintains a tolerant state at the T cell level but not in the B cells (see Figure 14-2). The natural unresponsive or tolerant state to antigens, such as thyroglobulin, is maintained because of a lack of T cell helper signal, and no autoantibody production is initiated. However, the B lymphocytes are able to respond to autoantigens suitably presented to them with a T cell helper signal. The T cell helper signal may be initiated by alteration of host tissue antigens via genetic mutation or viral transformation.

The mechanism of autoimmune thyroiditis involves a bypass of T cell specificity to initiate production of autoantibodies. When the T cell is bypassed, there is production of antithyroid antibodies with resultant thyroid tissue injury. The antigens involved in these reactions are thyroglobulin and thyroid epithelial microsomal antigen.

In severe forms of autoimmune thyroiditis, the glandular architecture is effaced, with destruction of thyroid tissue, and there are many large collections of lymphoid follicles. The lymphoid follicles may show active germinal centers, and the thyroid follicular cells may become enlarged, with eosinophilic cytoplasm. The gland may become enlarged to several times normal size and later show a progression of fibrosis and atrophy with a clinical picture of myxedema.

The presence of autoantibodies to normal thyroid antigens is the hallmark of thyroiditis. The production of autoantibodies is particularly related to the extent of lymphocytic inflammatory change within the gland. There are several milder forms of lymphocytic goiter that do not fit the clinical picture of classic autoimmune thyroiditis. Many of these milder forms demonstrate focal types of thyroid inflammation, which may lead to antibody formation to the same thyroid antigens.

Non-organ-specific
Autoimmune
Diseases

Autoimmune diseases that are not organ-specific are characterized by pathological changes in many different organs and tissues throughout the body, and the associated autoantibodies often lack organ and species specificity. In this group, the factors involved in the production of the autoimmune reactions are complex and are probably the result of abnormal imbalance and interaction of viral, genetic, and immunological factors.

The associated serum autoantibodies often lack organ and species specificity, and experimental lesions are not readily produced; however, similar diseases arise spontaneously in certain inbred animal strains. Examples of diseases in this group are systemic lupus erythematosus, rheumatoid arthritis, and various other connective tissue disorders such as progressive systemic sclerosis (scleroderma). One of the major mechanisms of injury is by immune complexes.

The reaction starts when immune complexes localize in tissue and fix complement. These complement-bound complexes elaborate a chemotactic factor that attracts polymorphonuclear leukocytes. The polymorphonuclear leukocytes enter the tissue at the sites of immune complex deposition and undergo a release reaction, during which lysosomal proteolytic enzymes escape. These enzymes cause necrosis and destructive damage of the surrounding tissues.

SYSTEMIC LUPUS ERYTHEMATOSUS (SLE). In systemic lupus erythematosus, there is a definite imbalance in the interaction of T and B cells due to abnormal interaction of factors that initiate and suppress autoantibody production. Systemic lupus erythematosus usually occurs in young females. It is a multisystem disease that often is associated with glomerulonephritis and shows the presence of antinuclear antibodies or DNA–anti-DNA complexes. In the typical case of systemic lupus erythematosus, there are numerous antinuclear antibodies and antibodies to other cellular constituents, such as anticytoplasmic antibodies. There are red cell antibodies, platelet antibodies, and lymphocyte antibodies. In patients with systemic lupus erythematosus, although many types of nuclear antibodies are in evidence, the major pathogenetic antibody is the DNA antibody. The patient forms DNA–anti-DNA immune complexes, which characteristically localize in the basement membrane of kidney glomeruli, in blood vessels, and in the synovial membrane of joints and other tissues.

The immune complexes will fix complement and release a chemotactic factor allowing polymorphs to be attracted. The polymorphonuclear leukocytes will attempt to clean up the complexes

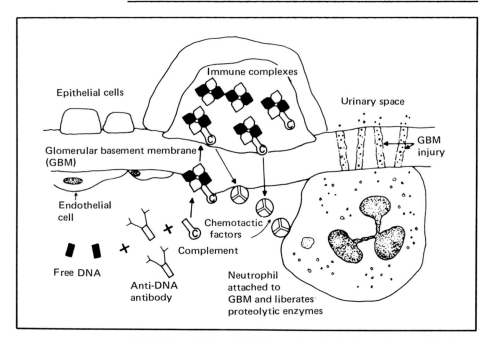

Fig. 14-12 : DNA–anti-DNA complexes in the glomerulonephritis of systemic lupus erythematosus. The immune complexes localize on the epithelial side of the glomerular basement membrane and will fix complement, with release of the chemotactic factor C5a, Polymorphs are attracted. In the process of removing and digesting the foreign material, the polymorphs will release proteolytic enzymes and cause destruction of the kidney basement membrane, with immune complex glomerulonephritis.

that localize on the epithelial side of the basement membrane of the glomeruli. In the process, there is proteolytic destruction of the glomerular basement membrane, initiating glomerulonephritis (Figure 14-12). Positive immunofluorescent staining shows localization of IgG in an irregular fashion along the basement membrane of the kidney, which is characteristic of immune complex disease. The third component of complement is localized in similar areas, thus providing further evidence that this is an immune complex glomerulonephritis (Figure 14-13).

Disorders with Non-organ-specific Autoantibodies with Lesions in One or Few Organs

By definition, the third group of diseases combines the features of both organ-specific and non-organ-specific categories. Examples of this group are primary biliary cirrhosis and chronic aggressive hepatitis.

The autoimmune liver disorders are characterized by the production of non-organ-specific and non-species specific antibodies such as antimitochondrial and anti-smooth muscle cell antibodies. The relationship of these antibodies to immune injury

Fig. 14-13 :
Kidney glomeruli,
showing immuno-
fluorescent local-
ization of IgG along
basement membrane
and mesangium in
an irregular lumpy
pattern. The third
component of
complement is
localized in the
same pattern (X200).

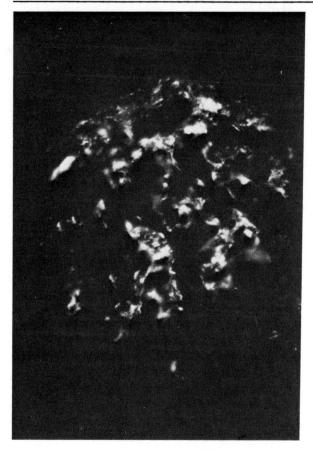

and tissue lesions is unknown. The levels of the antibodies do not have a correlation with the severity or duration of the disease. There is evidence that the mechanisms of immunological injury in liver disorders primarily involve a cellular immune mechanism via the suppressor cell and cytotoxic effector cell functions. In addition, there are humoral immunoregulatory factors that modulate the cellular functions of the immune system in the pathogenesis of the immunological liver disorders.

Laboratory Tests for Evaluation of Autoimmune Diseases

The tests most commonly used for the diagnosis of autoimmune disorders involve the detection of circulating antibodies. Tests for cellular sensitivity are done in larger medical centers primarily for clinical investigation.

Immunofluorescence, enzyme-labeled antibody, and radioimmunoassay methods utilize primary antigen-antibody binding reactions and, because of their high sensitivity, are preferred

Fig. 14-14 : Indirect immunofluorescence method for detection of autoantibody. The patient's serum, which contains the autoantibody, is first reacted with the substrate. The section is washed to remove excess proteins and then reacted with fluorescein-labeled antihuman immunoglobulin. The section is washed, mounted, and examined with a special fluorescence microscope.

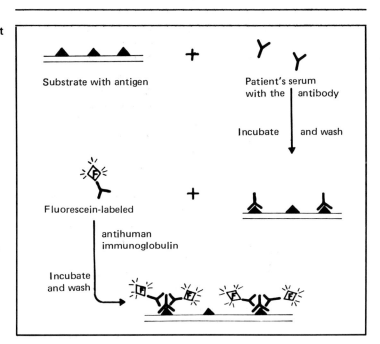

Substrate with antigen

Patient's serum with the antibody

Incubate and wash

Fluorescein-labeled

antihuman immunoglobulin

Incubate and wash

for the detection of circulating and tissue-bound antibodies and antigens.

Tests that involve secondary antigen-antibody preparations, such as complement fixation, agglutination, and precipitation in agar gel, may not be as sensitive as immunofluorescence or radio-immunoassay in some circumstances but may be technically more suitable for the identification of certain autoantibodies.

The immunofluorescence (IF) test and the more recently developed peroxidase-labeled antibody method are the most widely used immunohistochemical procedures for the detection of serum autoantibodies in the clinical laboratory. Both methods can be used to demonstrate autoimmune antibodies in serum, tissue localization, and fixation of autoantibody, and deposition of antigen-antibody complexes in the kidney, vessels, and other tissues.

In the indirect immunofluorescence test, the patient's serum is first reacted with a suitable substrate. The section is then washed and reacted in fluorescein-labeled antihuman globulin (Figure 14-14). The serum autoantibodies are detected by the indirect technique with use of a suitable substrate, and the highest titer of the serum that gives a positive reaction reflects the level of the autoantibody.

Serum autoantibody detection and quantitation is used for the diagnosis and evaluation of many of the autoimmune diseases.

In general, the level of antibody is high in patients with autoimmune disorders and low in apparently healthy persons. A very high titer of autoantibody is significant, while a low, or absent, titer of autoantibody does not rule out the possibility of an autoimmune disorder. For example, at the height of disease in severe thyroiditis, the gland may act as an immunoadsorbent and remove circulating antibody. In addition, thyroglobulin may be released into the circulation during the acute state and neutralize circulating autoantibody. Therefore, the level or titer of a given antibody must be interpreted in relation to the state or treatment of a particular disease.

In addition to tissue autoantibody detection, there are numerous other methods that have proved useful in the evaluation of patients with suspected autoimmune disorders. These include various assays for cell-mediated immunity that have potential usefulness in studying patients with autoimmune thyroiditis, certain liver diseases, and rheumatoid arthritis. Still other, less cumbersome, methods frequently are employed, such as those using rheumatoid factor, immune complexes in serum or joint fluid, quantitation of serum immunoglobulins, immunoelectrophoresis of serum and other body fluids, cryoglobulins, complement, and biopsy of kidney, vessels, or joints for immunofluorescence localization of antibody and immune complexes.

Summary

1. Autoimmunity can be defined as a failure of an organism to recognize self and includes any humoral or cellular immune response to self or host tissue.
2. a. Autoimmunity can also be defined as an apparent termination of the natural unresponsive state to self.
   b. An individual becomes tolerant or unresponsive to his own tissue antigens during early development of the immune system as a result of direct contact between self tissue antigens and the receptor sites of reactive specific lymphocytes. During fetal or early postnatal life, contact between antibody-forming cells and self antigen leads to the destruction or inactivation of the corresponding clones.
   c. Self tissue or autoantigen must be present to induce tolerance in the newly maturing lymphocytes. If the autoantigen is not present and not in contact with the newly arising lymphocytes, then tolerance may terminate.
3. a. The autoimmune reaction is the result of disruption of the normal pathways of interaction of T and B cells with self tissue antigens.
   b. Autoimmunity may arise whenever there exists a state of immunological imbalance in which B cell activity is excessive and suppressor T cell activity is diminished.

c. An imbalance of T and B cell interaction may occur as a consequence of genetic, viral, and environmental mechanisms, acting singly or in combination.

4. In the normal state, there is no T cell response to many autoantigens, such as thyroglobulin, protein hormones, and soluble membrane antigens, which circulate in very low doses. Tolerance to these antigens is found only at the T cell level; the B cells are not tolerant and are able to bind autoantigens. The nontolerant immunocompetent B cells can be stimulated by autoantigens if an appropriate T cell helper effect is present.

5. In the T cell specificity bypass mechanism of autoimmunity, there is a bypass of the normal need for specific T cells in the presence of immunocompetent B cells capable of reacting with the autoantigen. The various types of reactions that bypass T cell specificity are:
   a. Binding of foreign haptens or drugs to host tissue.
   b. Exposure to altered or cross-reacting antigens, e.g., viral and bacterial infections and enzyme degradation.
   c. Nonspecific stimulation of T cells by Freund's complete adjuvant.
   d. Nonspecific stimulation of B cells by lipopolysaccharide adjuvant.
   e. Allogeneic cell stimulation of B cells (graft-versus-host reaction).

6. A sequestered antigen is not readily accessible to the immune system. In the *sequestered antigen release mechanism* of autoimmunity, the sequestered antigen released by inflammation or tissue injury is recognized as foreign, causes stimulation of the immunocompetent T and B cells to produce autoantibodies, and initiates an important cell-mediated reaction.

7. Suppressor T cells normally inhibit autoimmune responses by suppression of B cell activity. With loss of the suppressor T cells by aging, immune deficiency, or other mechanisms, the B cells that are reactive to self tissue antigens are allowed to initiate autoantibody production.

Bibliography and Selected Reading

General

Gell, P. G. H., Coombs, R. R. A., and Lachmann, P. J. *Clinical Aspects of Immunology.* London: Blackwell, 1975.

Miescher, P. A., and Müller-Eberhard, H. J. *Textbook of Immunopathology,* Vols. I and II (2nd ed.). New York: Grune & Stratton, 1976.

Nakamura, R. M. *Immunopathology: Clinical Laboratory Concepts and Methods.* Boston: Little, Brown, 1974.

Talal, N. *Autoimmunity: Genetic, Immunologic, Virologic, and Clinical Aspects.* New York: Academic, 1977.

392

Fudenberg, H. H., Stites, D. P., Caldwell, J. L., and Wells, J. V. *Basic and Clinical Immunology* (2nd ed.). Los Altos, Calif.: Lange, 1978.

Genetics and Autoimmunity

Bach, F. H. The Major Histocompatibility Complex and Its Relationship to Autoimmune Disease. In N. Talal (Ed.), *Autoimmunity: Genetic, Immunologic, Virologic, and Clinical Aspects.* New York: Academic, 1977. Pp. 3–32.

Sasazuki, T., McDevitt, H. O., and Grumet, F. C. The association between genes in the major histocompatiblity complex and disease susceptibility. *Annu. Rev. Med.* 28:429–452, 1977.

Zinkernagel, R. M. H-2 Restriction of Cell Mediated Virus Specific Immunity and Immunopathology: Self Recognition, Altered Self, and Autoaggression. In N. Talal (Ed.), *Autoimmunity: Genetic, Immunologic, Virologic, and Clinical Aspects.* New York: Academic, 1977. Pp. 363–381.

Tolerance

Allison, A. C. Self-tolerance and autoimmunity in the thyroid. *N. Engl. J. Med.* 295:821–827, 1976.

Allison, A. C., and Denman, A. M. Self-tolerance and autoimmunity. *Br. Med. Bull.* 32:124–129, 1976.

Weigle, W. O. Immunologic tolerance and immunopathology. *Hosp. Prac.* 12:71–80, 1977.

Mechanisms and Concepts of Pathogenesis

Allison, A. C. Autoimmune Diseases: Concepts of Pathogenesis and Control. In N. Talal (Ed.), *Autoimmunity: Genetic, Immunologic, Virologic, and Clinical Aspects.* New York: Academic, 1977. Pp. 91–139.

Lambo, T. A., Nossal, G. J. V., and Torrigiani, G. (Eds.). *First Symposium on Organ Specific Autoimmunity.* The Menarini Series on Immunopathology, Vol 1. Basel/Stuttgart: Schwabe, 1978.

Sell, S. Immunopathology. Teaching monograph. Bethesda, Md.: American Association of Pathologists. *Am. J. Pathol.* 90:215–279, 1978.

Stobo, J. D., and Loehnen, C. P. Immunoregulation and autoimmunity. *Mayo Clin. Proc.* 51:479–483, 1976.

Talal, N. Disordered immunologic regulation and autoimmunity. *Transplant. Rev.* 31:240–263, 1976.

Laboratory Tests in Evaluation of Human Diseases

Nakamura, R. M., Chisari, F. V., and Edgington, T. S. Laboratory Tests for Diagnosis of Autoimmune Diseases. In M. Stefanini (Ed.), *Progress in Clinical Pathology.* New York: Grune & Stratton, 1975. Pp. 177–203.

Nakamura, R. M., and Tan, E. M. Recent progress in the study of autoantibodies to nuclear antigens. *Human Pathol.* 9:85–91, 1978.

Nakamura, R. M., and Deodhar, S. *Laboratory Tests for the Diagnosis of Autoimmune Disorders.* Chicago: American Society of Clinical Pathologists, 1976.

Rose, N. R. Laboratory Diagnosis of the Autoimmune Diseases. In J. E. Prier, J. Bartola, and H. Friedman (Eds.), *Modern Methods in Medical Microbiology: Systems and Trends.* Baltimore: University Park, 1976. Pp. 127–141.

Rose, N. R., and Friedman, H. *Manual of Clinical Immunology.* Washington, D.C.: American Society for Microbiology, 1976.

15 : Immunodeficiency Diseases

W. Stephen Nicols, Jr.
Robert M. Nakamura

Definition and Classification of Immunodeficiency Diseases

Immunodeficiency diseases comprise an interesting group of disorders that demonstrate defective function of a segment of the immune system (Figure 15-1). These diseases may be broadly categorized as either disturbances in the synthesis of various components of the immunological system or as abnormalities of catabolism.

Four major components of the immune system which are involved in the defense against various viral, bacterial, and other microbial infections. These consist of (1) B cell, or antibody-mediated, immunity; (2) T cell, or cell-mediated, immunity; (3) phagocytic mechanisms; and (4) the complement system. Each of these systems acts somewhat independently or in conjunction with one or more of the others in orchestration of the immune defense of the host organism.

The immunodeficiency diseases may be categorized as primary or secondary disorders. Primary immunodeficiency diseases result from a failure of proper development of the humoral and/or cellular immune systems. Often excluded from the primary group of immunodeficiency diseases are hypercatabolic disorders and disorders of the complement system. The secondary, or acquired, immunodeficiency diseases may occur in certain patients in association with a variety of diseases, including intestinal lymphangiectasia, protein-losing enteropathy, lymphoreticular malignancies, and treatment involving x-irradiation and immunosuppressive or cytotoxic drugs.

Primary Immunodeficiency Diseases

The primary immunodeficiency disorders constitute an interesting group of diseases. They are rare, but their effects are profound. These disorders are congenital, and some have fatal effects. Study of these diseases—"nature's experiments with the immune system"—has led to an understanding of the compartmentalization of the immune system (Good and Zak, 1956).

Primary immunodeficiency diseases have generally been classified into B cell, T cell, combined B and T cell-related disorders, and phagocytic and complement deficiencies (Table 15-1).

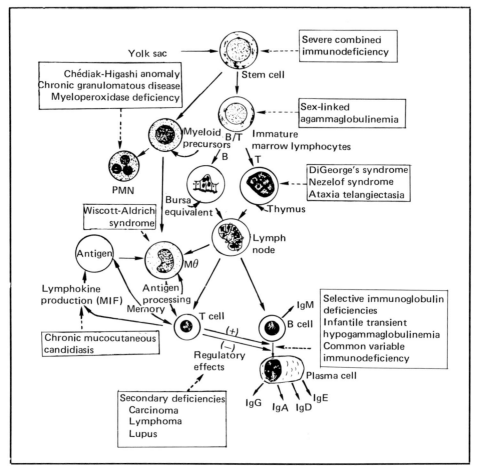

Fig. 15–1 : Defects in the immune system responsible for immunodeficiency syndromes: Defects (--->) at sites of differentiation in the sequence of maturational events lead to profound immunodeficiencies. Defects in the T cell compartment involve T and B cell functions through inappropriate regulatory effect(s). Several secondary (acquired) immunodeficiencies arise through malfunction of suppressor cells. Mθ = macrophage.

Primary B Cell Immunodeficiency Diseases

The stem cell differentiates, giving rise to precursor B cells, which are found in the marrow and spleen and which acquire an ability to express surface immunoglobulin. Mature B cells synthesize immunoglobulin and differentiate into cells that secrete antibody in response to an antigenic stimulation. B and T cells are identified by surface markers (listed in Table 15-2). The B cell is identified by surface Ig, Fc, and complement receptors. The mature, small B lymphocyte is a precursor to the plasma cell that appears upon antigenic stimulation (Figure 15-2). Immunodeficiency may result from the failure of terminal stages of B cell differentiation, even if normal-appearing small B lymphocytes are present.

Table 15-1 : Classification of Primary Immunodeficiency Diseases

Primary B cell immunodeficiency diseases
  Transient hypogammaglobulinemia of infancy
  X-linked hypogammaglobulinemia
  Hypogammaglobulinemia with normal or increased IgM
  Common variable, unclassifiable immunodeficiency
  Selective immunoglobulin deficiency

Primary T cell immunodeficiency diseases
  Congenital thymic aplasia
  Chronic mucocutaneous candidiasis

Primary T and B cell diseases
  Severe combined immunodeficiency
  Cellular immunodeficiency with abnormal immunoglobulin synthesis
    (Nezelof's syndrome)
  Wiskott-Aldrich syndrome
  Immunodeficiency with ataxia telangiectasis
  Immunodeficiency with enzyme deficiency

Disorders of the complement system

Disorders of phagocytosis

Source: Modified from Ammann, A. J., and Fudenberg, H. A. Immunodeficiency diseases. In H. H. Fudenberg et al. (Eds). *Basic and Clinical
Immunology.* Los Gatos, Calif.: Lange, 1976. P. 391.

Table 15-2 : Lymphocyte Surface Markers

Surface Marker	T Cell	B Cell
Rosettes with sheep erythrocytes (E)	+	−
Antithymocyte heteroantisera	+	−
Easily detectable surface immunoglobulin	−	+
Anti-B cell heteroantisera	−	+
Complement receptors (EAC rosettes)	−	+
Ig Fc receptor		
Ig-coated erythrocyte rosettes	±	+
Aggregated IgG	−	+

**Fig. 15-2 :
Maturation of
B cells.**

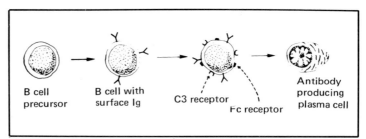

Fig. 15-2 : Maturation of B cells.

Table 15-3 : X-Linked Agammaglobulinemia

B cell deficiency (blood, lymphoid tissue)
Immunoglobulins decreased
Multiple bacterial infections
Normal cellular immunity
Family history (males)
Early onset

Deficient T helper function also comprises the humoral response. IgM production is relatively independent of T cell help, while production of IgA, IgG, and IgE requires T helper function.

There are several types of primary panhypogammaglobulinemia, involving all classes of immunoglobulins (IgG, IgA, IgM, IgD, and IgE).

TRANSIENT HYPOGAMMAGLOBULINEMIA OF INFANCY. Infants are born with maternal antibodies that have passed through the placenta. The maternal γ-globulin is catabolized during the first six months of life. Normally the infant's own immunoglobulin production is competent by this time. Some children have a prolonged physiological depression of the initiation of γ-globulin synthesis lasting up to two or three years. The number of B lymphocytes with surface immunoglobulin or complement receptors remains normal in this disorder. Such children are susceptible to bacterial respiratory infections and bronchitis, although the condition is relatively benign. This disorder must be distinguished from more serious immunoglobulin defects of poor prognosis.

X—LINKED HYPOGAMMAGLOBULINEMIA. The syndrome of X-linked hypogammaglobulinemia was recognized by Bruton in 1952 and is characterized by deficiency of B lymphocytes (Table 15-3). There is a failure of immunoglobulin production of all classes, with a very low concentration of circulating immunoglobulin. B cell immunoglobulin–producing cells are usually absent in the bone marrow, blood, lymphoid tissue, and gastrointestinal mucosal tissue. The lymph nodes show a paucity of germinal centers and plasma cells. Normal cellular immunity is present. The disorder is X-linked, affecting males predominantly.

During the first few months of life, infants with this disease are protected by maternal IgG antibody. After levels of maternal IgG begin to wane, patients become susceptible to severe recurrent infections, including pharyngitis, otitis media, and pneumonia secondary to streptococci, *Staphylococcus aureus, Hemophilus influenzae,* and *Neisseria meningitis.* The diagnosis of

Table 15-4 : Varieties of Common Variable Immunodeficiency

Absence of B cells

B cells present—decreased immunoglobulins

Defective immunoglobulin secretion

Increased suppressor cells present—decreased immunoglobulins

immunodeficiency is usually made by demonstration of pan-hypogammaglobulinemia, diminished number of circulating B cells, and maternal familial history of other males with the disease.

HYPOGAMMAGLOBULINEMIA WITH NORMAL OR INCREASED IgM. In another type of hypogammaglobulinemia, IgG and IgA are deficient, although IgM levels are normal or even increased, and B cells bearing IgM antibodies can be demonstrated. The cellular immune system is normal, and immunological abnormalities indicate arrest in the development of the switch from IgM to IgG production. There is also a high incidence of neutropenia, thrombocytopenia, hemolytic anemia, and B cell lymphomas. The disease is often X-linked.

An acquired form of this abnormality is probably a consequence of congenital rubella infection or transcobalamin II deficiency. Transcobalamin II is a transport protein involved in vitamin B_{12} metabolism. The hematological and immunological abnormalities arising from deficiency of the transport protein can be corrected by administration of large amounts of vitamin B_{12}.

COMMON VARIABLE, UNCLASSIFIABLE IMMUNODEFICIENCY. The most common type of panhypogammaglobulinemia affects both sexes, and the degree of immunoglobulin deficiency is less marked than in X-linked disorders. Clinical onset of the disease is usually delayed until late childhood or adulthood. The degree of associated T cell deficiency varies greatly. There has also been a high incidence of associated immunological abnormalities, such as systemic lupus erythematosus and hemolytic anemia. Several different types of defects have been identified in patients with common variable immunodeficiency (Table 15-4).

SELECTIVE IMMUNOGLOBULIN DEFICIENCY DISEASES. There are several combinations of defects of the three major immunoglobulins. Deficiencies of IgG subclasses have also been found.

Selective deficiency of serum IgA is the most common primary immunodeficiency found in humans: the incidence is about 5 to 6 per 1,000 individuals. Autosomal dominant as well as recessive inheritance patterns have been reported. Serum IgA levels are usually quite low or absent. IgA-producing cells are decreased, and secretory IgA is low to absent. Free secretory component is usually present. The defect appears to be located at the level of terminal differentiation of B cells to IgA-producing plasma cells. IgA deficiency may follow congenital rubella virus, cytomegalovirus, or *Toxoplasma gondii* infection.

Selective IgA deficiency has a striking association with autoimmune diseases and nontropical sprue. Ataxia telangiectasia is associated with an IgA deficiency about 80% of the time. There is no satisfactory treatment for IgA deficiency.

Selective IgM deficiency is the second most common selective immunodeficiency disorder. In most cases, the IgM serum levels are below 20 mg/dl. Normal individuals have IgM serum levels of 100 to 150 mg/dl.

Selective deficiencies of different combinations of IgG1, IgG2, IgG3, and IgG4 have been reported. Total IgG levels in these cases may be normal or slightly decreased. Diagnosis of this disorder is usually indicated by a restricted heterogeneity of the electrophoretic pattern of IgG, or by a lack of antibody production against certain antigens, and requires the quantitative measurement of IgG subclasses.

Primary T cell Immunodeficiency Diseases

Pure T cell disorders are encountered only rarely. The T cell immunodeficiency disorders are almost always associated with an aberration in the humoral immune system, since most antigens require both T and B cells for normal antibody production. Thus complete absence of T cells results in a defect of antibody production to all T cell-dependent antigens. A partial defect of the T cell system is more likely to result in a pure cellular immune deficiency syndrome. Patients with T cell immunodeficiency are susceptible to a variety of infectious agents that usually result in intracellular types of infections (virus, various bacteria, and protozoa).

CONGENITAL THYMIC APLASIA. The discovery of congenital thymic aplasia, or DiGeorge's syndrome (Table 15-5), is usually made shortly after birth, since affected patients often present with the clinical problems of hypoparathyroidism.

DiGeorge's syndrome results from failure of normal embryonic development at about 12 weeks of gestation. The thymus and parathyroid glands develop from epithelial evaginations of the third and fourth pharyngeal pouches. In many patients with DiGeorge's syndrome, the thymus is not absent but is hypoplastic or in an abnormal location. DiGeorge's syndrome can

Table 15-5 : DiGeorge's Syndrome

Absence of thymus

Decreased T cells (blood, lymphoid tissue)

Deficient, delayed type skin reactions

Tetany in some cases (hypoparathyroidism)

Infections (fungal, viral)

Normal to decreased immunoglobulin levels

Early onset

be either *complete* or *partial.* Complete absence of the thymus results in a defect of the humoral antibody system. The patient with a partial thymus gland, however, manifests a primary T cell deficiency. The peripheral lymphocyte count is low, and the number of T cells is low or absent at the time of birth. Studies of humoral immunity are difficult to interpret, since IgG in fetal serum is derived from maternal γ-globulin. IgM and IgA are normally present in very small amounts in newborns.

CHRONIC MUCOCUTANEOUS CANDIDIASIS. The majority of patients with chronic mucocutaneous candidiasis have minor defects in T cell immunity. The patients usually display a chronic candidal infection of the skin and mucous membranes associated with an endocrinopathy, the etiology of which has not yet been defined. There may be an autoimmune disorder associated with the T cell defect, and this may be related to the several endocrine abnormalities that have been described in this candidiasis. Hypoparathyroidism, Addison's disease, and diabetes have been observed in the disease. The total lymphocyte count and lymphocyte response to mitogens and the total number of T cells are normal. The hallmark of the disease seems to be an absent delayed hypersensitivity skin test response to candidal antigen in the presence of severe infection and, very often, lack of production of macrophage inhibition factor (MIF) in vitro in the presence of candidal antigen. Tests with other antigens are normal. Humoral immunity is intact in patients with chronic mucocutaneous candidiasis, and immunoglobulin levels are usually normal to elevated.

Primary T and B Cell Diseases

SEVERE COMBINED IMMUNODEFICIENCY. There are two forms of severe combined immunodeficiency disease. The X-linked recessive form was previously termed *X-linked lymphopenic agammaglobulinemia.* Both disorders are characterized by complete absence of T and B cell immunity (Table 15-6). Patients rarely survive beyond infancy because of poor resistance to infections. The etiology of severe combined immunodeficiency disease is

Table 15-6 : Severe Combined Immunodeficiency

Decreased T and B cells

Decreased response to T and B mitogens

Adenosine deaminase deficiency

Infections

Decreased immunoglobulin levels

History of other affected family members

Early onset

not understood. It is possible that the disorder is a result of a defect in stem cell differentiation, with absence of development of immunocompetent T and B cells. Other factors may also be responsible, however. Patients with manifestations of severe combined T and B cell immunodeficiency also may display deficiency of the lymphocyte enzyme adenosine deaminase.

The majority of patients with severe combined T and B cell immunodeficiency become symptomatic, with recurrent respiratory infections, candidal infections of the skin and mouth, and diarrhea. A certain number of infants with the disease appear quite normal at 6 to 9 months of age, however, and may not demonstrate an increased incidence of infection.

T cell abnormalities present in this disease include lymphopenia, decreased T cells, absence of peripheral blood lymphocyte response to mitogens and to mixed leukocyte stimulation, and absent thymic shadow. Studies of B cell immunity reveal a failure of antibody response following immunization. Biopsy of lymph nodes shows depletion of T- and B-dependent areas, and biopsy of the bowel demonstrates absence of plasma cells.

The treatment for patients with severe combined immunodeficiency is histocompatible bone marrow transplant. Patients who lack a histocompatible donor have been treated with fetal thymus or fetal liver transplant. Both forms of therapy have resulted in successful reconstruction of T cell immunity in several cases.

CELLULAR IMMUNODEFICIENCY WITH ABNORMAL IMMUNO-GLOBULIN SYNTHESIS (NEZELOF'S SYNDROME). Patients with Nezelof's syndrome demonstrate the following features: (1) susceptibility to viral, bacterial, fungal, and protozoal infections; (2) abnormally depressed T cell function; and (3) a varying degree of antibody immunodeficiency with various levels of immunoglobulins. The disease is sporadic, and no heritable pattern has been found.

The primary defect is a T cell deficiency. The accompanying B cell abnormalities are the result of failure of normal T and B cell interaction. The immunological defect in these cases has been treated with thymic transplantation and transfer factor.

WISKOTT-ALDRICH SYNDROME. Wiskott-Aldrich syndrome is a heritable, sex-linked recessive disorder. The primary defect may lie within the macrophages, although patients demonstrate T and B cell abnormalities and may show thrombocytopenia. The macrophages and immune lymphocytes are unable to process polysaccharide antigen normally. Consequently patients are unable to form antibody against polysaccharide-containing organisms such as *Hemophilus influenzae* and *Pneumococcus.* Older patients gradually manifest loss of both T and B cell functions.

Studies of T cell function during very early infancy may be normal. T cell and B cell dysfunction develop in varying degrees with progression of the disease. Blood group IgM isoagglutinins are absent. Often, there is a normal or elevated level of serum IgG, decreased serum IgM, and elevated IgA and IgE levels.

Treatment consists of platelet transfusions and antibiotics for thrombocytopenia and infections. The immune defect has been treated with partial success with bone marrow transplantation.

IMMUNODEFICIENCY WITH ATAXIA TELANGIECTASIA. Ataxia telangiectasia is an autosomal recessive disease that may involve a primary immunological defect with secondary involvement of other organs resulting from viral or perhaps autoimmune disease. About 80 percent of patients with ataxia telangiectasia lack both serum and secretory IgA. In these cases IgG may also be absent. Cell-mediated immunity is usually impaired, and the thymus is hypoplastic. There is lymphopenia with depressed response to T cell mitogens and to mixed leukocyte stimulation.

The primary T cell defect in ataxia telangiectasia could result in IgA and IgG deficiency through failure to facilitate B cell maturation.

IMMUNODEFICIENCY WITH SHORT–LIMBED DWARFISM. Immunodeficiency with short-limbed dwarfism presents as three different syndromes. The severe form (type I) is associated with cellular immunodeficiency disease. Type II is associated with cellular immunodeficiency, and Type III is associated with an antibody immunodeficiency. All three types display skeletal abnormalities, and these appear to be inherited in an autosomal manner. In short-limbed dwarfism associated with severe combined immunodeficiency, the patients become ill in infancy with viral, bacterial, fungal, or protozoal infections. Patients with

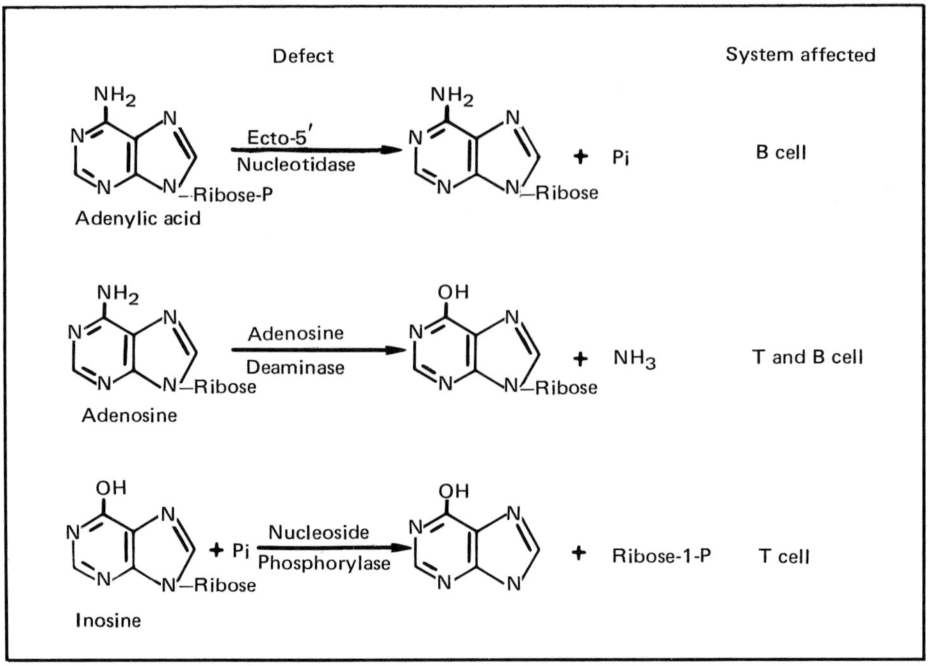

Fig. 15-3 : Postulated enzyme defects. (Modified from Seegmiller et al., Nucleotide and Nucleoside Metabolism and Lymphocyte Function. In E. W. Gelfand et al. (Eds.), Biological Basis of Immunodeficiency. New York: Raven Press, 1980. P. 252.)

short-limbed dwarfism and cellular immunodeficiency are susceptible to recurrent respiratory tract infections. Individuals with short-limbed dwarfism and antibody deficiency experience recurrent bacterial infections similar to those of congenital hypogammaglobulinemia.

IMMUNODEFICIENCY WITH ENZYME DEFICIENCY. There are three forms of enzyme deficiency that may exist in association with immunodeficiency (Figure 15-3). Adenosine deaminase deficiency is associated with a syndrome of both T and B cell immunodeficiency. Nucleoside phosphorylase deficiency is associated with a T cell immunodeficiency. Ecto-5'-nucleotidase deficiency is seen with B cell deficiencies. These enzymes are all necessary for the catabolism of adenylate purines. The exact mechanism by which a deficiency of the enzyme results in an immune defect is not known. It is thought that the immunodeficiency is the result of accumulation of adenine derivatives, with associated suppressive effects on lymphocyte functions. The mode of inheritance of these enzyme defects appears to be autosomal recessive. The carrier state can be shown in both sexes by decreased activity of the specific enzymes.

Table 15-7 : Complement Deficiencies

Deficiency	Inheritance	Symptom
C1r	Recessive	SLE-like syndrome
C4	Recessive	SLE-like syndrome
C2	Recessive	SLE-like syndrome
C3	Recessive	Pyogenic infections
C5	Recessive	SLE
C6	Recessive	Neisserial infections
C7	Recessive	Neisserial infections
C8	Recessive	Neisserial infections
C1 inhibitor	Dominant	Hereditary angioneurotic edema
C3b inactivator	Recessive	Pyogenic infections

The diagnosis of immunodeficiency with enzyme deficiency may be best established by enzyme assays of red cells. Tissue cells may also be deficient in these enzymes. An intrauterine diagnosis of adenosine deaminase has been made using cultured amniotic cells. Patients with nucleoside phosphorylase deficiency are unable to form uric acid. A rapid diagnosis of immunodeficiency disease associated with nucleoside phosphorylase defect may be made by measuring the serum and urine uric acid level which is extremely low.

Disorders of the Complement System

There are a few rare but significant defects of the complement system that may lead to an autoimmune syndrome or susceptibility to infection (Table 15-7). The genetically determined abnormalities of the complement system can be classified as follows: (1) defects in inhibitors, resulting in spontaneous consumption of complement components; (2) synthesis of defective complement components; and (3) absence of a complement component.

The most important of the complement-associated deficiencies is hereditary angioedema, which is caused by defective synthesis of C1 esterase inhibitor. In normal individuals, C1 esterase inhibitors block activity of C1s and thereby suppress the progression of the complement sequence beyond C1. Patients with hereditary angioedema suffer from spontaneous activation of the complement system and develop episodes of angioedematous reactions in the tissues, particularly within the upper respiratory tract. Recurrent attacks of edema usually involve the skin, gastrointestinal tract, and respiratory tract. Hereditary angioedema exists as two genetic variants. In one type there is absence of the C1 esterase inhibitor, and in the other there is formation of a nonfunctional C1 esterase molecule.

Patients with C3 deficiency may have repeated infections with pyogenic bacteria. The C3 deficiency leads to an absence of complement-mediated functions such as immunoadherence and opsonization. There is defective activation of the later components of complement. C3 deficiency may occur through failure of synthesis of C3 or through hypercatabolism of C3.

Several other rarely encountered, sometimes familial, complement deficiency syndromes have been described. Autosomal recessive deficiencies may be associated with diseases such as systemic lupus erythematosus.

Disorders of Phagocytosis

Phagocytic disorders are divided into extrinsic and intrinsic defects. The extrinsic disorders may arise secondary to (1) deficiency of antibody and complement factors; (2) suppression of phagocytic cells; (3) interference with phagocytic function by corticosteroids; or (4) suppression of circulating neutrophils by autoantibodies.

Intrinsic phagocytic disorders are related to enzymatic deficiencies within the metabolic pathway that is involved in killing bacteria. Such disorders include chronic granulomatous diseases with deficiency of NADPH or NADH oxidase, myeloperoxidase deficiency, and glucose-6-phosphate dehydrogenase deficiency.

Chronic Granulomatous Disease (CGD)

The major features of chronic granulomatous disease include susceptibility to infection by organisms of low virulence such as *Staphylococcus albus* and *Serratia marcescens*; onset of symptoms before 2 years of age with pneumonia and splenomegaly, and a diagnosis established by the quantitative nitroblue tetrazolium test and/or quantitative bacteria killing assay. The disease is usually X-linked.

The enzymatic deficiency in CGD is often NADH or NADPH oxidase. In a specifically female variant of this disease, glutathione peroxidase is apparently deficient. With enzymatic deficiency, the intracellular metabolism of neutrophils and monocytes is abnormal. Decreased oxygen consumpton and decreased utilization of glucose by the hexose monophosphate shunt are seen. There is resultant loss of production of antimicrobial hydrogen peroxide and superoxide radical production with decreased halogenation of bacteria. There is decreased intracellular killing of bacteria and fungi.

The in vitro screening test for diagnosis of chronic granulomatous disease is the quantitative nitroblue tetrazolium (NBT) test (Figure 15-4). Normal leukocytes reduce NBT dye during in vitro phagocytosis of particles such as latex. The leukocytes of patients with CGD show absent nitroblue tetrazolium dye reduc-

Fig. 15-4 : The nitroblue tetrazolium reduction test.

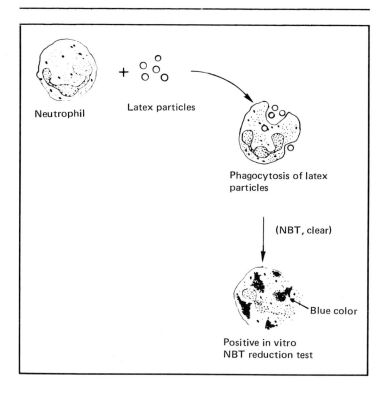

Neutrophil

Latex particles

Phagocytosis of latex particles

(NBT, clear)

Blue color

Positive in vitro NBT reduction test

tion. Carriers may reveal normal or decreased nitroblue tetrazolium reduction.

The peripheral white count is usually elevated, even if the patient does not have active infection. Cellular immunity is normal, and complement factors may be elevated.

Chédiak-Higashi Syndrome

The Chédiak-Higashi syndrome is a multisystem autosomal recessive disorder. Symptoms include recurrent bacterial infection with a variety of organisms, hepatosplenomegaly, partial albinism, central nervous system abnormalities, abnormal chemotaxis of neutrophils, and a high incidence of lymphoreticular malignancy.

The characteristic abnormality is a giant cytoplasmic granular inclusion in white blood cells and platelets, which is observed in peripheral blood smears. There is abnormal microtubular function of the affected cells, possibly related to cyclic nucleotide metabolic abnormalities. This results in abnormal chemotaxis of phagocytes and diminished intracellular killing of organisms such as pneumococci. The defect is one of delayed killing time. Oxygen consumption, hydrogen peroxide formation, and hexose monophosphate shunt activity are apparently normal. There is no altogether satisfactory treatment for the disease.

Table 15-8 : Secondary Immunodeficiencies

Disorder	T Cells	B Cells	Phagocytosis
Hodgkin's Disease	↓	N	±
Chronic lymphocytic leukemia	(↓)	↓	N
Acute lymphocytic leukemia	↓	↓	N
Sarcoidosis	↓	±N	?
Myeloma	N	↓	N
Lupus erythematosus	↓	↑	N
Tuberculosis	↓	N	?

↓ = depressed; ↑ = increased; N = normal; ? = unknown.

Job's Syndrome

Job's syndrome is described as a disease of recurrent staphylococcal abscesses of the skin, lymph nodes, or subcutaneous tissue. No abnormal immunological test results are associated with this disorder. There are indications that Job's syndrome is a variant of chronic granulomatous disease. Treatment consists of appropriate antibiotic therapy.

Tuftsin Deficiency

Tuftsin deficiency has been reported as a familial deficiency of a phagocytosis-stimulating tetrapeptide that is cleaved from immunoglobulin molecules in the spleen. Two families with tuftsin deficiency have been described. Tuftsin is also absent in patients who have been splenectomized. γ-globulin therapy has been found to be beneficial.

Secondary Immunodeficiency Diseases

Immunodeficiencies are observed to accompany certain infections, malignant conditions often involving the lymphoid system, loss of proteins from the body, drug therapy, aging, and debilitating diseases. An immunodeficiency accompanying another disease is called a *secondary immunodeficiency.* Secondary immunodeficiencies may affect both the humoral and the cellular immune systems. Examples of such disorders are shown in Table 15-8. In most cases both T cell and B cell systems are involved, although to varying degrees.

Many lymphoproliferative disorders are accompanied by a profound secondary immunodeficiency state. These diseases include multiple myeloma, Waldenström's macroglobulinemia, and other lymphoproliferative diseases. Myeloma disorders are called *monoclonal gammopathies,* because excessive amounts of monoclonal immunoglobulin are produced. Patients with multiple myeloma often suffer recurrent infections with various bacterial and fungal organisms.

Patients with Hodgkin's disease develop a progressive immunodeficiency of the cellular immune system, while the humoral immune system appears to be relatively intact. The etiology of immunosuppression in Hodgkin's disease may arise from increased suppressor cell phenomena.

Patients with chronic lymphocytic leukemia develop a deficiency of both T and B cell immune systems. Both systems are essentially normal in the early stages of acute lymphocytic leukemia, but in the late stages of this condition, recurrent infections take place.

Protein losses from the intestinal or urinary tract during certain acute and chronic diseases lead to hypogammaglobulinemia and relative humoral immunodeficiency.

Diagnosis and Laboratory Evaluation of Immunodeficiency Diseases

Recurrent infection is the bane of the immunodeficient patient. Recurrent infection caused by bacteria of high or low virulence, or by unusual organisms, and infections caused by fungi or vaccines (usually viruses) may suggest an immunological defect.

In evaluating patients suspected of having immunodeficiency disease, a detailed history should be obtained, with particular attention paid to allergy, previous treatment, other diseases, and family history (Table 15-9).

Evaluation of T cell Deficiency

The kind of immune deficiency determines the type of infections that arise. A T cell deficiency usually leads to increased susceptibility to intracellular infection by fungi, viruses, and acid-fast organisms. These organisms include *Candida albicans,* vaccinia and mumps viruses, *Mycoplasma,* and *Pneumocystis carinii. Pneumocystis* frequently causes infections in immunosuppressed individuals and exhibits characteristic accumulations of foamy, pink-staining pleural exudate containing many *Pneumocystis* organisms. Table 15-9 lists tests useful in documenting T cell deficiency. Defects in the lymphocyte transformation test are often suggestive of cellular immunodeficiency. Very recently, analysis of suppressor cell function has become useful in documenting and probing secondary immunodeficiency in diseases such as Hodgkin's disease and carcinoma.

Skin tests for evaluation of delayed type hypersensitivity to common antigens may be of little help in the case of children, who may not have had the opportunity to develop immunity to the antigens. However, a negative skin test to *Candida* antigens in children suffering from infection with this fungus is useful. Morphological analysis of the small lymphocytes in the peripheral blood and the deep cortical areas of biopsies of lymph nodes provides information as to the adequacy of the cellular immune system.

Table 15-9 : Evaluation of Patients with Immunodeficiency

History	T Cells	B Cells	Phagocytosis	Complement
Allergy	Lymphocyte count	Lymphocyte count	In vitro bactericidal tests	C1-9 components
Surgery	Skin test results (PPD, etc.)	Isoagglutinins	NBT test	C1 esterase inhibitor
Radiation	LBT (PHA)	IEP	Leukocyte enzymes	CH_{50}
Infections	MIF assay	Secretory immunoglobulins	Chemotaxis test	
Immunizations	T cell markers	LBT (PWM)		
Family history	X-ray (thymus)	B cell markers		
Other diseases	Lymph node biopsy	Lymph node biopsy		
	Suppressor cell assay	Skin test results (Schick test, etc.)		

PHA = phytohemagglutinin; LBT = lymphoblastic transformation; MIF = macrophage inhibition factor; IEP = immunoelectrophoresis; PWM = pokeweed mitogen; NBT = nitroblue tetrazolium reduction test; CH_{50} = complement hemolysis (50%) test.

Evaluation of B Cell Deficiency

Deficiency of the humoral immune system usually leads to frequent infections with pathogenic bacteria, causing otitis media, pneumonia, meningitis, and other infections. Such organisms include *Pneumococcus, Streptococcus, Hemophilus,* and *Meningococcus.* The tests for humoral immunity can be divided into tests for the presence of existing antibodies to common antigens and tests for antibody formation following immunization. Immunoglobulin levels are commonly quantitated by any of the various methods, including immunoprecipitin techniques. Absent or low serum levels of one or more immunoglobulins may have three possible causes: (1) absent or decreased B cells; (2) defective immunoglobulin synthesis and secretion; or (3) increased rate of immunoglobulin catabolism.

Tests that can distinguish among these possibilities include immunofluorescent staining of the membrane of lymphocytes to analyze the B cell population. In addition, a search for germinal centers and plasma cells in lymph nodes may be performed.

Tests for T Cell Function

ABSOLUTE LYMPHOCYTE COUNT. Infants should show a count of more than 1,500 small lymphocytes per cubic millimeter. The count in normal children is usually around 3,500 per cubic millimeter. The lymphocyte count declines during maturation of individuals to an average of 2,500, with a lower limit of about 1,000 per cubic millimeter.

DELAYED TYPE SKIN REACTIONS. Several antigens may be employed to test delayed type skin reactions: purified protein derivative (PPD), *Trichophytin, Candida,* streptokinase-streptodornase and mumps are the most common. Normal individuals respond to one or more of these antigens. If skin reactions to a variety of delayed type hypersensitivity antigens are negative, then de novo sensitization with substances such as 2,4-dinitrochlorobenzene may be attempted.

LYMPHOCYTE TRANSFORMATION TESTS. In vitro tests of lymphocyte transformation are especially useful in evaluating T cell reactivity to mitogens and antigens. Lymphocytes are obtained from peripheral blood and cultured with cell mitogens, such as phytohemagglutinin (PHA), for T cell competence. Transformation of lymphocytes in response to such stimuli is usually measured by lymphocyte incorporation of radiolabeled thymidine into DNA. This test is used to document reactivity of the T cell system. Failure of lymphocytes to undergo transformation in this test indicates probable immunodeficiency.

MIGRATION INHIBITION FACTOR ASSAY. Previously sensitized T lymphocytes release lymphokines in the presence of sensitizing antigen. One of the factors released is migration inhibitory factor (MIF), which inhibits migration of macrophages. Measurement of MIF release in vitro is an indicator of previous cell-mediated sensitization.

EXAMINATION OF CIRCULATING LYMPHOCYTES FOR T CELL MARKERS. Cell markers of peripheral blood and lymph node lymphocytes are examined for quantitation of T and B cells. Normally, 65 to 85 percent of circulating lymphocytes are T cells. A diminished number of T cells suggests immunodeficiency of the T system. Sheep red blood cell rosetting of T cells and/or heterologous antisera to T cells are used to enumerate T cells. Recently, surface Fc receptors on T cells have been used to count helper T cells (IgM Fc receptors) and suppressor T cells (IgG Fc receptors).

LYMPH NODE BIOPSY. Depletion of paracortical lymphoid cells suggests a T cell defect.

Tests of B Cell Function

TESTS FOR EXISTING ANTIBODIES. *Schick Test.* If a patient has previously been immunized with diphtheria toxoid, the Schick test will be negative. The Schick test consists of injecting diphtheria toxin into the skin. If immunization has been successful, antibody blocks a toxic erythematous skin reaction, and the test is said to be negative. A positive Schick test in an immunized individual is presumptive evidence of IgG immunoglobulin deficiency.

Isohemagglutinin Test. Isohemagglutinins are normally present after 1 year of age and primarily consist of IgM antibodies. The absence of isohemagglutinins is evidence of an IgM deficiency, although the isoagglutinin titer during the first two years of life is low.

Immunoelectrophoresis. To determine qualitative aspects of immunoglobulins IgG, IgM, and IgA, immunoelectrophoresis of the sera of suspected immunodeficient patients is carried out. Quantitative measures are performed for absolute levels of antibodies. An IgG concentration of less than 200 to 300 mg/100 ml is usually considered consistent with B cell immunodeficiency. An IgA deficiency shows less than 5 mg/100 ml of serum. Patients with normal levels of immunoglobulins may have a history of recurrent infections associated with selective IgG subclass deficiencies.

Biopsy. A biopsy may be taken for histological examination of lymphoid tissue and for immunofluorescent localization of IgG,

IgM, and IgA immunoglobulins. Infants over 1 month of age have many plasma cells in the lamina propria of the rectal mucosa, and immunofluorescence is an excellent confirmatory test for evidence of antibody production.

TESTS FOR ANTIBODY FORMATION FOLLOWING ACTIVE IMMUNIZATION. Diphtheria toxin is given weekly for three weeks. The Schick test is then administered. A positive Schick test occurs in agammaglobulinemia. Typhoid immunization can also be given, with antityphoid agglutinins determined in the laboratory. The antibody titer following three injections of the vaccine should be 1/160 or greater. Patients with antibody deficiencies have very low titers.

QUANTITATION OF B LYMPHOCYTES. The presence of surface immunoglobulin as determined by staining with fluorescent antisera to heavy chain determinants has been used to identify B cells. Problems related to Fc receptors and possible nonspecific antibody uptake are avoided by use of Fab and $(Fab')_2$ fragments of antisera. The surface immunoglobulin determinants on the B cells of normal individuals are usually IgM and LgD. B cells may carry both these determinants. The number of circulating B cells with surface immunoglobulin in normal adults ranges from 3 to 15 percent, depending on the laboratory.

B cells are also commonly identified by the presence of a surface receptor for the third component of complement. The most widely used method for quantitating C3 receptors on B cells makes use of ox erythrocytes sensitized with purified IgM red cell antibodies reacted with complement. These sensitized cells (EAC) can then be shown to adhere to B lymphocytes, forming rosettes through the complement receptor. Peripheral blood lymphocytes in normal individuals with EAC receptors usually have surface Ig markers. B cells also have receptors for the Fc portion of IgG and may be identified using IgG-coated erythrocytes or fluorescein-tagged aggregated IgG. Such receptors are also present on monocytes.

LYMPHOCYTE TRANSFORMATION TESTS. Lymphocyte transformation may be carried out with B cell mitogens, such as pokeweed mitogen, which stimulates mostly B cells to undergo division. Nonspecific production of immunoglobulins following such stimulation may also be used to indicate B cell competence.

Bibliography and Selected Reading

General

Fudenberg, H. H., Stites, D. P., Caldwell, J. L., and Wells, J. V. (Eds.). *Basic and Clinical Immunology* (2nd ed.). Los Gatos, Calif.: Lange, 1978.

Gelfund, E. W., and Dosch, H. (Eds.). *Biological Basis of Immunodeficiency,* New York: Raven, 1980.

Nakamura, R. M. *Immunopathology: Clinical Laboratory Concepts and Methods.* Boston: Little, Brown, 1974.

Rose, N. R., and Friedman, H. (Eds.). *Manual of Clinical Immunology.* Washington, D.C.: American Society for Microbiology, 1976.

Primary Immunodeficiency Diseases

Ammann, A. J. T-cell and T-B cell immunodeficiency disorders. *Pediatr. Clin. North Am.* 24:293, 1977.

Ammann, A. J., and Fudenberg, H. H. *Immunodeficiency Diseases.* In H. H. Fudenberg, D. P. Stities, J. L. Caldwell, and J. V. Wells (Eds.), *Basic and Clinical Immunology* (2nd ed.). Los Gatos, Calif.: Lange, 1978. P. 391.

Cooper, M. C., Lawton, A. R., Préudhomme, J. L., and Seligmann, M. Primary antibody deficiencies. *Springer Sem. Immunopathol.* 1:265, 1978.

Gelfund, E. W., and Dosch, H. (Eds.). *Biological Basis of Immunodeficiency.* New York: Raven, 1980.

Goldman, A. S., and Goldblum, R. M. Primary deficiencies in humoral immunity. *Pediatr. Clin. North Am.* 24:277, 1977.

Good, R. A., and Zak, J. J. Disturbances in gammaglobulin synthesis as "experiment of nature." *Pediatrics* 18:109, 1956.

Hayward, A. R. *Immunodeficiency: Curr. Topics Immunol.* Baltimore: Williams & Wilkins, 1977.

Hitzing, W. H., Dooren, L. J., and Vossen, J. M. Severe combined immunodeficiency diseases. *Springer Sem. Immunopathol.* 1:283, 1978.

Immunodeficiency: Report of a WHO Scientific Group. Geneva: World Health Organization, 1978.

Morito, T., Bankhurst, A. D., and Williams R. C. Studies of T- and B-cell interactions in adult patients with combined immunodeficiency. *J. Clin. Invest.* 65:422, 1980.

Walkmann, T. A., and Broder, S. T-cell disorders in primary immunodeficiency diseases, *Springer Sem. Immunopathol.* 1:239, 1978.

Enzyme Defects in Immunodeficiency

Ammann, A. J., and Fudenberg, H. H. Immunodeficiency Diseases. In H. H. Fudenberg, D. P. Stites, J. L. Caldwell, and J. V. Wells (Eds.), *Basic and Clinical Immunology* (2nd ed.). Los Gatos, Calif.: Lange, 1978. P. 391.

Hirschhorn, R., and Martin, D. W. Enzyme defects in immunodeficiency diseases. *Springer Sem. Immunopathol.* 1:299, 1978.

Seegmiller, J. E., Thompson, L., Bluestein H., Willis, R., Matsumoto, S., and Carson, D. Nucleotide and Nucleoside Metabolism and Lymphocyte Function. In E. W. Gelfand and H. M. Dosch (Eds.), *Biological Basis of Immunodeficiency.* New York: Raven, 1980. P. 251.

Phagocytic and Complement Disorders

Ammann, A. J., and Fudenberg, H. H. Immunodeficiency Diseases. In H. H. Fudenberg, D. P. Stites, J. L. Caldwell, and J. V. Wells (Eds.), *Basic and Clinical Immunology* (2nd ed.). Los Gatos, Calif. Lange, 1978. P. 391.

Lachmann, P. J., and Rosen, F. S. Genetic defects of complement in man. *Springer Sem. Immunopathol.* 1:339, 1978.

Nakamura, R. M. *Immunopathology: Clinical Laboratory Concepts and Methods.* Boston: Little, Brown, 1974.

Quie, P. G., Mills, E. L., McPhail, L. C., and Johnson, R. B. Phagocytic defects. *Springer Sem. Immunopathol.* 1:323, 1978.

Rose, N. R., and Friedman, H. (Eds.). *Manual of Clinical Immunology.* Washington, D.C.: American Society for Microbiology, 1976.

Secondary Immunodeficiency Diseases

Ammann, A. J., and Fudenberg H. H. Immunodeficiency Diseases. In H. H. Fudenberg, D. P. Stites, J. L. Caldwell, and J. V. Wells (Eds.), *Basic and Clinical Immunology* (2nd ed.). Los Gatos, Calif.: Lange, 1978. p. 391.

Bergsma, D., Good, R. A., Finstad, J., Paul, N.W. (Eds.). *Immunodeficiency in Man and Animals.* Sunderland, Mass.: Sinauer, 1975.

Gell, P. G. H., Coombs, R. R. A., and Lachmann, P. J. (Eds.). *Clinical Aspects of Immunology.* London: Blackwell, 1975.

Waldmann, T. A., Broder, S., Blaese, R. M., Durm, M., Goldman, C., and Maul, L. Role of Suppressor Cells in Human Disease. In E. W. Gelfand and H. M. Dosch (Eds.), *Biological Basis of Immunodeficiency.* New York: Raven, 1980.

Laboratory Diagnosis and Treatment

Ammann, A. J., and Fudenberg, H. H. Immunodeficiency Diseases. In H. H. Fudenberg, D. P. Stites, J. L. Caldwell, and J. V. Wells (Eds.), *Basic and Clinical Immunology* (2nd ed.). Los Gatos, Calif.: 1978.

Nakamura, R. M. *Immunopathology: Clinical Laboratory Concepts and Methods.* Boston: Little, Brown, 1974.

Pahwa, R., Pahwa, S., O'Reilly, R., and Good, R. A. Treatment of the immunodeficiency diseases—progress toward replacement therapy emphasizing cellular and macromolecular engineering, *Springer Sem. Immunopathol.* 1:355, 1978.

Rose, N. R., and Friedman, H. (Eds.). *Manual of Clinical Immunology.* Washington, D.C.: American Society for Microbiology, 1976.

Taubman, S. B. Screening tests for cell-mediated immunodeficiency diseases. *CRC Crit. Rev. Clin. Lab. Sci.* 11:207, 1979.

16 : Immunology of Cancer

The etiology of cancer in man is presently unknown. The disease is affected by the interactions of a variety of factors, such as genes, viruses, and chemical and physical agents. In experiments with chemically induced tumors, it has been shown that tumor development occurs as a result of an *initiator* and a *promoter*. Chemicals such as methylcholanthrene act as initiators and are referred to as *carcinogens*. On the other hand, compounds such as croton oil are promoters and are not carcinogens. Promoters do not initiate carcinogenesis but, when applied with a carcinogen, enhance or promote tumor development. Tumors induced by these chemical carcinogens may elicit an immune response in the host. This chapter will encompass the response of the host to tumor cells.

Over the past two decades, there has been a resurgence of interest and research in the immunology of cancer. These recent studies have aided our understanding of the host's immunological response to tumor antigens. As far back as the turn of the century, following Jenner's development of smallpox vaccination, attempts were made at immunization (autologous and homologous) with tumors and tumor extracts in man. A few cases were fairly successful; in others, surprisingly, enhancement of tumor growth was reported. Immune enhancement and the major histocompatibility complex (MHC) (see Chapter 12) antigens were unknown factors in these earlier experiments. Thus, in general, these attempts at immunization fell in disrepute.

The tremendous advances that have been made in transplantation, and the recognition of the MHC, including HLA antigens, have clarified some of the uncertainties encountered in the earlier immunization attempts in man. The establishment of inbred strains of mice (syngeneic) has contributed much to our understanding of the immunological phenomenon in cancer. These inbred strains have eliminated the problem of allogeneic transplantation rejection due to noncompatibility of antigens in the H-2 complex (see Chapter 10).

This chapter discusses tumor antigens; the immune response in individuals with the disease; the concepts of immune surveillance and enhancement; the mechanisms of the tumor escape

415

phenomenon; and the relevant approaches to immunotherapy, both specific and nonspecific. Although much has been learned about the immunology of cancer in the past decade, much remains to be elucidated as to the nature of the host response to tumors and the ability of the tumor to proliferate.

Tumor Antigens

Tumors are associated with various antigens and can be generally separated into three categories: (1) those associated with embryonic tissues; (2) those related to viruses antigenically and to virus-distinct antigens; and (3) the tumor-specific antigens, which are unique to the tumor only and not present in normal tissues. In addition, the tumor cells, when compared with their normal cellular counterparts, may show (1) deletion of normal susrface antigens, especially the ABO group antigens; (2) membrane changes in composition and immunochemical reactivity; and (3) elaboration of oncofetal isozymes, which can be readily detected in the plasma of cancer patients.

Definitions

Tumor-associated antigens (TAA) are antigens that are associated with the tumor and can be qualitatively, quantitatively, or transiently differentiated from normal cells. *Tumor-specific antigens* (TSA) are antigens present only in the tumor cells and not in normal cells. *Tumor-specific transplantation antigens* (TSTA) are able to induce an immune response or resistance to the specific tumor growth in the *autochthonous* host. TSTA are membrane surface antigens. *Tumor-associated phase-specific antigens* (TAPSA) or *oncofetal antigens* are embryonic or fetal antigens expressed on many tumor cell surfaces. These antigens occur in high levels in the plasma of cancer patients and in fetal tissues (see Table 16-2) during the first and second trimester of fetal life.

Membrane Alterations of Tumor Cells

Changes in the membrane surfaces of tumors have been examined in vitro, both in normal cells *transformed* into malignant cells and by direct examination of tumor membranes with specific antibody by immunological procedures, comparing the tumor membranes with normal tissue counterparts. Membrane alterations include *deletion* of normal determinants or specific residues as specified by gene derepression or mutation and/or *membrane changes* due to chemical inversion, rearrangement, and/or addition of cover layers (Figure 16-1).

DELETION. Among the earlier deletions demonstrated in tumor cells was the absence of the ABO blood group antigens in many human epithelial cancers, such as squamous cell carcinoma of the cervix, head, and neck. This presence or absence of the A, B, and H antigens has been used in histological and immuno-

Fig. 16-1 : Mechanisms of membrane alterations following transformation of a normal cell to a malignant cell.
A. Dislocation of a cytoplasmic structure to the surface of membrane;
B. Dislocation of an antigen molecule from the interior to the exterior surface of the membrane. C. Rearrangement of the terminal residues on the membrane surface. (Ext = exterior, Mem = membrane, Int = interior.

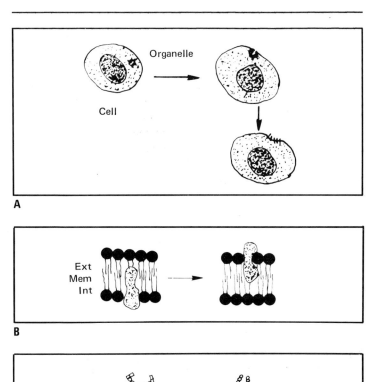

logical diagnosis of carcinoma. The precise mechanism associated with the deletion of normal cell markers on tumor cells is presently not determined. One postulated mechanism is that the cell surface may combine with the carcinogen (chemical or viral) to form a neoantigen, which induces antibody production. This "autoantibody" then combines with the neoantigens to induce the deletion of the surface antigens. Alternatively, absence of normal antigenic determinants or residues may be dependent on lack of gene expression or lack of the terminal enzyme regulated by the gene. For example, residues generally absent or decreased on membrane surfaces include carbohydrates such as fucose, galactose, N-acetylglucosamine, N-acetylgalactosamine, and N-acetylneuraminic acid (sialic acid). These are gene-regulated via the glycosyltransferases. It is interesting to note that in many patients with carcinoma of the gastrointestinal tract, an increase in A, B, and H blood group antigens, dependent on the secretor status (see Chapter 11) of the individual, can be demonstrated in the serum.

MEMBRANE ALTERATION. In contrast to their normal counterparts, the surface membranes of tumor cells demonstrate many physicochemical and immunochemical differences. Membrane changes involve differences in the distribution and density of normal membrane macromolecules. This is compatible with the present concepts of the fluid mosaic nature of the bilamellar membrane of mamallian cells. Tumor cells tend to agglutinate with plant agglutinins or lectins such as concanavalin A and wheat germ agglutinins more readily than normal cells. In this regard, it has been demonstrated that an isomeric form of carcinoembryonic antigen CEA-P (Table 16-1), in the free isolated state reacts with Con A in agar gel immunodiffusion. Tumor cell membrane alterations have involved lipids, carbohydrates, proteins and glycoproteins, and glycolipids. That is, changes have been associated with all macromolecules. The mechanism of membrane changes discussed here may be due to (1) dislocation from one part of the cell to another; (2) dislocation from one layer of membrane to another; and (3) rearrangement of residues of the macromolecule on the membrane surface.

Tumor-Specific Antigens (TSA) and Tumor-Specific Transplantation Antigens (TSTA)

The area of tumor immunology dealing with tumor-specific and tumor-specific transplantation antigens has been thoroughly documented by experiments in mouse models and has been the impetus for study of cancers in humans.

CHEMICAL CARCINOGENS AND VIRALLY INDUCED TUMORS. Tumors can be induced experimentally by chemical or physical agents and by viruses. Tumors induced by a chemical carcinogen, such as methylcholanthrene, or by a physical agent (x-irradiation) in mice have specific antigens which, even though similar in morphology, show no relationship in cross-immunization studies. This is illustrated in Figures 16–2 and 16–4. Chemical carcinogens may induce several individual specific neoantigens in the animal. These neoantigens and other chemical carcinogen–induced tumor antigens are demonstrated best by in vitro serological techniques such as immunodiffusion and immunofluorescence.

In contrast to chemical carcinogen–induced tumors, viral-induced tumors display identical tumor antigens, which are related and specific antigenically, even though induced in xenogeneic strains of mice (see Figure 16–2). There are two major categories of TSA in viral-induced neoplasias: (1) viral-specific antigens and (2) newly acquired antigens, which were absent in normal cells prior to neoplastic transformation. The viral-specific tumor antigens are expressed in the tumor cells via their viral genome, while the newly expressed tumor antigens reflect the specific interactions of the viral genome. Fetal antigens in tumor cells may be an

Table 16-1 : Comparison of the Pysicochemical Properties of the Carcinofetal Antigens and TennaGen Used as Tumor Markers in Cancer Patients

Antigen*	MW	PI	Mobility in IEP	Carbohydrate Content (%)	Mole (%)					
					Fucose	Mannose	Gal	Nac-Glu	Nac-Gal	SA
CEA	201,000	V	β	45-57	14.20-18.90	17.10-10.60	17.50-39.80	32.90-23.30	3.70-11.40	2.4-2.9
CEA-M	200,000	4.5-5.5	γ-β	48.8-87.7	22.20	15.70	19.60	9.18	trace	0.7
CEA-P	170,000	4.3-5.3	β	69.9-70.3	14.70	2.40	26.40	20.2	trace	6.3
CEA-S	181,000	4.5	β	—	—	—	—	—	—	—
α₁FP	70,000	4.9	α	4.0	—	—	—	—	—	0.8
TennaGen	100,000	3.84.2	β	51.3	2.54	16.37	22.80	20.91	9.49	19.88

*Con A reacts with CEA-P in immunodiffusion reactions in agar but not with CEA-M.
MW = molecular weight; PI = isoelectric point; Gal = Galactose; Nac-Glu = N-acetylglucosamine; NacGal = N-acetylgalactosamine; SA = sialic acid (neuraminic acid); IEP = immunoelectrophoresis. CEA-P, CEA-M, and CEA-S refer to antigens that are similar immunologically, but having different properties.

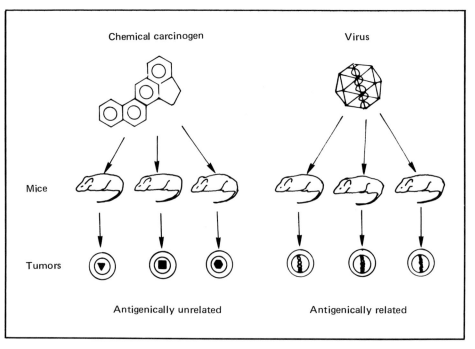

Fig. 16-2 : Comparison of chemical carcinogen–induced and viral–induced tumor antigens in animals. Chemically induced tumors are distinct and unrelated, even though stimulated by the same carcinogen in the same animal, whereas virally induced tumors are antigenically related, even though induced in allogeneic or unrelated strains.

example of the action of viral genomes on repressor genes, resulting in the suppression of differentiation of generating cells or the dedifferentiation of a normal differentiated cell (Figure 16-3).

Tumor antigens have been distinguished by their location or position in the tumor cell as (1) intracellular or (2) cell surface antigens. The intracellular antigens of virally induced tumors are usually formed in the nucleus and are part of the initial viral proteins of the DNA viruses. Thus, they are the products of the viral genes, although not incorporated into complete viruses. These antigens may continue to be produced within the tumor cells in the absence of the complete infectious viral agent. An example of this is the T antigen discovered in the nucleus of cells infected with the papovaviruses (polyomavirus, SV 40, papillomavirus). The group-specific antigens (gs 1 and gs 3) of RNA oncogenic viruses of the leukovirus group provide another example of intracellular viral antigens. In this case, however, the antigens are components of the complete virion and, like the T antigen of DNA viruses, are not known to play a significant part in the

Fig. 16-3 : Concept of derepression or dedifferentiation in tumors which results in the reexpression of fetal and neoantigens following carcinogenesis.

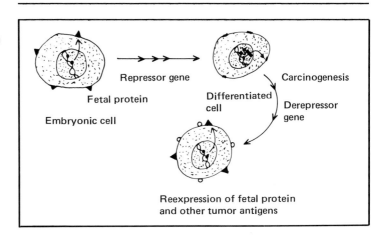

Repressor gene

Carcinogenesis

Fetal protein

Differentiated cell

Derepressor gene

Embryonic cell

Reexpression of fetal protein
and other tumor antigens

rejection of the tumor cells. These specific viral antigens can elicit an immune response following their release upon lysis of the tumor cells and can be detected by various immunological procedures intracellularly or by serological means from extracts of infected tumor cells.

The tumor antigens responsible for the rejection reactions and of importance to immunotherapy are at the cell surface, where they are accessible to the receptors of the effector cells and antibodies. These cell surface antigens are referred to as TSTA, because the usual procedure for their demonstration involves the transplantation rejection phenomenon, when the tumor cells are transplanted from one syngeneic host animal to another.

The capsid viral antigens of DNA viruses and the envelope surface antigens of the RNA viruses have been shown to possess TSTA properties. In addition, tumors induced by the same virus or family of viruses in different strains of mice have been demonstrated to share common TSTAs. This is true even for tumors arising from different tissues (Figure 16–4). These TSTAs are distinct from the antigens of the virus itself, at least for DNA viruses, SV 40, and polyoma, since cells transformed by the viruses lack the complete viral particles. Immune responses to tumors induced by viruses are often stronger than those generated by chemically induced tumors. Recent examinations have demonstrated weak distinct TSTAs for each separate tumor in virally induced tumors, as has been strongly demonstrated for carcinogen-induced tumors. As indicated in Chapter 17, in vitro distinction of tumor cells induced through the murine leukemia virus (MuLV) system by specific cytolytic T lymphocytes (CTL) appears to be restricted to tumor cells which are transformed by the appropriate virus and that also share the H-2 region (I genes) with the CTL. Tumor cells induced by MuLV, but in mice of different

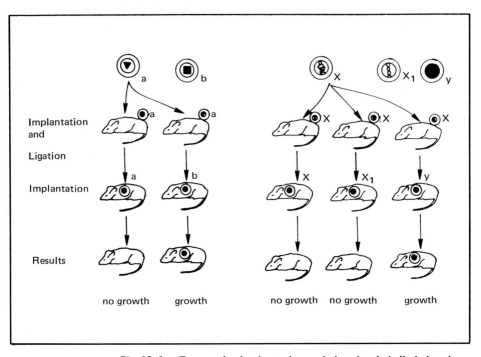

Fig. 16-4 : Tumor rejection in carcinogen-induced and virally-induced tumors examined in syngeneic mice. Results suggest common antigenic tumors related to the membrane tumor-specific transplantation antigens (TSTA). A. Mice implanted with chemically induced tumor #1(a) and then ligated are protected against challenge with tumor #1(a), but not against an unrelated chemically-induced tumor #2(b). B. Mice implanted with viral-induced tumor X and then ligated and rechallenged with tumors X, X_1, and Y showed no tumor growth when challenged with virally induced tumors X and X_1, but growth with tumor Y. This suggests a common TSTA antigen between X and X_1 virally induced tumors.

H-2 (I gene) composition, are not efficiently lysed by the CTL. Chemical carcinogen-induced tumors, even within syngeneic strains, have been shown to possess antigenically distinct TSTAs as determined by cross-immunization–transplantation experiments (Figure 16-4). Thus tumors induced in two different animals by the same carcinogen, or in one animal by the same carcinogen, or even different parts of a single tumor induced by a carcinogen, have been demonstrated to be *immunologically distinct* from one another in transplantation procedures. That is, the *immunodominant* determinants of TSTAs of chemical carcinogen-induced tumors are distinct (Figure 16-4). However, recent evidence has also shown that these tumors share weaker TSTAs. These TSTAs may be associated with the oncogenic RNA viruses demonstrated in certain carcinogen-induced carcinomas. Thus any distinction that could be made between carcinogen-induced tumors, each possessing a unique TSTA, and virally induced tumors, which share TSTA, is relative rather than absolute.

TUMOR, VIRUS, AND MAN. One of the best examples of the association of a human tumor with a virus is the relationship of the Epstein-Barr virus (EBV), a DNA virus (herpes), and Burkitt's lymphoma. EBV has also been shown to be closely associated with infectious mononucleosis and nasopharyngeal carcinoma. It is believed to be the etiological agent for infectious mononucleosis. Recent evidence demonstrated the presence of the EBV genome in tumor biopsies of Burkitt's lymphoma and nasopharyngeal carcinoma. This EBV genome has not been demonstrated in other lymphoproliferative diseases such as myeloma, heavy chain diseases, and IgM gammopathy.

Another possible viral association in human cancer is suggested by indirect evidence that cervical carcinoma may occur as the result of herpes simplex type 2 virus infection. A preliminary search for herpes simplex type 2 viral genome in cervical biopsies through nucleic acid hybridization has given both positive and negative data.

RNA tumor viruses of the leukovirus group have been associated with etiology of mouse mammary carcinoma, mouse leukemia, and mammary carcinoma in rhesus monkeys. Mouse mammary carcinoma is associated with B-type virus particles, which have a dense, eccentric core separated from the outer coat by electron-lucent space and are 1,000 Å in size as demonstrated by electron microscopy. Mouse leukemia, on the other hand, is associated with C-type virus particles of 1,000 Å and spherical and pleomorphic in shape, with a dense central core (helical nucleoid), giving some particles a bull's-eye appearance as observed by electron microscopy.

These various animal studies have suggested a possible viral etiology for human breast cancer, although concrete evidence for this hypothesis is still unavailable. Viral particles have not been isolated from nor established in human breast cancer tissue, nor have viral-like particles isolated from human milk demonstrated tumor-inducing capacity. Similarly, although the experimental data support the hypothesis that RNA viruses may be involved in the pathogenesis of human leukemia, conclusive evidence has not been established. Support for an RNA virus etiology in human leukemia is based on isolation of reverse transcriptase from human leukemic cells and observation of C-type particles in some cases. C-type particles have been observed in normal cells also, however. These observations are similar to the dilemma posed by EBV viruses.

Tumor-Associated Phase-Specific Antigens (TAPSA)

During carcinogenesis and the development of malignant tumors, there is a tendency to retrogressive dedifferentiation, normally repressed in the mature normal cell, which leads to reexpression of repressed genetic information. This process brings about an increased formation of fetal components of the cell, expressed as embryonic proteins detectable in increased levels in the plasma of cancer patients. These reversionary tumor antigens have been referred to as *carcinoembryonic antigen* (CEA) and α_1-fetoproteins (α_1FP). These tumor antigens are tissue constituents that are normally present in utero during fetal and embryonic life and whose synthesis is entirely or almost entirely repressed in the mature differentiated organism. The derepression or restoration of synthesis of these trace constituents may be reinstituted by a variety of tumors. The advent of sensitive immunological assay methods has shown that carcinofetal proteins are present in normal adults in trace amounts—usually < 2.5 ng/ml for CEA. The isomeric forms of enzymes such as Regan's antigen (placental alkaline phosphatase) and other acid and alkaline phosphatases have been also demonstrated in various tumors and are also considered as *carcinofetal proteins*. The enzyme acid phosphatase has been shown to be a useful marker for prostatic cancer. Table 16-1 summarizes the physicochemical properties of the various glycoproteins recognized as carcinofetal proteins and associated with tumors. These fetal antigens are referred to as *tumor-associated phase-specific antigens (TAPSA)*. The exception is TennaGen (Tennessee antigen), which as yet has not been demonstrated in normal fetal tissue extracts. These antigens are found in high levels in normal fetal tissues and in tumor tissues and in low concentrations in normal adult tissues.

CARCINOFETAL AND OTHER GLYCOPROTEINS. Carcinoembryonic antigen (CEA) was originally isolated from human colonic carcinoma, was found in the entodermally derived digestive tract epithelium, and subsequently was discovered to be present in the normal embryonic fetal gut, pancreas, and liver in high concentrations. These high levels are prevalent in the first two trimesters in fetal life. Several isomeric forms of CEA have been isolated. With the exception of CEA-A, all the others have been shown to cross-react with certain antigens of the ABO group (see Chapter 11). In addition, the carbohydrate residues show high levels of fucose and low levels of sialic acid (*N*-acetylneuraminic acid). When the accepted method of RIA (see Chapter 7) is used in the clinical laboratory, CEA levels of less than 2.5 ng/ml are considered normal in adult individuals. Elevated levels of CEA have been demonstrated in about 20 percent of normal smoking individuals, while fewer than 5 percent of nonsmoking individuals have demonstrated greater than 2.5 ng/ml CEA. Again by an RIA procedure, CEA-S, (an isomeric form of CEA) has shown greater specificity than CEA in that fewer than 7 percent of smokers examined have shown elevated levels of CEA-S.

Antibodies to CEA have been demonstrated in limited numbers of cancer patients and in pregnant women and appear to be of the IgM class. Purified CEA in the specific CMI responses in vitro has shown no responses (no ^{3}H-thymidine uptake by lymphocytes in presence of CEA). The effect on the nonspecific mitogen responses in vitro has been inconclusive.

The importance of CEA assessment in cancer patients, especially in cases of GI tract carcinoma, is in management postoperatively and during therapy. Elevated levels of CEA postoperatively would indicate the persistence of tumor residue. Generally a prolonged remission of CEA postoperatively carries a better prognosis.

TENNA GEN. TennaGen is also used in the assessment of cancer patients for therapy and postoperatively. The normal value in adults is < 5.0 μ/ml. The assay method involves a hemagglutination inhibition procedure. The purified TennaGen is coated onto red blood cells, and the degree of inhibition by the individual's serum (containing TennaGen) against standard goat anti-Tenna-Gen is compared with known standards of purified TennaGen.

TennaGen differs from CEA in its fucose and sialic acid residue contents and in its concentrations of the various amino acid residues. It does not cross-react with CEA nor α_1FP and as yet has not been demonstrated in fetal serum. Like CEA-S, it has shown greater specificity among smokers, that is, fewer false positives in smokers.

α_1-FETOPROTEIN. When α_1FP was first seen, it was presumed to arise from a selective derepression of protein synthesis that resulted from the complex formation between metabolite (carcinogenic) and the specific repressor gene. α_1FP was demonstrated initially in rats with hepatoma and subsequently in the plasma of human hepatomas. Like CEA, it is a fetal protein found in high levels in fetal liver and normal cord blood and in pregnant mothers' plasma, especially during the last trimester. α_1FP persists in the newborn's plasma for several months after birth. It has demonstrated immunosuppressive effects in the CMI, both specific and nonspecific responses, in vitro. Nonspecific studies have been shown with highly purified nanogram concentration of α_1FP in the in vitro CMI using adult female lymphocytes suppression in the mitogen response. A dose response effect on lymphocyte responses to mitogen is shown in Figure 16–5. Normal adult levels of α_1FP are in the range of 1 to 16 ng/ml. Nevertheless, as

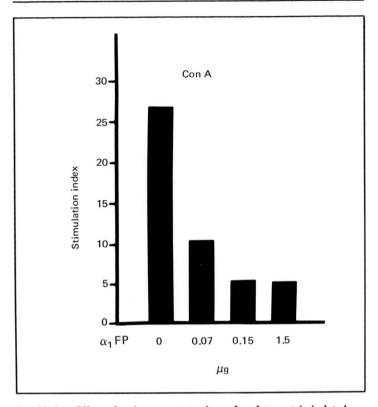

Fig. 16-5 : Effect of various concentrations of α₁-fetoprotein isolated from cord blood on concanavalin A-stimulated blastogenesis of human lymphocytes in vitro. Stimulation index (y axis) represents the ratio of ^{3}H-thymidine uptake between Con A-stimulated lymphocytes and the unstimulated lymphocytes in the presence of varying concentrations of Con A (x axis). A significant suppression of blastogenesis is demonstrated.

with CEA, the role of elevated α_1 FP in newborns and pregnant mothers is still undetermined. α_1 FP is also a glycoprotein but does not cross-react with CEA. High levels of α_1FP in the amniotic fluid during the twentieth week of gestation ($\sim$ 5 months) would suggest a neural tube defect in the fetus (spinal bifidus or anencephaly). A rapid rise in α_1 FP at 24 weeks would signal impending death of the fetus. Thus measurement of α_1 FP in the amniotic fluid could be of diagnostic value.

The physicochemical properties of the carcinofetal proteins and TennaGen and summarized in Table 16-1. The fetal and placental antigens associated with human tumors are summarized in Table 16-2.

The major value presently of the fetal antigens is their use as tumor markers by sensitive immunological procedures. α_1 FP, in addition to the detection of neural tube defects, has demon-

Table 16-2 : Human Carcinofetal and Placental Antigens Associated with Tumors in Adults

Carcinofetal Antigen	Fetal Tissue of Origin	Found in Adult Tumors
1. Fetal Antigens		
Carcinoembryonic Protein CEA CEA-S CEA-M CEA-P	GI tract	GI tract and variety of endodermal tumors
β-oncofetal	Fetal organs	Carcinoma—all types
γ-fetoprotein (γFP)	GI tract, spleen, thymus	Various tumors
α_1-fetoprotein (α_1 FP)	Liver, plasma (newborns and pregnant mothers)	Hepatomas, teratomas
α_2H-ferroprotein	Liver	Leukemia, Hodgkin's disease
Fetal sialoglycoprotein	GI tract	Stomach cancer
Pancreatic oncofetal protein	Pancreas	Pancreatic tumors
2. Placental Antigens		
Human chorionic gonadotropin (β-HCG)	Trophoblasts	Choriocarcinomas, teratocarcinomas
Placental alkaline phosphatase (Regan's antigen)	Placenta	Various tumors
3. Others		
Acid phosphatase	Prostate	Prostate carcinoma

strated a high binding affinity to estrogens and may be associated as a hormonal carrier, thus a regulator. There is some evidence for α_1 FP as an immunoregulatory property for T cell–dependent antigens in both the primary and the secondary response in vitro (plaque-forming assay examinations). The effect may be directly on the T cell, since a suppressive effect has been demonstrated with PHA in vitro. Nevertheless, the exact physiological role of the fetal proteins is not known. However, they serve a useful purpose as tumor markers in the management of tumor growth and therapy. Thus the carcinoembryonic antigen or TAPSA may be an expression of (1) genetic derepression with synthesis of a new gene product; (2) changes in gene regulation of protein synthesis; and/or (3) postsynthetic changes in protein or antigen structure in the altered cell metabolic environment. The second of the three postulates appears to be the most acceptable.

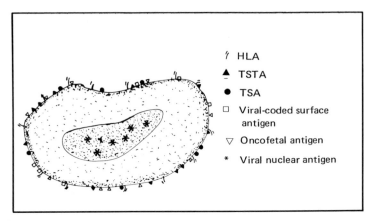

Fig. 16-6 : Composition of antigens in a tumor cell. A single tumor cell may have all these antigens, only some, or perhaps only one of the many potential tumor-associated antigens described. TAA may be in close relationship to the HLA or may be alone, as indicated in the diagram.

Specific tumor antigens (TSA) unrelated to TAPSA or viruses have been reported from melanoma and ovarian carcinomas. A schematic representation of tumor-associated antigens and the MHC antigens is given in Figure 16-6.

Immune Response to Tumor

The existence of a host response to tumors is established and has been strengthened by studies in mouse models and by the recent delineation of the nature of the tumor antigens involved (discussed in the preceding section of this chapter).

The rejection of chemically and virally induced tumor antigens by in vivo experiments in inbred strains of mice was presented in Figure 16-2. In addition, it is interesting to observe that the ability of the host to reject is dependent on the length of its exposure to the initial priming tumor cells. Rejection appears to represent a typical primary immune response. This is summarized in Table 16-3 and in Figure 16-7. Groups of mice were implanted with 1×10^6 tumor cells at or near the tip of the tail. At varying intervals after the initial implant, the tails were amputated. The animals were immediately challenged again with viable tumor cells. The percentage of tumor rejection is plotted against the time exposure to the initial tumor implant. It can be readily demonstrated that a great percentage, 80 to 100 percent of the animals rejected the challenge following exposure to the tumor for 6 to 16 days, respecitvely, before amputation. Further experiments using a longer period of tumor implantation and subsequent surgical amputation beyond 16 days should be of benefit for understanding of the host response in human tumors of advanced cancer patients. Deterioration of some aspects of the host immune response would be expected.

Table 16-3 : Mouse Immunological Rejection Phenomenon

Group[a]	Total No. Mice	Days Exposed to 1st EAT	No. Rejected/ Total Mice[b]
A	15	—	—
B	25	—	3/25
C	10	1	2/10
D	10	2	2/10
E	10	3	3/10
F	10	6	8/10
G	10	9	9/10
H	10	14	10/10

[a]Group A consisted of normal untreated control mice; group B represents the positive control mice given only the second EAT injection after amputation of tails.
[b]In group B spontaneous regression of 3 out of the 25 was noted.

Fig. 16-7 : Percentage (y axis) of tumor growth in mice rechallenged with the same tumor after initial implantation of the tumor in the tail. X axis shows length of exposure to the initial tumor and day of surgical removal of tail. EAT = Ehrlich ascites tumor.

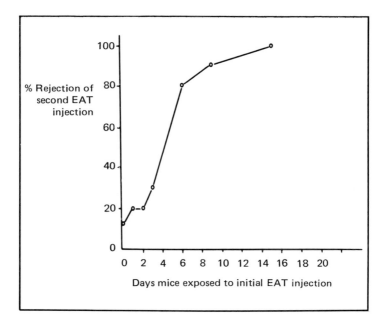

A major role as a positive defense against tumor cells has been attributed to the cell-mediated system, although it is generally accepted that the humoral immune response also participates in the host-tumor relationship. In part, evidence for the participation of the immune response in the host's defense against tumors has been demonstrated by histological observations associated with infiltration of several types of mononuclear inflammatory cells in the region of the lesion (tumors and allografts) and proximal lymph nodes. The increased cellularity includes

Fig. 16-8 : Active
adoptive immunity.
A. Significance of
the number of sensi-
tized (spleen) cells
that can be mar-
shaled against a
constant number of
tumors. B. Evi-
dence for specific
immunity in pro-
tection against
tumors.

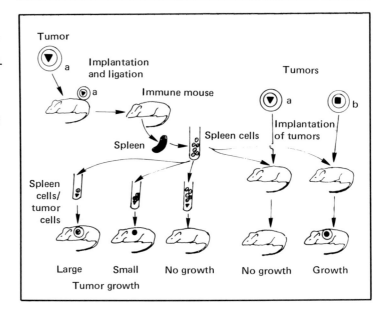

lymphocytes, monocytes, macrophages, and in some cases plasma
cells. These observations of cellular infiltration have led to the
formulation of the immunosurveillance theory. This concept was
established experimentally as follows: (1) Tumor cells were
neutralized with spleen cell suspension from an immune mouse
admixed with viable homologous tumor (tumor cells used to
immunize the animal) in vitro and subsequently transferred to
normal syngeneic strains; and (2) The immune spleen cells were
adoptively transferred to normal syngeneic mice and then challenged with the appropriate homologous tumor, resulting in
suppression of tumor growth. Thus, spleen cells from immune
animals have been shown to protect the recipient normal host
against subsequent challenge with the appropriate tumor. This
has been demonstrated with both chemically and virally induced
tumors. These types of immunity are presented schematically in
Figure 16-8A. Specificity in the rejection of the tumors has been
demonstrated. When specific antibodies to tumors have been
passively administered to a host, they have generally shown a
disappointingly small ability to inhibit the appropriate tumors.
In only a few cases have antisera from tumor-immune animals
been able to protect nonimmune animals from tumor growth.
Protection has been demonstrated mainly in certain types of
leukemia, particularly those of viral etiology, in animal models.
In most cases of solid tumors, antisera either had no effect or
enhanced tumor growth, for reasons to be discussed later. However, specific antibodies may function via killer and macrophage
cells, as will be discussed.

Cell-Mediated System in Tumor Cytotoxicity

Tremendous progress, especially in inbred mice, has been made in understanding the diverse cells involved in resistance to tumors. As discussed in Chapters 3 and 13, several cells act to protect the host against tumors: T lymphocytes; B lymphocytes; K cells; NK, or natural killer cells; and macrophages, Ia$^+$ specifically and Ia$^-$ nonspecifically.

CYTOLYTIC T LYMPHOCYTE (CTL). The cytolytic T lymphocyte (CTL), as demonstrated in the mouse, is derived from the thymus. It shows antigen-specific effector activity, is specifically regulated by the MHC, and has immunological recall. CTL consists of Thy-1$^+$, Ly-1$^+$,2$^+$,3$^+$, and Ly-2$^+$,3$^+$ markers and Fc$^+$ receptor. It has no Ia, C3, and/or immunoglobulin surface markers. The mechanism of action of CTL is a direct lysis of specific target cells during cell-to-cell contact mediated through a genetically determined receptor.

The importance of CTL in the adoptive transfer of tumor immunity and in the mediation of in vitro tumor cell destruction is well established in animal models. The CTL involved in specific tumor target rejection and that associated with CTL in alloimmune CTL (MLC reaction in humans) are indistinguishable except for the antigenic determinants to which they are directed. In adoptive immunity studies, CTL may be the important cell in protection because of its specificity to the tumor target cells and possibly because of its numbers. This same CTL population mediates the in vitro cytolysis of tumor target cells labeled with ^{51}Cr (Figure 16-9). Restimulation in vitro of the sensitized CTL with homologous tumor cells or TSA antigen increases CTL activity for destruction of target cells. In vivo secondary increases in CTL have been observed within animals restimulated with the same tumor cell or with tumor antigenic determinants. These same secondary responses have been demonstrated in alloantigenic rejections in multiple kidney transplantations. The characteristic secondary response of shorter induction period, higher peak activity, and longer duration of immunity has been demonstrated for the CTL in tumor immune response studies.

The precise nature of the tumor antigenic target determinants on the cell surface of the tumor to which CTL is directed is presently unknown. They are known to be surface determinants, however, and are most likely the antigens associated with TSA and TSTA.

In viral tumors the H-2 complex plays an important role in destruction by immune CTL. The infected viral tumor cell must possess an H-2 product (Ia) identical to that of the immune CTL cell in order for the latter to destroy the tumor cells (Figure 16-9). This H-2 restriction has been interpreted as follows: the

Fig. 16-9 : Effector lymphocyte action in cell-mediated immunity against tumors.

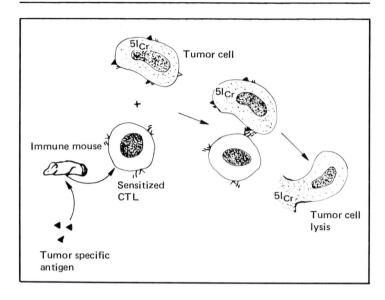

Fig. 16-9 : Effector lymphocyte action in cell-mediated immunity against tumors.

formation of a neoantigen by interaction of H-2–regulated cell surface molecules with viral proteins (or viral genomes affecting H-2 gene loci); and/or associated with a two-receptor function for the immune CTL target cell to recognize the viral infected cell, one receptor for self H-2 product (both cells must have same Ia) and another for the viral-specific antigen (see Chapter 17). Although the experimental studies have established a significant role for CTL or T cells in tumor immunity, the absolute relationship of CTL and degree of tumor immunity have not been established firmly, and studies in man are insufficient.

B LYMPHOCYTE. The characteristics of B lymphocytes have been presented in Chapters 1 and 3. The primary positive role of B lymphocytes in tumor immunity resides in the production of specific antibodies to tumor surface antigens. These antibodies can help to kill target cells in the following manner (Figure 16-10): (1) antibody + complement lyse tumor target cells; (2) antibodies act with K and macrophage cells; and (3) in animal viral tumors, antibodies neutralize infective viral antigens. The negative effect of free antibodies is achieved via their contribution through the blocking phenomenon. They can also block K cells, CTL, and ADCC macrophages to protect tumors through formation of soluble complexes with circulating tumor antigens. These mechanisms are depicted in Figure 16-15. Tumor cell killing in these studies can be demonstrated by dye exclusion or ^{51}Cr release assays.

KILLER CELLS. The K cell is characterized by (1) unknown lineage; (2) specific determination by available antibody; (3) no

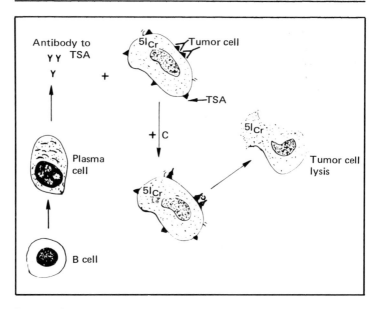

Fig. 16-10 : The B lymphocyte's role in immunity against tumor cells. Its primary function is the production of specific antibodies to the tumor and the subsequent binding of the antibodies to tumor surfaces and activation of complement. The lytic action on the tumor cell is attributed to classic pathway activation of C.

evidence of memory; (4) no evidence of Thy-1$^+$, Ia, and Ly surface markers; and (5) possession of Fc receptor—a major factor. It acts by arming with specific antibody through the Fc receptor during direct contact of the mediating antibody bound to tumor target surface antigen. The precise action in the killing processes is not known. The K cell is also called *antibody-dependent cytotoxic cell* (ADCC). Immunization is not required for expression of K cells. They are present in nonimmune animals and can be distinguished from K cells of immune animals. The cytolytic effect of K cells from immunized and nonimmunized animals depends on the antibody they attach to via their Fc receptor. Whether $K\mu$ or $K\gamma$ cells exist remains to be determined, that is, differentiation of K cells on the basis of $Fc\mu$ or $Fc\gamma$ receptors. The role of K cells in tumor rejection is presently unclear, and few data are available on the ability of these cells to affect tumor growth in vivo. The adoptive transfer of K-enriched cells by depletion of B cells and T cells from immunized animals to syngeneic normal animals afforded no protection against rechallenge with the same tumor as had been used in immunization. This suggests that a specific antibody is also required for K cell function. Correlative studies of K cell activity and tumor fate are needed to begin to establish an in vivo role for this type of host response in tumor rejection. Figure 16-11 depicts K

Fig. 16-11 : The killer cell (K cell) is an antibody-dependent cytolytic cell and requires specific antitumor antibody for the specific killing of tumor cells.

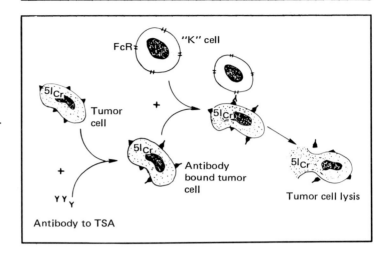

Fig. 16-11 : The killer cell (K cell) is an antibody-dependent cytolytic cell and requires specific antitumor antibody for the specific killing of tumor cells.

cell action on a tumor target cell in combination with specific antibody derived from plasma cells.

NATURAL KILLER CELL (NK CELL). The natural killer NK cell is characterized by the following: (1) its lineage is unknown; (2) its specificity may be programmed; (3) its specific memory potential is not known; (4) it is potentiated by interferon, increase in K cell number or activity, thus its activity to kill is increased by specific T cell release or nonspecific macrophage release of interferon; (5) its effector activity is regulated by MHC; it possesses no Thy-1$^+$, Ly, la, C3, or surface Ig markers; and (6) Fc receptor is present. Its mechanism of action is lysis of tumor cells by direct contact via its own receptors. The nature of these receptors is unknown, although Fc receptors have been shown on human NK cells. Free TSA or anti-TSA–TSA complexes do not affect the cytotoxic effect of the NK cell. The control of NK appears to reside in the MHC, since variation in mean levels of NK activity have been demonstrated in different strains of inbred mice.

Recent studies in man suggest that the NK cell plays a significant part in protection against viral infections, especially those due to herpes (DNA viruses). It has been shown to be low in patients with leukemia and in transplant recipients under immunosuppressive therapy who are highly vulnerable to viral infections. In this regard, studies of viral tumors in mice have shown that a correlation exists between resistance to tumor virus–induced tumors (small inoculum) and levels of natural killer cells. Thus, it has been suggested that the NK cell may be the truly relevant one in the in vivo control of tumor growth, at least of growth of tumor cells arising from viral oncogenesis.

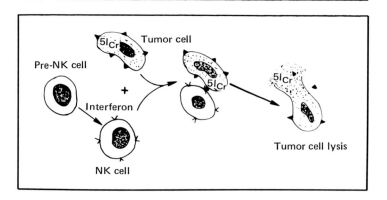

Fig. 16-12 : Natural killer cell (NK cell) attaches to tumor cell via a receptor (unknown) and kills directly (mode unknown).

This effector system, its relationship to interferon, and its possible control of tumor growth requires serious study. The action of the NK cell on tumor target cells is shown in Figure 16-12. Human NK cells possess Fc receptors, but their mode of killing is direct and does not require antibodies. In this respect NK cells differ from K cells.

Although the mechanism of destruction of tumor cells differs between K and NK cells, as shown in Figures 16-11 and 16-12, recent findings suggest that the two cell types are closely related, since Fc receptor has been shown to be present in both cells. In addition, it has been suggested that, at least in man, the K/NK cells constitute a heterogeneous group of cells of the null cell population and may be subsets of closely related cells of simlar stem cell origin. Ganglio-N-tetraosylceramide is a possible unique surface marker for murine natural killer cells. Such a marker would be useful in delineating NK and K cell relationships in man.

MACROPHAGE. Perhaps the most important nonlymphoid mononuclear effector cell in host resistance against tumors is the macrophage ($M\theta$). The significance of this cell in cellular immunity has been appreciated in bacterial infections and in delayed hypersensitivity (Chapter 13). Nevertheless, the precise role of $M\theta$ in tumor resistance is still unclear. The characteristics of macrophages are as follows: (1) they are derived from monocytic lineage; (2) they are activated directly by antigens, microorganisms, etc.; (3) they are affected by lymphokines elaborated by T cells; (4) reactivation may be more rapid due to T cell memory; (5) they lack Thy-1+ and Ly antigens and possess Fc and C3 receptors; and (6) two subsets have been demonstrated and separated into Ia+ and Ia−. Macrophage functions involve (1) phagocytosis, which is enhanced by opsonizing antibody; (2) lysis of target cells during direct contact mediated by nonspecific

436

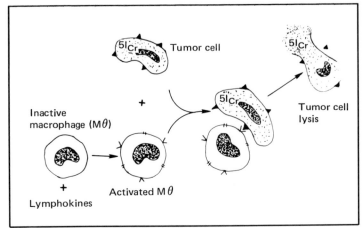

A

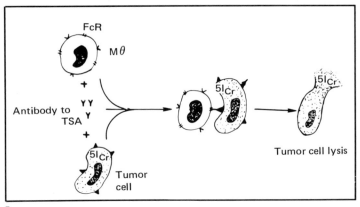

B

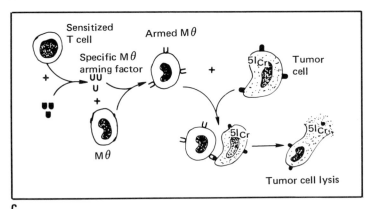

C

Fig. 16-13 : The manner in which macrophages protect against tumor growth. A. Both the Ia$^+$ and Ia$^-$ macrophages can be activated by lymphokines from sensitized T cells to attack tumor cells directly via their receptors. B. Macrophages can be attached to the Fc portion of specific tumor

membrane receptors; (3) lysis of target cells during direct contact mediated via the Fc receptor through specific antibody bound to the target cells; and (4) secretion of various monokines (see Chapter 5). In addition to those listed in Table 5-3, Chapter 5, a thymocyte differentiation factor of 40,000 daltons has also been demonstrated by Mθ. Macrophage involvement in tissue repair and reorganization is associated with production of *angiogenesis factor.*

In a functional sense, macrophages can be separated into an inactive and an active state with regard to cytotoxicity potential. Thus, the exposure of "normal" or inactive macrophages to lymphokines such as MAF or MIF, as well as to certain substances such as lipopolysaccharides or double stranded DNA that affect their membrane without a lymphoid intermediary, results in the activation of the macrophages and acquisition of an enhanced cytotoxic activity. This activated state is characterized by the following: (1) changes in morphological appearance, especially on the membrane surface; (2) more extensive spreading in the substrate, with increased vacuolation; and (3) enhanced adherence to surfaces, with increased phagocytosis and pinocytosis. Biochemical changes include (1) an increase in energy; (2) an overall increase in synthesis of the content of the lysosomal enzymes, reflected in an increase in protein synthesis and a cytocidal effect on target cells. In vivo nonspecifically activated macrophages obtained from animals stimulated by BCG or another adjuvant were found to be cytotoxic for tumor cells in vitro. This type of cytotoxicity was exercised via direct contact between the activated Mθ and tumor target cells. Macrophage-soluble factors were not involved. These Mθs differentiated between tumor cells and "normal" cells. This ability of activated Mθ to differentiate has not always been clear-cut, however. Lymphokines obtained from immune lymphocytes have been shown to be capable of activating macrophages. A schematic representation of a macrophage activated by lymphokines and its cytotoxic effect on tumor target cells is given in Figure 16-13A.

Peritoneal macrophages can become specifically cytotoxic after being armed with antibodies (anti-TSA) or with a specific arming factor (SMAF) elaborated by sensitized T lymphocytes. This is illustrated in Figures 16-13B and 16-13C. SMAF is believed to

antibodies bound to tumor cells and in this manner also destroy tumor cells. C. Macrophages may be activated by an arming factor released by sensitized T cells, which acts as a specific receptor for tumor surface antigenic determinants. The macrophage destroys the tumor cells upon contact. The mode of macrophage killing may be similar to that demonstrated for PMNs (see Chapter 8).

be smaller than the immunoglobulin and has a specific reactive site for the TSA. The T lymphocyte associated with the release of SMAF is presently undetermined. These demonstratrations were carried out in mice.

In vivo studies in syngeneic mice with passively administered anti-TSA antibodies and macrophages have suggested that macrophages armed with anti-TSA will increase significantly the protection of the animals challenged with high concentrations of tumor (from 10^4 to 10^6 tumor cells). Higher concentrations of anti-TSA or macrophages given alone did not increase resistance to the tumor. Nevertheless, in vivo evidence for the participation of macrophages in tumor rejection is meager. Attempts to block the reticuloendothelial system (RES) with agents such as carbon and silica have indeed enhanced tumor growth. However, substances of this sort may also block other functionally important cells involved in tumor resistance, and thus any interpretation should be made with reservation. Injection of BCG intralesionally results in an increase in macrophages in the region of the necrotic tumor cells, as observed microscopically or electron microcscopically. The function of macrophages under these circumstances may be one of repairing and reorganization and not necessarily of cytotoxicity. At this stage the role of macrophages in tumor rejection requires further examination. Nonetheless, macrophages undoubtedly must play a significant role, if not directly, then indirectly, via their association with T and B lymphocytes.

Recent studies (Trofather and Daniels, 1979) have suggested that PGE_2 at high levels suppresses the ADCC function of macrophages by keeping the Fc receptor from binding to the Fc portion of the antibody bound to tumor cells. PGE_2 interferes with the killing depicted in Figure 16-13B.

Immune Surveillance

The demonstration of specific immunity in experimental tumor studies has led to the expounding of the immune surveillance theory. This theory states that the immunological action associated with rejection in transplantation of normal tissue grafts evolved as a means of distinguishing "self" from "nonself". Nonself or altered self results from transformation of normal cells to malignant cells (whatever the cause) bearing TSA. The immune system maintains "surveillance" over the organism and rejects small clones of these malignant cells (altered self) as they arise, provided the malignant cells are sufficiently distinct from their normal counterpart.

This simplistic and logical concept is generally accepted, but there is considerable controversy as to whether the surveillance involves immune rejection or rejection by nonspecific nonimmunological means. Both supporting and nonsupporting data from animal experiments and observations in man have been obtained in attempts to test the validity of the immune surveillance theory. Evidence contrary to support of the theory is demonstrated by the following observations: (1) The frequency of spontaneous or induced solid tumors in animals whose immunity is suppressed by antilymphocyte serum (ALS) or in congenitally immunodeficient animals (nude mice with thymus deficiency) is no different from that in immunologically intact animals, although it would be expected that the frequency of tumors would increase in the immune-compromised groups if the theory is valid; (2) normal cells in spontaneous transformation in vitro in the absence of immunoselection have poor immunogenicity in vivo, although the theory would predict a good immunogenic tumor; (3) the ability of a small tumor inoculum to escape the immune defenses of the immunocompetent host, while a larger tumor inoculum is rejected, is contrary to the concept of immune surveillance; and (4) some patients with selective immune deficiency disease show no evidence of increase in tumors. An example is the lepromatous leprosy patients, who appear to have severely depressed T cell functions.

The evidence for the presence of immune surveillance in tumor rejection is as follows: (1) patients under immunosuppressive drug therapy, as in renal transplantation, have an increased incidence of tumors; (2) there is an increase in incidence of both lymphoreticular and solid tumors in patients with immunodeficiency diseases; and (3) stimulation of the immune response by specific tumor antigen immunization or by nonspecific methods results in a decreased incidence of tumors following infection with certain oncogenic viruses. Further support for immune surveillance comes from the notable increase in cancer incidence with aging.

It is well established that immunological competence diminishes with old age. However, exceptions to cancer in older individuals are the increased incidence of germ cell tumors of the testes seen in young men and the nodular sclerosing Hodgkin's disease seen mostly in young women. The incidence of malignancy is increased in patients with congenital immunodeficiency diseases (see Chapter 15). For example, the incidence of cancer is approximately 10 percent for patients with Wiskott-Aldrich Syndrome, common variable immunodeficiency, or ataxia telangiectasia and is about 5 percent for patients with Bruton type agammaglobulinemia or with severe combined immunodeficiency. The risk of developing cancer is greater for patients with respiratory sarcoidosis (depressed T lymphocyte function) than for the normal immunocompetent population.

Further evidence supportive of the immune surveillance concept comes from studies of patients in transplantation. These patients are exposed to chemotherapy for prolonged periods to maintain the transplanted organ and in all cases are severely immunosuppressed. For example, the incidence of lymphoma in a group of kidney transplant patients was found to be 35 percent higher than in the general population. The majority of these tumors were the reticular cell sarcomas. In the same group of patients, the risk of skin cancer was four times higher than normal, and other types of malignancy were also higher than in the normal population. The majority of immunosuppressed patients are also more susceptible to infections with herpes viruses. In this regard, the higher incidence of cervical carcinomas in females with kidney transplants is of interest, since herpes type 2 virus has been associated with cervical carcinoma.

Although these findings tend to support the immunosurveillance theory, it is of interest to observe the high incidence of lymphoreticular malignancy in immunodeficient and iatrogenically immunosuppressed patients. This is especially true of patients defective in the T cell system. This aspect is not compatible with the immune surveillance concept, since the theory states that spontaneous tumors (all kinds) that appear in the body should be rejected by the immune system. The increased incidence in the lymphoreticular type of tumor may be associated with an inability of the regulatory cells (suppressor regulators) of the lymphoid system to control or terminate the proliferation of the lymphoid cells. It is suggested also that patients with suppressed T cell function are more susceptible to virus infections and virally related tumors (leukemias, sarcomas, and lymphomas).

The relevance of the MHC products (immune surveillance) with respect to recognition of self and nonself relative to virus infections is of significance, although this relationship may have no importance with respect to tumor transformation unless the tumor is of viral origin.

Mechanism of Tumor Escape and Immunological Enhancement

It remains an enigma how a small number of tumor cells circumvent the myriad of potential defense mechanisms at the disposal of the host, proliferate, and eventually cause the demise of the host. Numerous factors appear to facilitate the escape of tumors from the host immune surveillance mechanism. Several of these mechanisms have been documented, but undoubtedly others are still undetermined. It has been suggested that tumors generally lack TAAs recognizable by the host's immune response as foreign. A few examples of tumors that appear to meet this criterion have been reported. Inability to detect the immune response in the host may, however, be due to the inability of the methods used to detect a weak response. The vast majority of all tumors tested in active immunizations elicit some responses, however, although often weak. Animals bearing tumors almost always demonstrate some reactivity to their tumors. Thus an undetectable immune response cannot explain a successful tumor growth in most situations. Under certain circumstances, however, due to a lack of certain Ir genes, the animal may be incapable of responding to the TAA. A state of tolerance to the TAA is thus suggested. Any mechanism of tumor escape attributable to lack of recognizable TAA is at best weak, since essentially all tumors examined can be shown to be immunogenic to some degree.

A second possibility of tumor escape from the host defense mechanism is that the maximum immune response elicited by the host may be quantitatively insufficient to cope with the tumor growth rate. It is assumed in this case that weakly immunogenic tumors escape destruction by producing new cells faster than these new cells can be killed by the limited number of immune effector cells that respond to the weakly immunogenic TAA. In this situation, the tumor burden overrides the antitumor effectors quantitatively. Evidence for this concept comes from experiments in the ability of actively immunized or adoptively immunized animals to resist graded doses of viable tumor cells. Thus, in an actively immunized animal, a larger tumor burden is required for tumor growth. The evidence for this mechanism of tumor escape is fair. A schematic representation of this concept is shown in Figure 16-14.

A third possible mechanism of tumor escape is through an increase in specific T suppressor cells and release of T suppressor factors (TsF, Chapter 5). Evidence for this mode of suppression of the immune response to tumor cells is good and has been demonstrated in several model systems both in vivo and in vitro. These T suppressor cells appear to inhibit the specific antitumor CTL effector cells, and they also have a suppressive effect on the T helper cells, which are necessary for the stimulation of the specific antitumor antibodies required by K cells or macrophages. These two cells destroy target cells via the ADCC mechanism. T suppressor effect has been demonstrated by transfer of T cells from mice bearing actively grown tumors into normal mice, the growth of the freshly implanted tumor cells was enhanced. These suppressor T cells have been shown to bear I-J antigens and Ly-2^+,3^+ markers on their membranes. Reversal of the T suppressive effect can be demonstrated by treatment of the animals with xenogeneic anti-T lymphocytes, anti-I-J, or anti-Ly-2^+,3^+ antibodies. In enhancement of tumor growth T

Fig. 16-14 : Sensitized lymphocyte expansion as compared with tumor expansion. Presumably tumor expansion is quantitatively greater than lymphocyte expansion and thus a certain number of tumor cells escape surveillance.

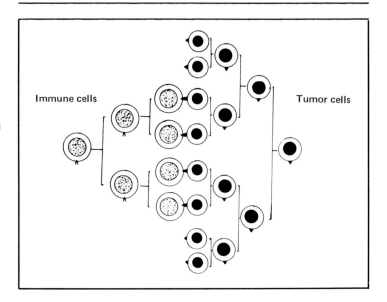

Immune cells

Tumor cells

T suppressor cells act by suppressing the immune response through their specific soluble factor, TsF. The FcγR T cell has been implicated as the T suppressor cell in man.

A fourth possibility for tumor escape from host surveillance is through the modulation of the tumor surface (deletion, rearrangement, inversion, etc.) and/or secretion of inhibiting substances such as prostaglandins. The latter in high concentrations have been demonstrated to suppress immune responses in general as well as the ADCC function of K cells. Evidence supporting this mechanism of escape is fair and is based on morphological observations and some in vitro experiments.

Finally, the most widely examined mechanism and one with good supporting evidence from experimental studies in animals and findings in man is the blocking phenomenon attributed to serum factor(s). These specific factors are free specific antitumor antibody and tumor-associated antigen and the complexes formed by their interactions in vivo. Thus, blocking and enhancement of tumor growth may occur through the following mechanisms, categorized as afferent, efferent, and central inhibitions depending on the site of blockage of the immune system.

1. *Efferent blockade.* Free soluble tumor antigens or that portion of the immune complex that binds to the receptors on the effector CTL can mask the receptor sites on the viable CTL cells, preventing the recognition of the viable tumor cells by the effector CTL cells (Figure 16-15B).

2. *Afferent blockade.* Tumor sites are masked by the free antibody and/or antibody portion of the complexes and thus mask

Fig. 16–15 : The mode by which tumor enhancement occurs. A. Afferent blocking of the CTL cells due to excess soluble tumor antigens and tumor-antitumor complexes that attach to the CTL receptors. B. Efferent blocking due to excess antibody and antitumor-tumor complexes that attach to the tumor surfaces and protect tumors against the CTL. In both cases the tumor escapes destruction and proliferates.

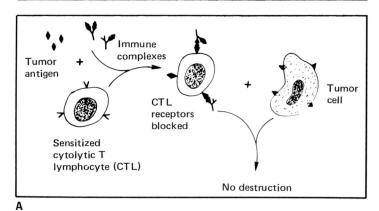

A

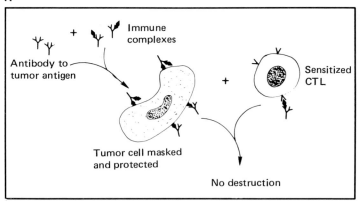

B

the antigenic determinants of the viable tumor cells against the effector CTL receptors (Figure 16-15A).

3. *Central blockade.* Tolerogenic soluble serum factors and/or suppressor cells could induce a state of tolerance and thus prevent an immune response that could be mounted against the tumor by the host.

Afferent blockade or masking is an important mechanism for the enhancement of tumor growth in vivo. Enhancement can be achieved with a single injection passively of an antitumor antibody. The binding of the antibody to tumor is transient but allows sufficient time for the tumor burden in the host to increase and overcome the elicited immune response. Nevertheless, the masking phenomenon also observed in human tumors, especially in neuroblastoma, for the enhancement of tumor growth is difficult to explain with the observation that very small quantities of antiserum are sufficient to induce enhancement. The more plausible explanation for tumor enhancement appears to be that of the efferent and control blockade discussed above.

Another factor to be considered is that normal donor allogeneic spleen cell transplants induce angiogenesis in normal recipients.

In contrast, a normal allogeneic spleen transplant to a tumor-bearing recipient interferes with angiogenesis in the recipient. Tumor survival may be associated with an ability to interfere with immune effector cells, as demonstrated by inhibition of angiogenesis.

Finally, to attribute tumor escape from surveillance to a single system of the multifaceted complex interacting host response would be unwarranted, since all the factors discussed here may play a part in the tumor escape phenomenon. Obviously some systems may play a greater role than others.

Immunological Evaluation

Several immunological procedures have been established as a supplement for the diagnosis of cancer in patients. Obviously the simplest and most applicable way is to examine the serum for the presence of tumor-associated antigens. Several such assays have been developed, although their usefulness and specificity remain to be evaluated.

Assays for Tumor-Associated Antigens

TAAs may be found in higher concentrations in tumor cells than in their normal counterparts and thus may also be found in higher quantities in plasma. Ideally, to be of practical value in immunodiagnosis, the tumor antigens should be common to a variety of tumors, particularly those of similar tissue origin, and appear in body fluids as long as the tumor persists. The common antigens of tumors that have been identified and used in immunodiagnosis are classified as follows: (1) *virus-induced or associated antigens* of tumors induced by the same virus, which generally share all or some of the same common TAAs, even when the tumors differ in morphology; (2) *fetal antigens* of tumors, which are present in normal fetal cells and in a variety of tumors, regardless of etiology. Fetal antigens (carcinofetal proteins) are found in high levels in body fluids of patients with persistent tumors; and (3) *tissue antigens* of normal cells, which may be expressed in larger amounts in tumor cells. Some of these may be specific for the organ from which the tumor is derived. These include HLA, ABO, enzymes, and hormones, which may be increased in cancer patients.

The circulating TAAs useful for immunological evaluation in cancer have been summarized in Tables 16-1 and 16-2. These antigens are generally TAPSA and include the oncofetal proteins such as CEA, α_1FP, isomeric enzymes, and hormones. A potentially useful assay would have features of high *specificity* with high *sensitivity*. Presently the immunological assays used for tumor markers are useful for the management of patients known to have tumors. These tests have not proved useful for the early detection of tumors in patients prior to metastatic lesions.

A carcinoembryonic antigen, a glycoprotein of endodermal cell origin of colorectal carcinomas, did not fulfill its initial expectation of a specific antigen and thus lost its diagnostic value. Nonetheless, CEA radio immunoassay is routinely used for its value in the management and prognosis of colorectal and other gastrointestinal tract carcinomas. The weakness of CEA assay lies in its high false positives in benign gastrointestinal tract and other noncancerous diseases. Furthermore, patients with *localized* gastrointestinal tract carcinomas tend to have low values of CEA in their plasma. Nevertheless, the discovery of CEA has initiated further impetus for search of specific tumor antigens. Several isomeric forms of CEA have been found (Table 16-1), and an RIA procedure for CEA-S has been developed (Edgington, et al, 1975). This assay has detected a higher proportion of patients with gastrointestinal tract carcinomas with a lower incidence of false positives in noncancer patients and smokers.

Another RIA for the detection of carcinofetal protein (α_1 FP), has been made available for use in the differential diagnosis and monitoring of patients with hepatoma, choriocarcinoma, and testicular tumors. This assay for α_1 FP in amniotic fluid has also been useful for detection of neural tube defects of the fetus in pregnancy at about 20 weeks' gestation. Recently, a glycoprotein tumor antigen from colonic carcinoma called Tennessee antigen (TennaGen) has been used in the hemagglutination inhibition assay. This assay has demonstrated specificity similar to that reported for CEA-S, although no immunological cross-reactivity has been shown with CEA. Thus far this glycoprotein has not been found in fetal tissue (see Table 16-1).

Hormones have also been found to be useful tumor markers. For example, human chorionic gonadotropin (HCG) and human placental lactogen (HPL) may be ectopically produced by a small proportion of the tumors arising in regions outside the reproductive tract. HCG has been useful for the assessment of choriocarcinoma and certain testicular tumors known to produce HCG. A highly specific radio immunoassay has been developed for the assessment of βhCG. In this procedure the antibody to β-polypeptide of the HCG molecule has been used, since HCG has been shown to cross-react strongly with the luteinizing hormone (LH). Pro-ACTH (adrenocorticotropic hormone) may be useful in the diagnosis of lung cancer, since a high percentage of lung cancer patients have elevated ACTH. Similarly, abnormal levels of thyrocalcitonin have been demonstrated in lung cancer patients.

Elevated enzymes demonstrated in cancer patients include acid phosphatase in plasma of prostatic cancers and alkaline phosphatase in leukemias.

The immune systems to be examined for the evaluation of immunocompetency of individuals and of patients with cancer and other diseases have been described in Chapter 6, Table 6-1. In patients with malignancies, a correlation exists between general immunocompetence and level of specific tumor immunity and extent of disease and prognosis. Changes in the clinical status of cancer patients tend to parallel the changes in general immunocompetence. That is, cancer patients with poor, depressed immune status tend to have a poor prognosis. Immunocompetence also declines with progression of the tumor, with the patients becoming more immunodeficient in several areas of function. These have been observed in Hodgkin's disease, leukemia, lymphoma, and solid epithelial tumors such as carcinomas of the breast, lung, colon, head, and neck. In Hodgkin's disease there is often a depressed cell-mediated immunity, which appears to be brought about by altered macrophages that produce high levels of prostaglandin E_2. The latter compound, at high levels, has shown suppression of T cell responses to PHA. Removal of the macrophages restores the mitogenic response of the T cells to PHA in patients with Hodgkin's disease. Patients with chronic lymphocytic leukemia have shown impairment of the humoral antibody responses with milder suppression of the cell-mediated responses. In general, cell-mediated immunity and inflammation may be markedly suppressed in patients with solid tumors, while antibody responses may be mildly impaired.

Impaired immune functions in cancer patients are reflected by (1) depressed delayed hypersensitivity responses to tumor antigens, DNCB, PPD, and other skin test antigens; (2) low levels of T and B lymphocytes in the peripheral blood; (3) decreased lymphocyte blastogenic responses; (4) changes in serum immunoglobulins and complement levels; (5) generally depressed primary and secondary antibody responses; (6) suppressed specific antitumor levels; and (7) decrease in cytotoxic T lymphocytes as examined by in vitro procedures.

The immune responses to specific TAAs have been examined in man. Partially purified and purified extracts of autochthonous tumors have been examined by a delayed type hypersensitivity skin test similar to that employed for PPD and coccidioidin. Routine hypersensitivity skin test reactions have been examined for leukemia, colon cancer, breast carcinoma, lung carcinoma, and cancer of the cervix. Skin test reactivity to leukemia-associated antigens has been shown to have a correlation with the clinical status of the patient. In general, delayed hypersensitivity skin tests to specific tumor-associated antigens reflect the clinical condition of the patients. Skin tests with specific TAAs have been useful for monitoring of the response to therapy. The potential use of skin testing as used in tuberculosis detection for cancer screening and diagnosis is limited, due to the hazards of inoculation of allogeneic specific tumor antigens into normal healthy individuals.

Assessment of the levels of activity of cytotoxic T lymphocytes may have a possible application in immunodiagnosis. Differentiation of sensitized and nonsensitized T lymphocytes can be performed in vitro. For example, T lymphocytes removed from patients with cancer and mixed with viable tumor cells in vitro would demonstrate cytolysis or cytostasis of the tumor cell, while T lymphocytes from a normal nonsensitized individual under similar condition would exhibit growth of the tumor cells.

Leukocyte migration inhibition assay has been carried out on patients' cells mixed with extracts of tumor tissues. Such examinations have been successful for breast cancer, malignant melanoma, lymphoma, and leukemia patients.

Potential fruitful approaches are practical tests for the detection of specific antibodies to specific tumor-associated antigens. In this regard, antibodies to common tumor antigens in melanoma and osteosarcoma have been described. However, the specificity of this reaction requires further study. If specificity exists, a highly sensitive and specific immunological procedure can be developed for the early diagnosis of cancer.

Immunotherapy

Any immunotherapeutic approaches utilizing antigens must take into consideration the immunocompetent status of the patient. It is necessary to examine all the parameters of the patient's immune system: the status of the T and B cells, including their subsets, such as T helper and T suppressor levels; the levels of NK, K, and $M\theta$ and their functions; and the quality and quantity of the levels of the important humoral factors, such as complement, immunoglobulins, tumor-associated antigens (CEA, α_1 FP, enzymes), acute phase proteins, and prostaglandins.

Current methods used in specific immunotherapy with tumor antigens present many problems. The major drawback appears to be a lack of isolation of highly purified specific tumor antigen (TSA) or TSTA. The human tumor antigens thus far isolated for immunotherapy have not been defined with regard to (1) their origin (nuclear, cytoplasmic, or surface membrane); (2) their immunogenicity; (3) their cross-reactivity with normal tissues; and (4) their interaction with the host immune surveillance system.

The success of immunotherapy obviously will depend on the immune competency of the patient. If a deficiency of a key immune cell is observed, antigen administration will be of no value. Immunotherapy purports to enhance the immune system to combat and contain the growth of cancer cells by (1) increasing cell-mediated immunity; (2) augmenting antibody immunity; and (3) stimulating the general host defense with nonspecific reagents (adjuvant).

Immunorestoration

Nonspecific and specific immunorestorations have been attempted to increase the cell-mediated immune response. Nonspecific immunopotentiating drugs (see Chapter 6) such as levamisole have been administered to cancer patients with depressed T lymphocyte functions. Levamisole acts through secondary messengers such as the cyclic nucleotides or prostaglandins on lymphocytes and in this manner may help to restore cell-mediated responsiveness in the anergic host. The possible mechanism of levamisole action has been presented in Chapter 6.

Specific immunorestoration has been attempted with the administration of xenogeneic thymic hormones into immunodeficient and immunosuppressed patients in order to increase the maturation and/or function of the circulating lymphocytes. Thymosin administration in vivo or treatment in vitro has demonstrated an increase in the number of E-rosette T cells. The probability that thymic factors will augment the cell-mediated response of cancer patients has been suggested by the enhancement of T cell functions by thymosin in in vitro studies. Thymosin in conjunction with Ia$^+$ macrophages has been implicated in the maturation of thymocytes to functional T lymphocytes. A *thymocyte-stimulating differentiation factor* (TSDF) has been shown to be elaborated by Ia$^+$ macrophages. Preliminary in vivo results have demonstrated some clinical improvement in cancer patients given thymosin. However, further studies are necessary for establishment of its true therapeutic benefits.

Active Immunotherapy

NONSPECIFIC THERAPY. This mode of therapy involves the use of adjuvants such as BCG and *Corynebacterium parvum.* These adjuvants increase nonspecifically the general immunocompetence of the host through augmentation of the cell-mediated and humoral responses. Adjuvants have demonstrated one or more of the following immunological effects: (1) increase in general immunocompetency, which includes the cell-mediated and humoral systems; (2) activation of macrophages and stimulation with increase of the T lymphocyte population; and (3) general enhancement of the reticuloendothelial system. Immunoadjuvant therapy has been used in the therapy of patients with various tumors, including melanoma, leukemia, and colorectal, lung, and breast carcinomas, with variable success.

SPECIFIC THERAPY. Specific therapy includes the use of purified specific tumor-associated antigens or intact killed tumor cells for immunization. The antigens may first be modified by viral or chemical means to increase their immunogenicity and hence, presumably, to enhance specific cell-mediated and humoral immunity. Specific stimulation of immunity has been attempted by several methods:

1. Unmodified killed allogeneic cancer cells or cell membrane extracts have been used as immunogens. For example, allogeneic leukemia cells have been used for immunotherapy in leukemic patients. Leukemic cells were x-irradiated prior to immunization to inhibit cell division. These cells were injected periodically into recipients in remission from acute lymphocytic leukemia induced by chemotherapy. BCG was administered concurrently with the x-irradiated leukemic cells. This combined immunotherapy, specific and nonspecific, with the leukemic cells, had a synergistic effect, since either modality alone was ineffective.

2. Detection by the host of a specific functional residue from the tumor membrane surface may contribute to the enhancement of immunogenicity of the tumor cells. In experimental studies, tumor cells treated with neuraminidase, an enzyme that removes sialic acid residues from membrane surfaces, have shown increased immunogenicity. Animals immunized with tumors treated with neuraminidase have demonstrated a marked increase in survival and protection when challenged with the allogeneic viable tumor. However, the efficacy of treatment of patients with autologous or allogeneic tumors subjected to neuraminidase hydrolysis has not been established.

3. Another way to enhance the immunogenicity of tumor cells is to alter their membrane surface by infection with virus. The infected tumor cells may produce strong immunogenic viral tumor antigens on their surface and thus enhance the immunogenicity of the weak tumor-specific antigens. Immunization with tumors infected with virus results in immune responses directed to viral antigens as well as to the tumor-specific antigens. Rejection of challenged uninfected tumor cells has been demonstrated in animals immunized with the viral infected tumors. This approach has been used in humans with malignancy, but on a limited scale. When patients with osteogenic sarcoma were given injections of influenza virus–infected autologous or allogeneic osteogenic tumor cells, no therapeutic benefits were seen.

4. Chemically modified membranes on tumor cells can enhance the immunogenicity of the tumor cells. This has been demonstrated in experimental models by using haptens such as 2,4-dinitrophenol or NIP (3-iodo-4-hydroxy-5-nitrophenyl acetic

acid). Hapten-modified tumor membrane antigens have been shown to stimulate cell-mediated cytotoxicity in experimental studies.

This kind of therapy uses the transfer of viable sensitized cells or cell products from a specifically immunocompetent donor to a tumor-bearing recipient. The therapy may involve the transfer of lymphocytes, transfer factors, and immune RNA extracted from sensitized lymphocytes. Interferon produced in vitro may also be transferred. This would be of significance in the enhancement of natural killer cells, especially for viral infections and for possible viral tumors.

1. *Transfusion of normal T lymphocytes.* The therapeutic infusion of normal T lymphocytes into cancer patients with depressed primary or secondary T cell function will often initiate or augment an antitumor response. In T lymphocyte transplantation, the donor and recipient should be closely matched for HLA compatibility (see Chapter 12). This appears to be a major obstacle to adoptive immunotherapy. HLA incompatibility generally results in GVH reactions in the immunosuppressed recipient.

2. *Transfusion of sensitized T lymphocytes.* The transplantation of allogeneic sensitized T lymphocytes in the form of total leukocyte transfusion was one of the first methods used in adoptive immunotherapy in cancer patients. Donors and recipients are matched for the ABO blood group and HLA antigens. This mode of therapy has been partially successful in humans. It has also been used for control of infections in highly immune-suppressed patients.

3. *Treatment with cellular components and elaborated factor(s).*
   a. *Transfer factor* has been used to activate the immune response in cancer and other immune-deficient patients. This dialyzable low molecular weight (see Chapter 3) compound derived from sensitized lymphocytes appears to program recipients' lymphocytes to certain specific cellular immune functions, for example, to T cell–mediated cytotoxicity (a T cytotoxic effector cell). Transfer factor therapy has been used in the treatment of malignant melanomas. It has prolonged remission and thus delays the clinical recurrence of the disease.
   b. *Immune RNA* is an extract from sensitized immune lymphocytes. Experimental observations have suggested that the injection of immune RNA inhibits tumor growth most effectively if the extract is administered when the tumor mass is small and in the early stages of proliferation. As a clinical treatment of cancer patients, this type of immuno-

therapy is still in its infancy. The mode of immune RNA action and its beneficial effects in humans have yet to be examined.

c. *Interferon.* The therapeutic use of interferon for cancer patients is presently nil due to the limited supply of the substance. In experimental models, interferon has shown great promise in control of virus infections through its stimulatory action on specific and nonspecific immune cells. For further discussion of interferon see Chapter 3.

Passive Immunotherapy

Passive immunotherapy is the transfer of cytotoxic antitumor antibodies from an immune donor to a recipient with a malignant tumor. Tumor growth has been controlled successfully with tumor-specific antibodies in experimental animals. In humans this approach has not been adequately examined because of the potential danger from the enhancing effect (blocking phenomenon). However, the limited reported studies in man have been successful. An added approach to this type of immunotherapy would be to use the passively administered allogeneic tumor-specific antibodies as carriers for an effective chemotherapeutic agent such as adriamycin or bleomycin.

Local Immunotherapy

Active nonspecific or adoptive immunotherapeutic agents can be injected directly into a tumor site in order to induce local killing and presumably to enhance the specific tumor immunity of the host's immune system. This type of approach is especially applicable to easily accessible tumors such as skin cancers. BCG, for example, has been injected directly into melanoma of the skin.

Combinations of the various models of immunotherapy discussed in the preceding paragraphs have been used in the treatment of cancer patients, and results have been variable. In general, immunotherapy by itself has not been very effective but has had some benefit when administered in conjunction with other therapeutic modalities (x-irradiation, chemotherapy, or surgery).

Summary

This chapter discusses various aspects of the immune response of host to malignant tumor cells. Information gleaned from experimental animals and from human studies is presented.

1. Tumor-associated antigens include all the tumor antigens and can further be categorized specifically as (a) *tumor specific antigens* (TSA), which are unique to tumor cells and not present in normal cells; (b) *tumor specific transplantation antigens* (TSTA) which specify the membrane antigens of tumors and are recognized by rejection of the tumor within a syngeneic or autochthonous host; and (c) *tumor-associated*

phase-specific antigens (TAPSA), generally referred to as carcinofetal or fetal proteins, which are normal embryonic antigens reexpressed in many tumor cells in large quantities, in contrast to their very low levels in normal adult tissues.

2. Antigenic variation in the tumor cell surface may be associated with deletion of determinants and rearrangement of surface layers.

3. Chemically induced tumors have unrelated antigenic determinants even within the same syngeneic strains, while viral-induced tumors have similar or related antigenic determinants, even if growing in different species of animals. These findings, however, are not absolute and depend on the sensitivity of the immunological procedures.

4. Both specific and nonspecific host immune responses have been established in patients with cancer. Experimental mouse models have strongly established the existence of the immune response, but extrapolation of these models to human studies has not been as successful. Nevertheless, five major cells and humoral factors and perhaps some undetermined factor(s) appear to play major roles in the host defense against malignant cells. The cells examined include (1) T lymphocytes, (2) B lymphocytes, (3) macrophages (monocytes), (4) killer cells, and (5) natural killer cells. The polymorphonuclear granulocytes may also contribute to the defense against tumors, but their precise role is undetermined. The humoral factors include (1) nonspecific acute phase proteins (C-reactive protein, fibrin products, etc.) and tumor antigens and (2) specific antibodies and antigen-antibody complexes. The mechanism of killing by specific and nonspecific cells may be via the free radical generation, the myeloperoxidase-H_2O_2-halide mechanism, enzymatic degradation of tumor cells, and/or complement activation and lysis.

5. The immune surveillance theory states that the immunological action associated with the rejection in transplantation of normal tissue grafts evolved as a means of distinguishing *self* from *nonself*. The immune system maintains surveillance over alteration of self cells to nonself cells and causes the destruction of the latter. Both experimental data and observations in humans suggest the presence of the surveillance mechanism, but the host system involved in the immune surveillance function is not as simple as originally conceived.

6. Another intriguing facet of tumor immunology involves the ability of the tumor to escape the surveillance mechanism and to use the immune system itself to proliferate (enhancement phenomenon). Possible reasons for the ability of tumors to

escape the host defense mechanism can be summarized as follows: (1) Lack of recognizable tumor-associated antigens (weak immunogenic antigens). This suggestion is weak, since all tumors have shown immunogenicity under appropriate conditions. (2) A maximal immune response that is insufficient quantitatively to cope with the tumor growth rate. This suggestion is considered fair. (3) Inhibition of the host responses by increase in T suppressor cell function and humoral factor(s). Evidence for this concept is good. (4) Inhibition of the afferent or efferent arms of the host-tumor response by blocking antibodies and antibody-antigen complexes. Evidence for this concept is also good. (5) Protection of the tumor due to modulation of the malignant cell surface, resulting in secretion of inhibitory factor (a macrophage inhibitory factor elaborated by tumors has been demonstrated). This concept is fair to good, with further findings of antihost factors or increases in ectopic hormones to alter the normal metabolic processes of the host. It is most likely that a tumor escapes rejection because of these factors working simultaneously.

7. Immunological evaluation of cancer patients involves examination of the patient's immune profile by established laboratory procedures (see Chapter 6) and assessment of tumor-associated antigens in plasma. The carcinoembryonic antigens, CEA and CEA-S and α_1-fetoprotein assessment have proven useful in management in some patients.

8. Both specific and nonspecific immunotherapy studies involving whole tumor cells or chemically altered cells have been used in limited studies in humans. To date, BCG and/or adjuvant studies have been disappointing, although some patients have survived longer with these types of therapy. Specific immunotherapy with cells has been controversial, and again studies are limited. Passive immunotherapy is again being considered, with use of monospecific antibodies with cytotoxic properties. Nevertheless, this approach is limited by the lack of a universal tumor-specific antigen unique to malignant cells. Transfer factor and immune RNA have been examined. The limited studies have not shown any striking breakthroughs. The use of interferon awaits its availability and may be restricted to viral infections and/or tumors.

Bibliography and Selected Reading

General

Benacerraf, B., and Unanue, E. R. (Eds.). *Textbook of Immunology.* Baltimore: Williams & Wilkins, 1979.

Cinader, B. (Ed.). *Immunology of Receptors.* New York: Dekker, 1977.

Fishman, W. H., and Sell, S. (Eds.). *Onco-Development Gene Expression.* New York: Academic, 1976.

Green, I., Cohen, S. and McCluskey, R. T. (Eds.). *Mechanisms of Tumor Immunity.* New York: Wiley, 1977.

Harris, J., and Copeland, D. Impaired immunoresponsiveness in tumor patients. *Ann. N. Y. Acad. Sci.* 230:56–85, 1974.

Rosenthal, A. S. (Ed.). *Immune Recognition: Proceedings of the 9th Leukocyte Culture Conference.* New York: Academic, 1975.

Weisman, G., and Clairborne, R. (Eds.). *Cell Membranes, Biochemistry, Cell Biology and Pathology.* New York: H. P. Publishing, 1975.

Tumor-Associated Antigens

Becker, F. F., and Sell, S. Early elevation of α_1-fetoprotein in N-2-fluorenylacetamide hepatocarcinogenesis. *Cancer Res.* 34:2489–2494, 1974.

Bhattacharya, M., Barlow, J. J., Chu, T. M., and Pinea, M. S. Tumor associated antigen(s) from granulosa cell carcinomas of the ovary. *Cancer Res.* 34:818–822, 1974.

Burtin, P. Carcino-Embryonic Antigens. In L. Brent and J. Holbrow (Eds.). *Progress in Immunology II,* Vol. 3, Amsterdam: North-Holland, 1974.

Davidson, I., and Ni, L. Y. Loss of A, B, and H in carcinoma of the lung. *Am. J. Pathol.* 57:307–334, 1969.

Gallo, R. C., Yang, S. S., and Ting, R. C. RNA dependent DNA polymerase of human acute leukemic cell. *Nature* 228:927–929, 1970.

Herbeman, R. B. Immunogenicity of tumor antigens. *Biochem. Biophys. Acta* 473:93–119, 1977.

Joung, J. I., Hsu, R., Rochman, H., and Cifonelli, J. A. The isolation and characterization of carcinoembryonic antigen: An improved method for large scale purification. *Prep. Biochem.* 5: 359–374, 1975.

Nicolson, G. L., and Poste, G. The cancer call: Dynamic aspects and modifications in cell-surface organization. Part I. *N. Engl. J. Med.* 295: 197–203, 1976.

Saeed, S. M., and Fine, G. Excessive serum levels of A and H substances in a patient with gastric carcinoma. *Transfusion* 8:179–183, 1968.

Slayter, H. S., and Coligan, J. E. Characterization of carcinoembryonic antigen fractionated by Concanavalin A chromatography. *Cancer Res.* 36:1696–1704, 1976.

Steplewski, Z., Koprowski, H., Herlyn, M., and Herlyn, D. Human tumor antigens detected by monoclonal antibodies. *Proc. Am. Assoc. Cancer Res.* 20:283, 1979.

Immune Response to Tumor

Jensen, P. J., and Korn, H. S. Heterogeneity within the population of NK and K cells. *J. Immunol.* 124:315–398, 1980.

Haller, O., Hansen, M., Kiessling, R., and Wigzell, H. Role of non-conventional natural killer cells in resistance against syngeneic tumor cells in vivo. *Nature* (London) 270:609–611, 1977.

Herbeman, R. B. Cell-mediated immunity to tumor cells. *Adv. Cancer Res.* 19:207–263, 1974.

Hellström, K. E., and Hellström, I. The Role of Cell-Mediated Immunity in Control and Growth of Tumors. In F. H. Bach and R. A. Good (Eds.), *Clinical Immunobiology,* Vol. 2. New York: Academic, 1974. Pp. 233–264.

Klein, E., and Sjorgren, H. O. Humoral and cellular factors in homograft and isograft immunity against sarcoma cells. *Cancer Res.* 20:452–461, 1960.

Old, L. J., Benacerraf, B., Clarke, D. A., Carswell, E. A., and Stockert, E. The role of the reticuloendothelial system in the host reaction to neoplasia. *Cancer Res.* 21:1281–1300, 1961.

Poplack, D. G., Bonnard, G. D., Holiman, B. J., and Blaese, R. M. Monocyte-mediated antibody-dependent cellular cytotoxicity: A clinical test of monocyte function. *Blood* 48:809–816, 1976.

Santoli, D., Trinchieri, G., and Koprowski, H. Cell-mediated cytotoxicity against virus-infected target cells in humans. II. Interferon induction and activation of natural killer cells. *J. Immunol.* 121:532–538, 1978.

Unanue, E. R. The macrophage as a regulator of lymphocyte function. *Hosp. Pract.* 14:61–74, 1979.

Young, W. W., Jr., Hakamori, S., Durdils, J. M., and Henney, C. S. Identification of ganglio-N-tetraosylceramide as a new cell surface marker for murine natural killer cells. *J. Immunol.* 124:199–201, 1980.

Immune Surveillance

Burnet, F. M. *Immunological Surveillance.* Oxford: Pergamon, 1970.

Burnet, F. M. The concept of immunological surveillance. *Prog. Exp. Tumor Res.* 13:1–27, 1970.

Kurpke, M. L., and Borsos, T. Immune surveillance revisited. *J. Natl. Cancer Inst.* 52:1393–1395, 1974.

Prehn, R. T. Immunological Surveillance: Pro and Con. In F. H. Bach and R. A. Good (Eds.), *Clinical Immunobiology,* Vol. 2. New York: Academic, 1974. Pp. 191–204.

Mechanism of Tumor Escape and Immunological

Hellström, K. E., and Hellström, I. Lymphocyte-mediated cytotoxicity and blocking serum activity to tumor antigens. *Adv. Immunol.* 18:209–277, 1974.

Kamo, I., and Friedman, H. Immunosuppression and the role of suppressive factors in cancer. *Adv. Cancer Res.* 25:271–324, 1977.

Kersey, J. H., Spector, B. D., and Good, R. A. Primary Immunodeficiency and Malignancy. In D. Bergsma, R. A. Good, J. Finstand, and N. W. Paul (Eds.), *Immunodeficiency in Man and Animals.* Sunderland, Mass.: Sinauer, 1975. Pp. 289–298.

Prehn, R. T., and Lappe, M. A. An immunostimulation theory of tumor development. *Transplant. Rev.* 7:26–54, 1971.

Sidky, Y. A., and Auerbach, R. Lymphocyte-induced angiogenesis in tumor bearing mice. *Science* 192:1237–1238, 1976.

Stutman, O. Immunodepression and malignancy. *Adv. Cancer Res.* 22:261–422, 1975.

Trofather, K. F., Jr., and Daniels, C. A. Interaction of human cells with prostaglandins and cyclic AMP modulators. I. Effects on complement-mediated lysis and antibody dependent cell-mediated cytolysis of Herpes simplex virus-infected human fibroblasts. *J. Immunol.* 122:1363–1370, 1979.

Whitehead, J. S., and Kim, Y. S. An inhibitor of lymphocyte proliferation produced by a human colonic adenocarcinoma cell line in culture. *Cancer Res.* 40:29–35, 1980.

Immunological Evaluation

Edgington, T. S., Astarita, R. W., and Plow, E. F. Association of an isomeric species of carcinoembryonic antigen with neoplasia of the gastrointestinal tract. *N. Engl. J. Med.* 293:103–107, 1975.

Kirkpatrick, A., Wepsic, H. T., and Nakamura, R. M. Comparison of double-antibody radioimmunoassay with Farr-technique radioimmunoassay and coupled antibody enzyme immunoassay for α-fetoprotein. *Clin. Chem* 23:50–59, 1977.

Krupey, J., Gold, P., and Freedman, S. O. Physiochemical studies of carcinoembryonic antigens of the human digestive system. *J. Exp. Med.* 128:387–398, 1968.

Potter, T. P., Jr., and Jordan, T. Evaluation of a hemagglutination-inhibition assay for carcinoembryonic antigen. *Am. J. Clin. Path.* 62:305, 1975.

Immunotherapy

Bekesi, J. G., Holland, J. F., Fleminger, R., Ystes, J., and Henderson, E. S. Immunotherapeutic Efficacy of Neuraminidase-Treated Allogeneic Myeloblasts in Patients with Acute Myelocytic Leukemia. In M. A. Chirigos (Ed.), *Control of Neoplasia by Modulation of the Immune System*. New York: Raven, 1977. Pp. 573–592.

Eilber, F. R., Morton, D. L., Holmes, E. C., Sparks, F. C., and Ramming, K. P. Adjuvant immunotherapy with BCG in treatment of regional lymph node metastases from malignant melanoma. *N. Engl. J. Med.* 294:237–240, 1976.

Nadler, S. H., and Moore, G. E. Immunotherapy of malignant disease. *Arch. Surg.* 99:376–381, 1969.

Rosenberg, S. A., and Terry, W. D. Passive immunotherapy of cancer in animals and man. *Adv. Cancer Res.* 25:323–388, 1977.

Schmidtke, J. R., and Simmons, R. L. Experimental Models of Tumor Therapy. In F. H. Bach and R. A. Good (Eds.), *Clinical Immunobiology*, Vol. 2. New York: Academic, 1974. Pp. 267–285.

Simmons, R. L., and Rios, A. Immunotherapy of cancer: Immunospecific rejection of tumors in recipients of neuraminidase-treated tumor cells plus BCG. *Science* 174:591–593, 1971.

17 : Immunity and Infections

Lucille H. Kimura

Historically, the rudimentary concepts of immunity emerged from observations of host responses to infectious agents. For example, the idea of acquired immunity was suggested by the observation that individuals who had recovered from acute infections often had resistance to reinfection upon later exposure to the same causative microorganism. Vaccines of killed or attenuated microorganisms were found to be effective in inducing immunity against infectious diseases. Thus early principles of immunity were applied to control the spread of transmissible diseases long before the actual mechanisms of antimicrobial immunity were deciphered. Through the years, knowledge acquired about immune responses to infectious agents has contributed greatly to the general understanding of concepts in immunology.

The response of the host to an infectious agent involves both nonspecific immunity and specific acquired immunity. Nonspecific immunity encompasses defense mechanisms that operate independently of the particular antigens of the invading organism. Examples of nonspecific mechanisms include the barrier function of intact skin, mucosae, and mucosal fluids; antibacterial and antiviral activities of humoral factors such as lysozymes and the antimicrobial functions of the professional phagocytes, polymorphonuclear leukocytes (PMN or neutrophils), and macrophages. The characteristics and biological functions of these phagocytic cells have been described in Chapter 8. Often nonspecific immune mechanisms alone are ineffective in limiting the growth and spread of pathogens, and the development of specific acquired immunity is necessary for arresting the disease process. Specific acquired immunity refers to resistance that develops upon exposure to the infectious agent and is mediated by specific antibodies or by specifically activated T lymphocytes and macrophages. Specific immunity is acquired either by contact with the infectious agent (active immunity) or by the transfer of serum or cells from an immune donor to a nonimmune recipient (passive immunity). The general types of antimicrobial immunity are summarized in Table 17-1.

This chapter focuses on the primary host defense mechanisms of nonspecific and specific immunity against bacteria, viruses,

Table 17-1 : Types of Immunity against Microbial Infections

Type of Immunity	Characteristics
A. Nonspecific immunity	Innate (inborn) resistance to infection
B. Specific acquired immunity	
1. Natural active immunity	Develops following natural infection by microbial agent; disease need not develop.
2. Induced active immunity	Develops following vaccination with dead or attenuated agent, or with inactivated microbial toxin or extract.
3. Natural passive immunity	Acquired by transfer of maternal antibodies to the fetus through the placenta or to the newborn by colostrum or milk.
4. Induced passive immunity	Acquired by transfer of serum (passive immunity) or cells (adoptive immunity) from immune donors to nonimmune recipients.

fungi, and parasites. The interactions between infectious agents and host immune responses during the course of infections is discussed, including the contribution of host immune responses to the pathogenesis of certain diseases. In the following discussions, the term *infection* refers to the presence of viable microorganisms in host subepithelial tissues; an inapparent or silent infection exists prior to clinical evidence of host injury and may progress to a clinically apparent infection (disease) if host defense mechanisms are breached.

Immunity in Bacterial Infections

The host defense against any bacterial infection involves nonspecific and specific immune mechanisms, with the primary mechanism being dependent upon the properties of the invading organisms. Thus, humoral antibodies and phagocytes are more effective against extracellular bacteria, while cell-mediated mechanisms are required for resistance to intracellular bacteria.

Role of Phagocytes

The invasion of host subepithelial tissues by bacteria triggers an inflammatory response beginning with vasodilatation and increased vascular permeability and continuing with fibrin deposition, platelet aggregation, and the formation of leukocyte chemotactic factors, including kallikrein, C5a, C3a, and microbial secretion products (see Chapter 8). Circulating leukocytes (primarily neutrophils, followed by monocytes and lymphocytes) are attracted to the site of inflammation and adhere to the capillary and venule walls. By a process called diapedesis, the leukocytes pass through the blood vessel wall into the extra-

Fig. 17-1 : The phagocytic process in neutrophils and macrophages.

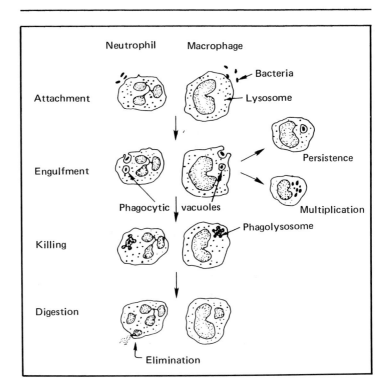

vascular tissue by squeezing between endothelial cells and penetrating the basement membrane. The phagocytic cells accumulated at the site of inflammation constitute the primary line of defense against invading bacteria prior to the development of specific immune mechanisms.

The effectiveness of phagocytes in controlling the infection depends upon the following events in the phagocytic process: attachment of bacteria to the phagocyte's surface, engulfment of bacteria by pseudopodia, killing of ingested organisms, and digestion of killed organisms (Figure 17-1).

ATTACHMENT OF BACTERIA TO PHAGOCYTES. Before engulfment is possible, the bacterium must first adhere to the phagocytic cell membrane. Although both phagocytic and bacterial surfaces are negatively charged, attachment can occur under certain conditions. Attachment is favored at normal host body temperature, occurs over a pH range of 6.5 to 7.2, and is enhanced in solutions of low ionic strength. Divalent cations such as calcium also increase attachment. A current hypothesis suggests that bacteria having surfaces that are more hydrophobic than the surface of the phagocyte are rapidly ingested, while bacteria with hydrophilic surfaces resist phagocytosis. Some bacteria, such as *Mycobacterium tuberculosis* and *Listeria monocytogenes*, have definite affinity for the surfaces of phagocytic cells, which readily ingest these organisms.

Phagocytes require additional mechanisms for the engulfment of bacteria that do not attach directly or that possess antiphagocytic surface factors, such as polysaccharide capsules. The deposition of fibrin at the inflammatory site aids in trapping the bacteria and provides surfaces against which phagocytes can corral bacteria for more efficient ingestion (surface phagocytosis). Engulfment of bacteria with antiphagocytic surface factors is greatly facilitated if the bacteria are coated with specific antibodies (IgG); this enhancement is called *opsonization,* a defense mechanism operative after the development of specific immunity against the infecting organism (discussed in detail in later paragraphs).

ENGULFMENT. Bacterial attachment stimulates phagocytic cell glycolysis, which provides energy for the engulfment process in human neutrophils, monocytes, and guinea pig peritoneal macrophages. In the presence of oxygen, there is a simultaneous increase in respiratory oxidative metabolism. With human neutrophils and monocytes, stimulation of oxidative metabolism is not required for the ingestion process, guinea pig alveolar macrophages, however, need energy generated by this process for ingestion of organisms.

Engulfment occurs with the surrounding of bacteria by pseudopodia, resulting in complete enclosure of the organisms within phagocytic vacuoles. When phagocytosis is initiated in neutrophils, actin-binding protein becomes activated by changes in the plasma membrane and causes polymerization of actin into microfilaments, which then contract, leading to pseudopodia formation. The divalent cations, calcium and magnesium, are required for the ingestion process; guinea pig alveolar macrophages, potassium ions have little effect.

Once formed, the phagocytic vacuole moves into the cytoplasm, where it collides with lysosomal granules. The lysosomal walls first adhere to, then fuse with, the walls of the phagocytic vacuole. Lysosomal contents are explosively released into the vacuole, which is now called a phagolysosome. Both the primary (azurophil) granules and the secondary granules of neutrophils can discharge their contents into phagocytic vacuoles. These granules and the lysosomes of macrophages contain numerous digestive hydrolases and potential bactericidal agents (see Chapter 8).

KILLING. The fate of bacteria within the phagolysosome depends upon their susceptibility or resistance to the phagocyte's arsenal of oxygen-dependent or oxygen-independent microbicidal mechanisms. As mentioned previously, initiation of phagocytosis in neutrophils activates oxidative metabolism, which is characterized by a surge in oxygen consumption, increased glucose utilization, stimulation of the hexose monophosphate (HMP) pathway, and increased production of hydrogen peroxide (H_2O_2). This oxidative metabolic burst represents one of the most critical events associated with the microbicidal activities of phagocytes, as reduction products of oxygen, including its reactive free radicals that are generated during this response, appear to be directly involved in killing mechanisms. In addition, the generation of lactic acid following the metabolic burst causes a drop in the vacuole pH to levels at which some bacteria are killed.

Two metabolic sequences have been suggested to explain the enhanced oxygen uptake in the metabolic burst (see Figure 8–12A). The first pathway begins with activation of a cyanide-insensitive NADH (nicotinamide adenine dinucleotide) oxidase localized in the neutrophil plasma membrane. This enzyme promotes the reaction $2NADH + O_2 \rightarrow 2NAD + H_2O_2$. Hydrogen peroxide is rapidly removed by the glutathione peroxidase and reductase reactions ($2GSH + H_2O_2 \rightarrow GSSG + 2H_2O$; $GSSG + NADPH \rightarrow 2GSH + NADP^+$). The $NADP^+$ generated enters into the HMP pathway, which oxidizes glucose while producing NADPH.

In the second pathway, activation of NADPH oxidase generates H_2O_2 as follows: $2NADPH + O_2 \rightarrow H_2O_2 + 2NADP$. By generating $NADP^+$ directly, this scheme of oxidative metabolism is closely linked to stimulation of the HMP pathway. The NADPH oxidase is associated with azurophil granules of neutrophils.

Oxygen-dependent microbicidal mechanisms of neutrophils (see Chapter 8) involve H_2O_2 as well as intermediate products of oxygen reduction such as superoxide anion (O_2^-), hydroxyl radical ($\cdot OH$), and singlet oxygen ($^1O_2$). An important bactericidal mechanism of neutrophils consists of the interaction of myeloperoxidase (MPO), an enzyme carried in azurophilic granules, H_2O_2, and halides (iodide or chloride), resulting in halogenation and killing of bacteria. Toxic aldehydes and ketones generated by this system are also microbicidal. Neutrophils from patients with chronic granulomatous disease (CGD) are unable to generate sufficient H_2O_2, and although the phagocytes cannot kill catalase-positive bacteria, they are able to kill H_2O_2-generating, catalase-negative bacteria such as lactobacilli, streptococci, and pneumococci. In the absence of catalase, which rapidly destroys H_2O_2, CGD neutrophils utilize H_2O_2 from bacteria in the MPO-H_2O_2-halide bactericidal system. In addition, it has been proposed that H_2O_2 itself functions directly as a bactericidal agent.

Suggestive evidence exists for the participation of intermediate oxygen reduction products in bactericidal mechanisms. The superoxide anion, a free radical formed by the univalent reduction of molecular oxygen or the univalent oxidation of H_2O_2, is a highly reactive oxidation reduction agent generated in stimulated phagocytes. The ubiquitous presence of superoxide dismutase (SOD), an enzyme that breaks down O_2^-, in all respiring cells suggests that O_2^- is a potentially toxic free radical. The inhibition of phagocytic killing by scavengers of hydroxyl ($\cdot$OH) radicals also suggests that these agents are microbicidal. Singlet oxygen, which may be generated by several pathways, including the MPO-H_2O_2-halide system, appears to mediate the chemiluminescence phenomenon observed in normal phagocytizing leukocytes. Leukocytes from CGD patients fail to produce chemiluminescence during phagocytosis, suggesting that singlet oxygen functions in microbicidal systems.

Although bactericidal mechanisms of macrophages have not been well defined, it has been found that oxidative metabolic changes accompany the engulfment process in some classes of macrophages. In addition to the release of lysosomal enzymes into the phagocytic vacuole, there are increases in oxygen consumption, glucose oxidation, H_2O_2 and O_2^- production, and chemiluminescence. The number of peroxidase-containing granules in human mononuclear phagocytes ranges from many in promonocytes, to fewer in monocytes, to essentially none in mature macrophages. In the absence of peroxidase, perhaps other factors such as toxic O_2^- reactivity assume more prominent roles in the bactericidal functions of macrophages.

Oxygen-independent antibacterial mechanisms in neutrophils and macrophages have also been described. Neutrophil and macrophage granules that fuse with phagocytic vacuoles contain lysozyme and lactoferrin in addition to numerous hydrolases. Neutrophil granules also store a group of highly cationic (basic) proteins, which are bactericidal for some organisms. Lysozyme (muramidase) hydrolyzes mucopeptide moieties in the cell walls of certain bacteria, which then become sensitive to osmotic lysis; lysozyme by itself, however, has only a limited bactericidal capacity and often functions synergistically with other agents such as H_2O_2 and ascorbic acid and antibody and complement in the killing of some bacteria. Lactoferrin, an iron-binding protein, is bacteriostatic rather than bactericidal; as such its role is limited in phagocytes. On the other hand, the cationic proteins of neutrophils exhibit bactericidal activity against *Escherichia coli, Streptococcus faecalis, Staphylococcus aureus,* and *Pseudomonas aeruginosa.* The bactericidal activity of the proteins is heat-stable and functions independently of their chymotrypsin-like property.

DIGESTION. If bactericidal mechanisms of the phagocyte are effective, the next step in the phagocytic process is degradation of killed bacteria by the numerous hydrolases (see Chapter 8) contributed by lysosomal granules. These enzymes include proteases, nucleases, phosphatases, lipases, and carbohydrases. Low molecular weight subunits or fragments are then eliminated from the phagocytic cell cytoplasm. Some bacterial polysaccharides, complex waxes, and lipids are more resistant to degradation and persist in macrophages for weeks or months. Macrophages serve the important function of removing excess foreign antigens while simultaneously processing antigen molecules to the appropriate immunogenic configuration and presenting these altered molecules to lymphocytes participating in humoral or cell-mediated immune responses (see Chapter 5).

PERSISTENCE OR MULTIPLICATION OF INGESTED BACTERIA. Engulfment is not necessarily followed by killing of the ingested microbes; some bacteria persist and multiply within macrophages. It must be emphasized that these are nonimmune macrophages, for once macrophages are activated by mediators from T cells in specific cell-mediated immune responses, they are much more resistant to these bacteria. In general, extracellular bacteria (obligatory multiplication outside of host cells) are usually susceptible to phagocytic killing mechanisms once they are ingested (Table 17-2). A notable exception is *Salmonella typhi,* which can survive and multiply within macrophages. When facultative and obligate intracellular bacteria are ingested, they resist killing mechanisms and either persist in low numbers for long periods of time within macrophages or multiply, eventually destroying the macrophage. Bacteria such as salmonellae, brucellae, tubercle bacillus, and *Listeria* organisms persist within macrophages that offer protection from the onslaught of humoral antibacterial factors and antibiotics. With highly virulent strains of mycobacteria, salmonellae, *Listeria* organisms, brucellae, *Pasteurella* organisms, some staphylococci, and streptococci, multiplication of the bacteria proceeds within macrophages. Experimentally it has been demonstrated that the extent of resistance to intracellular digestion and cytotoxicity towards phagocytes of staphylococci can be correlated with their degree of virulence.

Possible explanations for the resistance of ingested bacteria to microbicidal mechanisms include protection against lysosomal contents and prevention of the fusion of lysosomes with phagocytic vacuoles. An example of the first possibility is the resistance of *Mycobacterium lepraemurium* to killing and digestion within phagolysosomes. The bacterium is enclosed in capsular material

**Table 17-2 : Primary Host Defense Mechanisms against
Extracellular and Intracellular Bacterial Pathogens**

Bacteria	Phagocytes/ Opsonins	Ab-C- Mediated Bacterio- lysis	Anti- toxin	Cell- Mediated Immunity	Attachment Inhibition
Extracellular					
Bacillus anthracis	x				
Bordetella pertussis	x				
Clostridium botulinum			x		
Clostridium perfringens			x		
Clostridium tetani			x		
Corynebacterium diphtheriae			x		
Enteric gram- negative rods	x	x			
Haemophilus influenzae	x				
Neisseria gonorrhoeae	x				x?*
Neisseria meningitidis	x				
Salmonella typhi				x	
Shigella dysenteriae	x		x		x?
Staphylococcus aureus	x				
Streptococcus pneumoniae	x				
Streptococci, groups A and B	x				
Treponema pallidum		x		x	
Vibrio cholerae		x			x
Yersinia pestis	x			x?	
Facultative intracellular					
Actinomyces israelii				x	
Brucella abortus				x	
Franciscella tularensis				x	
Myobacterium tuberculosis				x	
Nocardia asteroides				x	
Obligate intracellular					
Myobacterium leprae				x	

*? = mechanism may be important.

composed primarily of a peptidoglycolipid, "mycoside C", which shields the organism from toxic agents in the phagolysosome. The second explanation is exemplified by the inhibition of lysosome-phagocytic vacuole fusion by virulent *Mycobacterium tuberculosis* surviving within vacuoles of mouse peritoneal macrophages. As will be discussed later, the effective control and eventual eradication of intracellular bacteria from macrophages requires specific activation of the cell-mediated arm of immunity.

In summary, initial nonspecific immune responses manifested by phagocytic cell activities are crucial as a first line of defense once bacteria gain entry into host subepithelial tissues. Phagocytic cells can effectively limit the numbers of multiplying bacteria, especially if the original infecting dose is small, thus giving the host time to mount specific humoral and cell-mediated immune responses to the foreign bacterial antigens.

Antibody-Mediated Immunity

Specific immune mechanisms mediated by antibodies are essential for successful defense against certain pathogenic extracellular bacteria, including exotoxin producers. Many of these bacteria possess antiphagocytic surface factors. Antibodies are produced against a variety of T-independent and T-dependent antigens on bacterial morphological structures or secreted molecules, including outer capsules, cell wall components, flagella, fimbriae, and exotoxins. Primary antibody responses to bacteria yield mostly IgM and some IgG antibodies, while secondary responses generate mainly IgG antibodies. Secretory IgA responses also occur when bacterial antigens gain access to mucosal lymphoid tissues. When specific antibody responses are the primary defense mechanism against certain bacteria, passive transfer of protection can be achieved by injecting immune serum into a nonimmune recipient following challenge by the infectious agent. Antibody-mediated antibacterial mechanisms include opsonization, bacteriolysis, exotoxin neutralization, and attachment inhibition.

OPSONIZATION. Obligate extracellular bacteria are rapidly killed when ingested by phagocytes; thus antiphagocytic surface factors represent major virulence determinants in these microorganisms. Many virulent bacterial strains possess polysaccharide capsules or other surface structures that are antiphagocytic as well as antigenic (Table 17-3). In some bacteria, such as *Streptococcus pneumoniae* and *Klebsiella pneumoniae,* the polysaccharide capsule is the major antigenic component of the cell and specifies numerous antigenic groups within each bacterial species. The development of group-specific antibodies that cause capsular swelling in vitro (quellung reaction) were vital to host survival prior to the advent of antibiotics. Once antibodies attach to antigenic determinants on the bacteria, they enhance phagocytosis by facilitating the binding of bacteria to phagocytic surfaces (opsonization).

Opsonization is mediated primarily by the IgG class of antibodies (IgG1 and IgG3 in humans), which attach to surface Fc receptors on neutrophils and macrophages (Figure 17-2A). Activation of the classic complement pathway by bacterial antigen-antibody complexes or activation of the alternative complement pathway by bacterial polysaccharides or endotoxin generates C3b, which optimizes phagocytosis. Maximal phagocytosis occurs when complement is activated, because neutrophils and macrophages

Table 17-3 : **Examples of Antiphagocytic Surface Factors of Pathogenic Bacteria**

Genus and Species	Antiphagocytic Factor	Composition
Bacillus anthracis	Capsular polypeptide	D-glutamic acid
Haemophilus influenzae	Capsular polysaccharide	Polyribophosphates
Klebsiella pneumoniae	Capusular polysaccharide	Various sugars
Neisseria gonorrhoeae	Pili	Protein
Neisseria meningitidis	Capsular polysaccharide	Sialic acid, hexosamines
Pseudomonas aeruginosa	Capsular polysaccharide	Various sugars
Staphylococcus aureus	Protein A	Variuos amino acids
	Capsular antigen (Smith strain)	2-amino-2-deoxy-D-glucuronic acid polymer
Streptococcus pneumoniae	Capsular polysaccharide	Various sugars, i.e., glucose, galactose, N-acetylyglucosamine
Streptococcus pyogenes	Hyaluronic acid capsule	N-acetylglucosamine, glucuronic acid
	M protein and fimbriae	Various amino acids
Yersinia pestis	V antigen	Protein
	W antigen	Lipoprotein
Other gram-negative species	Lipopolysaccharide	Lipid, protein, poly-saccharide

also have surface receptors for C3b. Phagocyte Fc and C3b receptors appear to function synergistically, as shown by the lower concentrations of specific antibody required for opsonization when complement is activated. The IgM class of antibodies indirectly functions as opsonins by activating complement. Complement activation also produces potent chemotactic factors that attract phagocytes (see Chapter 9), thereby further promoting the phagocytic process.

In addition to providing the link between bacteria and phagocytes via Fc receptors, it has been suggested that the binding of specific antibodies to encapsulated bacteria makes the bacterial surface more hydrophobic. As mentioned earlier, hydrophobic bacteria are more readily engulfed than hydrophilic organisms. Complement binding renders the bacteria even more hydrophobic. These studies have been done with encapsulated *S. pneumoniae, K. pneumoniae,* and *S. aureus* (Smith strain).

BACTERIOLYSIS. Antibodies against bacterial cell surface antigens activate complement, leading to the formation of a membrane attack complex that damages the cytoplasmic membranes of certain gram-negative bacteria, including *Salmonella* and *Shigella* species, *E. coli,* and *Vibrio cholerae* (Figure 17–2B). Although

Fig. 17-2 : Functions of antibodies in antibacterial immunity. A. Enhancement of phagocytosis by opsonic activity. B. Lysis of bacteria in concert with complement and lysozyme. C. Neutralization of exotoxins by blocking of binding site. D. Inhibition of bacterial attachment to host epithelial cells by specific secretory IgA.

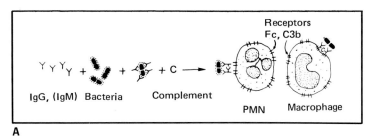

the mechanisms of complement action in the lysis of red blood cells have been studied in detail (see Chapter 9), the sequence of events in antibody-complement-mediated bacteriolysis is only partially understood. Gram-negative bacterial cell walls consist of inner and outer phospholipid-protein membranes separated by a thin layer of peptidoglycan (murein). This cell wall structure imposes requirements for complement lysis mechanisms different from those needed for red cell lysis.

One requirement for optimal lysis is the action of lysozome, which hydrolyzes the muramic acid–N–acetylglucosamine backbone structure of peptidoglycan. Current evidence indicates that lysozyme plays an accessory role in bactericidal events by facilitating the passage of complement components through the peptidoglycan layer to the inner cytoplasmic membrane. Recently it has been suggested that the lytic actions of lysozyme function independently of the bactericidal mechanisms of specific antibody and complement components that cause the actual cytoplasmic membrane damage. Apparently bacterial cell death, as determined by a reduction in viable cells, increased cytoplasmic membrane permeability, and inhibition of macromolecular synthesis, occurs well before final cell lysis resulting from extensive degradation of the cell wall by lysozyme.

As in other types of complement-mediated cell lysis, both IgM and IgG molecules participate. Complement activation requires only one IgM molecule or two adjacent IgG molecules on the cell surface. Therefore IgM antibodies are more efficient in this bactericidal mechanism.

EXOTOXIN NEUTRALIZATION. A major protective function of antibodies is their ability to neutralize potent bacterial exotoxins. In diseases such as diphtheria, tetanus, botulism, gas gangrene, and cholera, exotoxins are essentially responsible for pathogenesis (Table 17-4). Antibody neutralization of exotoxins is a crucial defense mechanism, and preventive immunizations with diphtheria and tetanus toxoids (inactive, but antigenic toxins) offer nearly complete protection against the diseases. For enterotoxins, such as cholera enterotoxin, however, the host target cell is the intestinal epithelial cell; so toxicity is confined to the intestinal tissues, with only a limited amount of toxin entering the systemic circulation. In this instance, the protective role of serum antitoxin antibodies is restricted, and the part played by antibodies present in the intestinal environment (such as secretory IgA) may be more important.

Presently the principal mechanism of antibody-mediated exotoxin neutralization appears to involve prevention of exotoxin binding to specific receptors on host target cells (Figure 17-2C). This has been suggested by studies on diphtheria and cholera toxins. As described in Table 17-4, each of these toxins consists of two subunits; the A subunit exerts toxic, biological effects on host cells, and the B subunit mediates exotoxin binding to target cells. With diphtheria toxin, the hydrophilic A subunit alone cannot get into host cells and requires assistance from the hydrophobic B subunit to facilitate this entry. Antibodies directed against the B subunit are more effective in neutralizing complete exotoxin than antibodies directed against just the A subunit,

Table 17-4 : Biological Activities of Some Bacterial Exotoxins

Bacteria	Toxin-Induced Disease	Biological Activities of Exotoxin
Clostridium botulinum	Botulism	Toxin blocks cholinergic nerve fiber transmission by preventing acetylcholine release.
Clostridium perfringens	Gas gangrene	Necrotizing and hemolytic exotoxins; major toxin is α-toxin or lecithinase C.
Clostridium tetani	Tetanus	Toxin binds to nerve tissues causing convulsive contractions of voluntary muscles.
Corynebacterium diphtheriae	Diphtheria	Target tissues include peripheral nerves, pericardium, diaphragm, heart muscle, liver, kidneys.
		A subunit—catalyzes ADP ribosylation of elongation factor 2 (EF-2), thus inhibiting protein synthesis.
		B subunit—binds toxin to target cells.
Vibrio cholerae	Cholera	Enterotoxin binds to intestinal epithelium.
		A subunit—activates adenylcyclase, resulting in cAMP increase, which affects water and electrolyte transport by mucosal cells.
		B subunit—binds toxin to GM_1-like receptor on cell surface.

suggesting that antibodies function by steric blocking of exotoxin binding to surface receptors on host target cells.

ATTACHMENT INHIBITION. The ability of bacteria to attach to host epithelial cells contributes to their success in colonizing mucosal tissues and to their pathogenicity. Different bacterial species normally colonizing mucosal areas such as the oral cavity show preferential attachment to different types of epithelial cells, thus demonstrating the role of attachment as an ecological determinant. Pathogenic strains of *E. coli* and *Neisseria gonorrhoeae* (colonial types 1 and 2) attach to epithelial cells to a greater extent than nonpathogenic strains. Other examples of selective attachment of pathogens include the binding of *Bordetella portussis* to respiratory epithelium, *Shigella dysenteriae* to colonic epithelium, and *Vibrio cholerae* to intestinal epithelium.

Antibody-mediated defense against these bacteria is probably most effective in the local mucosal environment. Secretory IgA (SIgA), the predominant immunoglobulin in mucosal secretions, becomes a critical factor in this type of defense (Figure 17–2D). Antidobies against *V. cholerae* have been detected in the feces (coproantibodies) of patients recovering from cholera. Copro-antibodies, most of which are probably SIgA have the ability to inhibit the attachment of *V. cholerae* to intestinal epithelial cells from experimental animals. Specific SIgA has also been shown to inhibit the attachment of other bacteria to epithelial cells, suggesting that attachment inhibition represents another defense mechanism of antibodies and that oral immunizations to induce SIgA formation may be beneficial in these diseases.

Cell-Mediated Immunity

During bacterial infections, both B and T lymphocytes are sensitized by bacterial antigens. Sensitized T lymphocytes not only provide helper activity to B cells in specific antibody production but also participate in cell-mediated reactions against bacteria. The latter reactions are necessary for controlling the spread of bacteria that escape other bactericidal mechanisms by finding shelter within macrophages. These bacteria include *M. tuberculosis, M. leprae, Brucella abortus, Listeria monocytogenes* and *Salmonella typhi.* Among the functions of T lymphocytes (see Chapter 3), the activities most important in defense against these bacteria are T cell recruitment and activation of macrophages participating in acquired immune and delayed hypersensitivity responses. The primary role of cell-mediated mechanisms in defense against certain bacteria is demonstrated by the passive transfer of protection with immune T cells but not with immune serum and is suggested by the lack of correlation between specific serum antibody levels and degree of resistance to infection.

ACQUIRED CELLULAR IMMUNITY. Development of cell-mediated immunity against bacteria can be divided into two stages, induction of immunity and the effector phase (Figure 17–3). The first stage begins with the engulfment of invading microorganisms by macrophages, which then process and present bacterial antigens to T lymphocytes located in thymus-dependent areas of regional lymph nodes and spleen. Specific sensitization of T cells requires identity at the major histocompatibility complex (MHC) between the T cells and macrophages, suggesting that antigens are presented by macrophages in association with an MHC-controlled gene product. Sensitized T cells undergo proliferation, then emigrate from lymph nodes or the spleen, enter the systemic blood circulation, and accumulate at the foci of infection. The

Fig. 17-3 : Development of cell-mediated responses against bacteria. MIF = migration inhibition factor; MAF = macrophage-activating factor; MCF = macrophage chemotactic factor.

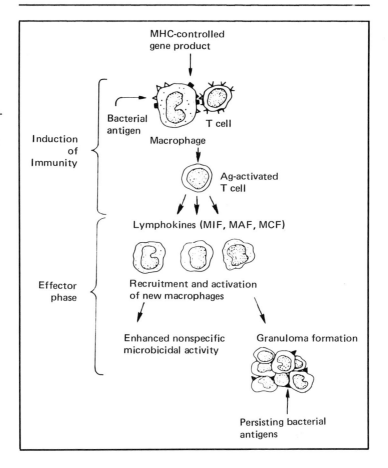

sensitized T cells release lymphokines, which are probably responsible for the recruitment and activation of macrophages, the effector cells in the response. Among the lymphokines released are migration inhibition factor (MIF), macrophage-activating factor (MAF), which may be the same as MIF, macrophage chemotactic factor (MCF), and monocyte growth factor(s) (MGF). Characteristics and functions of the lymphokines are described in Chapter 3.

The effector phase of immunity is characterized by the accumulation of macrophages (originally from a rapidly dividing stem cell pool in the bone marrow) and the functions of activated macrophages in the infectious foci. Compared to unstimulated macrophages, activated macrophages show increases in cell size, motility, spreading, phagocytic capacity, metabolic rate, glucose and oxygen consumption, and number and contents of lysosomal granules. Of critical importance is the enhanced capacity of activated macrophages for killing intracellular bacteria. Unlike the antigen-specific activation of T cells, effector macrophage killing is nonspecific; once activated, these macrophages are able to kill not only the inciting bacteria but other unrelated intracellular bacteria as well.

In the presence of discrete foci of bacteria, a granulomatous response often occurs in which bacteria are surrounded by activated macrophages that have transformed into elongated nonmotile cells exhibiting decreased phagocytic capacity but increased bactericidal activities. Called *epithelioid cells,* they adhere tightly to each other by interdigitations in their processes and form multiple layers, thus imprisoning bacteria. Centrally located in granulomas are often found multinucleated giant cells formed by the fusion of macrophages. Viable bacteria are sometimes present in these giant cells. Macrophages, lymphocytes, and a few plasma cells form the outermost layer of the infectious granuloma.

Formation of granulomas usually brings the infection under control; however, if the infecting dose of bacteria is too large, or if host cellular immune responses are too weak, the bacteria may override the restraints of granulomas and continue to multiply, eventually disseminating the disease. For example, intradermal injection of virulent tubercle bacilli into highly susceptible nonimmune guinea pigs often results in spread of the infection, leading to death of the animal. On the other hand, similar injections into immune guinea pigs (those surviving a primary challenge) result in granuloma formation, which effectively restrains the bacteria.

DELAYED HYPERSENSITIVITY REACTIONS. The state of specific T cell immunity to bacteria can be detected by intradermal injections of soluble bacterial products. If immune T cells are present in an individual, an inflammatory lesion forms at the injection site and peaks in intensity by 24 to 48 hours. Like the infectious granuloma, the lesion is characterized by macrophage and lymphocyte infiltration. This inflammatory reaction is called a *delayed hypersensitivity response* and reflects the existence of T cell immunity against particular antigens (discussed further in Chapters 3 and 13). The role of delayed hypersensitivity (allergic) reactions against bacterial antigens has not been clearly defined in terms of benefit to the overall cell-mediated defense against bacteria.

GENETICALLY CONTROLLED RESISTANCE. Recent studies strongly suggest that host genetic factors play a major role in cell-mediated defense against an intracellular bacterial pathogen,

L. monocytogenes. Experimentally induced infections with this organism have served as a reproducible model for intracellular bacterial infections. During the first three days following inoculation of viable bacteria into mice, the numbers of bacteria in various organs continue to increase. Host resistance at this time is conveyed by the innate ability of nonimmune macrophages to kill or inhibit the bacteria. In this early period, the numbers of bacteria in the liver or spleen are smaller in nude (thymus-deficient) mice than in their normal littermates. By the third or fourth day, the numbers of proliferating bacteria drop, signaling the onset of acquired T cell–mediated resistance. The numbers of activated macrophages increase, following by eventual elimination of the bacteria.

Different strains of mice vary in their resistance to infection by *L. monocytogenes.* For example, C57B1 and related sublines, NZB and SJL mice are resistant to infection; BALB/c, CBA, A, DBA/1 and C3H mice are susceptible to infection. Resistance was found to be related to the ability of nonimmune macrophages to kill bacteria early in infection and to the effector role of macrophages in the acquired immune response. Macrophage resistance appears to be controlled by genes clearly distinct from the H-2–linked immune response genes (at loci other than H-2).

Bacterial Immunosuppression

A number of bacterial products have been identified which cause suppression of specific antibody production or cell-mediated responses to infectious agents, tumors, or tissue grafts (Table 17-5). Other suppressive activities involve cytotoxicity for cells such as macrophages (exotoxin A from *Pseudomonas aeruginosa*) and cleavage of SIgA1 (proteases from *Haemophilus influenzae, Streptococcus pneumoniae, S. sanguis,* and *Neisseria meningitidis*). Possible mechanisms of immunosuppression by bacterial products include (1) interference with macrophage processing or orientation of antigen, (2) stimulation of suppressor T cells, (3) suppression of T or K cytotoxic cells, (4) direct toxic effects on lymphocytes or macrophages, (5) synthesis of blocking antibodies and (6) alterations in cell cAMP levels resulting in inhibition of mediator release. Immunosuppressive properties of bacteria may contribute to their inventory of virulence factors.

Bacterial Immunopathology

Antibody and cell-mediated immune responses in bacterial infections are basically beneficial to the host; however, sometimes immune mechanisms contribute to the pathogenesis of infections. For example, the formation of soluble antigen-antibody complexes during the course of infection may lead to problems such as poststreptococcal glomerulonephritis, vasculitis, and arthritis (see Chapter 13). In diseases such as lepromatous leprosy, chronic

Table 17-5 : Examples of Bacterial Immunosuppressive Agents

Bacterial Agent	Immunosuppressive Effects			
	Decreases Ab Responses	Decreases CMI Responses	Cytotoxic for Phagocytes	Cleaves SIgA
Staphylococcus aureus				
α-toxin			x	
Leukocidin			x	
Group A *Streptococcus*				
Membrane-associated				
immunosuppressant (SF)	x			
Pyrogenic exotoxin (SPE)	x			
Exotoxin A	x	x		
Escherichia coli	x	x		
Pseudomonas aeruginosa	x	x		
Pseudomonas aeruginosa exotoxin A			x	
Vibrio cholerae enterotoxin	x	x		
Bacterial enzymes				
IgA1 proteases				x
L-Asparaginase	x	x		
L-Glutaminase	x	x		
Ribonuclease	x	x		
Mycobacterium leprae		x		
Listeria monocytogenes		x		

antigenemia frequently occurs, making immune complex pathology a major concern. Delayed hypersensitivity reactions are also responsible for host injury, as shown by the formation of chronic granulomas causing local disruption of surrounding tissues or by severe delayed-type inflammatory lesions in contact sensitivity reactions (such as with poison ivy). Occurrence of immunopathology in association with defense mechanisms illustrates the complex nature of the host's immune response to bacterial infections.

Immunity in Viral Infections

Host resistance in viral infections involves mechanisms intimately associated with certain viral characteristics, notably the obligate intracellular manner of replication, expression of viral antigens on host cell surfaces, and mode of transmission among host cells. Intracellular viral replication means that effective humoral defenses are limited to occasions when mature viruses pass between host cells and that mechanisms preventing either viral entry into cells or replication within cells are very effective. Expression of viral antigens on host cell surfaces allows for antigen-directed attack by humoral and cell-mediated immune

Table 17-6 : Viral Infections in Humoral and Cellular Immunodeficiencies

Cellular Immunodeficiencies	Humoral Immunodeficiencies
Papovaviruses	Myxoviruses
Herpesviruses	Enteroviruses
Simplex	Polio
Varicella-zoster	Coxsackie
Zoster	Arboviruses
CMV	
Poxviruses	
Vaccinia	
Paramyxoviruses	
Measles	

mechanisms on infected cells. Modes of virus transmission include extracellular dissemination of progeny virus after host cell destruction; intercellular transmission through adjacent host cell walls having virally-induced surface changes; and vertical transmission, in which the viral genome is passed from mother to daughter cell. Intercellular transmission restricts certain humoral mechanisms and necessitates cell-mediated mechanisms for optimal resistance. Vertical viral transmission may lead to persistent host infections. In addition, viral infection of lymphocytes and macrophages complicates an already complex system of host defenses.

Nonimmune defense mechanisms either prevent viral entry into cells or inhibit intracellular replication. Perhaps the best defense against viral infections is the lack of specific membrane surface receptors on host cells for certain viruses, a deficiency conferring genetically determined, species-specific resistance to infections. For example, mouse cells lack receptors for poliovirus and are resistant to these viruses. Another host barrier is intact keratinized skin, which is less penetrable than mucosal epithelium. The next line of defense consists of macrophages, which engulf and kill many viruses, as will be discussed shortly.

The importance of antibody-mediated and cell-mediated mechanisms against viral infections in humans has been demonstrated by the susceptibility of immunodeficient or compromised patients to these infections (Table 17-6). Cell-mediated immunodeficiencies predispose patients to infections by poxviruses, herpesviruses, papovaviruses, and some myxoviruses; humoral immunodeficiencies predispose patients to infections with enteroviruses, arboviruses, and other myxoviruses. The study of immune mechanisms in experimental viral infections are discussed in this section. Immunity against viral-induced tumor cells is not described here but is discussed in Chapter 16.

Role of Macrophages   Viruses gaining entry into the host via the lungs or other tissues, or traveling in the blood stream, are readily taken up by macrophages in the lungs, lymph nodes, liver, spleen and other blood sinuses. The effectiveness of macrophages in limiting viral infections depends upon their ability to prevent intracellular replication of viruses. This property functions independently of T cells (in the absence of acquired immunity or in nude mice) and appears to be genetically controlled by a single medelian dominant factor in mice. Thus, strains of mice susceptible to a particular virus have macrophages that support viral replication, while resistant strains have macrophages that fail to support viral replication. Concomitantly, the ability to replicate in macrophages correlates with the virulence of different viral strains. Genetically determined resistance in mice does not apply to all types of viruses, and resistance factors appear to segregate independently.

Age-dependence of macrophage resistance has been demonstrated with herpesviruses, which grow most rapidly in neonatal macrophages. This may explain the high susceptibility of newborns, unlike adults, to disseminated herpesvirus infections.

Antibody-Mediated   ANTIBODY RESPONSES TO VIRAL ANTIGENS. The kinetics of
Immunity   antibody production against viruses have been examined in experimental and natural infections with poliovirus in humans. In natural infections, IgM antibodies increase rapidly to maximal levels by 3 or 4 weeks after infection, then decline to preinfection levels by 3 months, just about the time of peak IgG responses and peak serum neutralizing capabilities. Significant levels of serum neutralizing antibodies persist for many years. Specific IgA titers appear between 4 and 6 weeks and continue to increase for the next two months. Oral immunizations stimulate specific SIgA responses, which prevent mucosal infection and excretion of viruses; however, parenteral immunizations have proved to be equally capable of preventing paralytic disease in humans and spread of the virus among individuals.

Although preferable, it is difficult to induce sufficient titers of antibodies against all cross-reacting types of a particular virus, such as influenza A virus and various paramyxoviruses and enteroviruses. Antibody production is dominated by the type of antibody induced against the particular antigens involved in the first exposure to virus (phenomenon of "original antigenic sin").

ANTIBODY-MEDIATED NEUTRALIZATION OF VIRUSES. Antibody neutralization (elimination of infectivity) of viruses may occur either prior to or following virus contact with host cells (Figure 17-4). Antibody-mediated mechanisms functioning on free

Fig. 17-4 : Various mechanisms of antibody-mediated neutralization of viruses. A. Neutralization before virus contacts target cell. B. Neutralization at target cell level. Ab = antibody; C = complement; PMN = polymorphonuclear leukocyte.

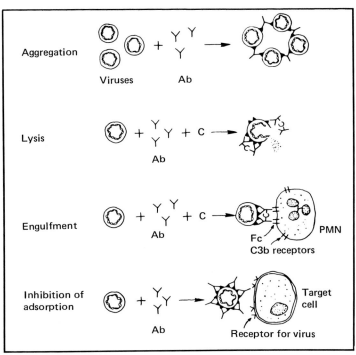

A

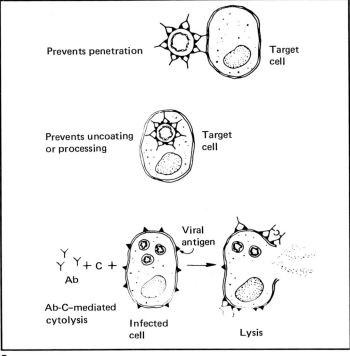

B

viruses include virus aggregation, lysis, engulfment, and inhibition of adsorption. Aggregation effectively reduces the number of infectious particles and may promote phagocytic engulfment of the viruses, especially if complement has been activated. Antibody and complement also cooperate in the lysis of enveloped viruses that have host-derived lipid coats (rubella virus, influenza virus, coronaviruses and Gross leukemogenic virus). Antibody enhances the uptake of viruses by neutrophils and certain macrophages that restrict intracellular viral replication. Prevention of viral adsorption to host cell receptors by the blocking effects of antibodies has been demonstrated with influenza and polioviruses.

Antibodies may also neutralize viruses at the target level by preventing viral penetration of host cell membranes; inhibiting uncoating or further processing of viruses within cells, as with adenoviruses; and by mediating lysis of infected cells in conjunction with complement, as shown with herpesviruses.

Inhibition of viral adsorption to host receptors, penetration of cell membranes, and intracellular uncoating or processing may involve the covering of "critical sites" on viruses by antibodies. For example, antibodies directed against the hemagglutinin on influenza viruses are most efficient in neutralizing infectivity; they do this by preventing viral attachment to host cells. Antibodies against influenza virus neuraminidase may prevent release of virus from infected cells but do not prevent viral adsorption to cells and are much less effective in offering protection. Hemagglutinin represents a critical site on the virus, and antigenic variations at this site have been responsible for influenza epidemics (minor antigenic variations) and pandemics (major antigenic variations). Other critical sites include the vertex antigens of foot-and-mouth disease virus and the hexon antigens of adenoviruses, which may be unable to undergo uncoating or processing in the presence of antihexon antibodies. Some virus-antibody complexes remain infectious and may indicate inadequate covering of critical sites on the virus. In this respect the addition of complement or rheumatoid factors may help to neutralize viruses by covering these sites.

Cell-Mediated Immunity

Cell-mediated mechanisms against viruses involve cytotoxic T lymphocytes, T cell–macrophage interactions, antibody-dependent cellular cytotoxicity, and natural killer cells.

CYTOTOXIC T LYMPHOCYTES. During acute viral infections in mice, a T cell subset exhibiting specific toxicity for virus-infected cells is induced (Figure 17-5A), the effector cells are called *cytotoxic T lymphocytes* (CTL or Tc). Both the induction and the effector activity of CTL against certain viruses require H-2 compatibility between the CTL and virus-infected target cell. For example, cytomegalovirus (CMV) infected target cells are destroyed by immune spleen CTL expressing the same H-2 haplotypes. The CMV-immune CTL show little lytic activity against CMV-infected cells of unrelated H-2 haplotypes (Figure 17-6). This H-2 restriction of CTL activity is further illustrated by data presented in Table 17-7. These results suggest that induction and effector mechanisms require presentation of viral antigens in association with an MHC-gene product. The H-2 restriction phenomenon has been observed with a number of viruses, including lymphocytic choriomeningitis virus, vaccinia, ectromelia, Sendai virus, adenoviruses, herpes simplex virus (HSV), and CMV (but not influenza virus).

It is not known if CTL induction results from direct presentation of viral antigen and the MHC gene product to CTL precursors or occurs indirectly through the activities of mediators from helper T cells. The increase in CTL activity against HSV when animals are treated with cyclophosphamide suggests that suppressor mechanisms may operate in vivo.

T CELL–MACROPHAGE INTERACTIONS. Antiviral activities are also exerted by macrophages that have been activated by mediators from viral antigen–stimulated T cells (Figure 17-5B). As mentioned in the discussion on bacterial infections, these mediators include MIF, MAF, and MCF. In addition these T cells release interferon, a protein preventing viral replication in other host cells. Recently studies have shown that T cell–macrophage interactions are important in varicella-zoster infections.

ANTIBODY-DEPENDENT CELLULAR CYTOXICITY. Leukocytes having Fc receptors may participate in antibody-dependent cellular cytotoxicity (ADCC) reactions against antibody-coated virus-infected cells (Figure 17-5C). Murine peritoneal and spleen effector cells having the characteristics of macrophages are able to mediate ADCC against HSV-infected cells. Neutrophils have also been shown to exert ADCC against herpesvirus-infected cells. In addition, lymphocytes having characteristics of null cells or K cells destroy virus-infected cells by this mechanism.

NATURAL KILLER CELLS. Populations of lymphoid cells from normal human donors or mice exert natural cytotoxicity against virus-infected cells. These cells are called *natural killer* (NK) cells and are nonadherent, nonphagocytic cells, lacking conventional concentrations of B or T cell surface markers (see Chapter 3)

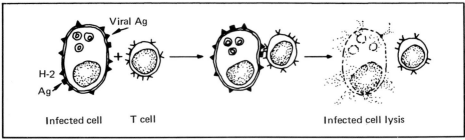

A

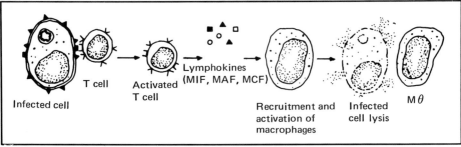

B

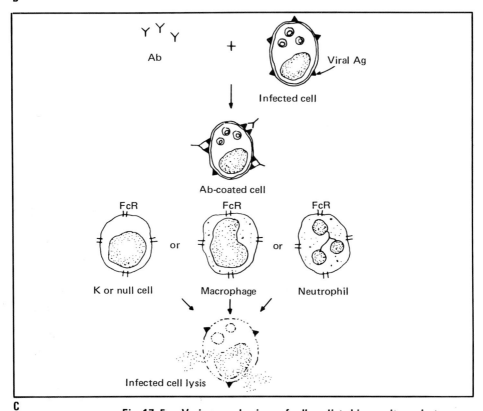

C

Fig. 17-5 : Various mechanisms of cell-mediated immunity against
viruses. A. Cytotoxic T cells. B. T cell–macrophage interaction:

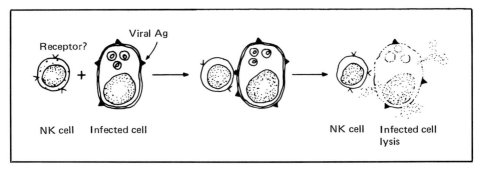

Fig. 17-5 (Continued) : macrophage-mediated cytotoxicity (nonspecific). C. antibody-dependent cellular cytotoxicity. MIF = migration inhibition factor; MAF = macrophage-activating factor; MCF = macrophage (monocyte) chemotactic factor; Ab = antibody; Ag = antigen.

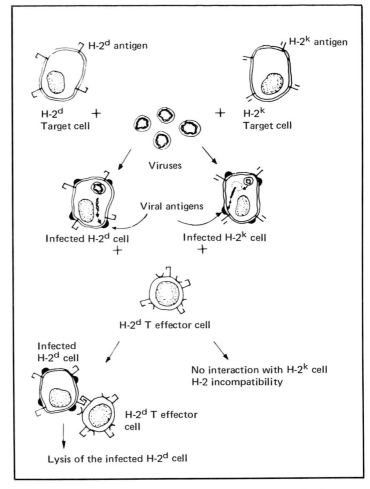

Fig. 17-6 : Mechanism of H-2 restriction on induction and effector activities of cytotoxic T lymphocytes.

Table 17-7 : H-2 Restriction of Target Cell Recognition by Cytomegalo-virus (CMV) Immune Spleen Cells in the Cytotoxic T Lymphocyte Response

H-2 Haplotypes			
Immune Effector T Cell	Target CMV-Infected Cells	% Lysis	P*
d	d	19.3	<0.01
d	d	10.1	<0.01
d	k	6.5	N.S.
k	d	3.3	N.S.
k	k	21.4	<0.01

*Significance of difference between test and spontaneous lysis; N.S. = not significant.
Source: Modified and adapted from Quinnan et al., *Nature* 273:541, 1978.

but possessing detectable Fc receptors for IgG. Murine NK cells are cytotoxic for vaccinia virus and HSV-infected cells; the interactions are species-specific, requiring syngeneic or allogeneic (not xenogeneic) target cells, unlike ADCC reactions, which are not species-restricted.

Interferon

Another antiviral mechanism involves interferon, a protein released by lymphocytes, macrophages, epithelial cells, and fibroblasts in response to virus infections or by lymphocytes stimulated with nonviral antigens or mitogens. Released interferon enters uninfected cells and, by mechanisms not fully understood, prevents viral replication in these cells. One mechanism may involve host cell production of an antiviral protein that inhibits virus replication (see Figure 3-8). Recent studies on murine leukemia virus–infected cells suggest that the major inhibitory effects of interferon are exerted on the late stages of virus maturation. If interferon is present during the first cycle of virus replication, inhibition occurs before virus assembly, decreasing the numbers of assembled virus particles and buds in the host cell. If the viral infection has already been established in a cell, interferon may not prevent viral assembly but leads to virus accumulation on the cell surface. A high percentage of these viruses are noninfectious. Because interferon action is rapid in this system, it has been suggested that some effects of interferon may not require the induction of antiviral protein. Interferon may also affect oxidative phosphorylation in host cells. Not all viruses induce interferon production; levels are decreased in infections with herpes virus, which appears to be resistant to interferon action.

Table 17-8 : Examples of Viral Immunosuppression

Effects on Host Immunity	Viruses Mediating Effects
Depressed RES clearance	Lactate dehydrogenase virus (LDV) Ectromelia LCM Dengue virus
Decreased antibody production	Most leukemogenic viruses CMV
Prolonged skin graft rejection	LDV Newcastle disease virus
Decreased DTH reactions	Measles virus Polio virus
Depressed T cell mitogen responses	CMV
Selective depletion of T cell subpopulations	Dengue virus
Depletion of thymus cortex	Herpesvirus

Chronic Viral Infections

Chronic infections may occur with slow viruses such as those causing scrapie, visna, Aleutian mink disease and kuru, or with latent viruses such as herpes simplex, varicella-zoster, and a measles variant causing subacute sclerosing panencephalitis (SSPE). In latent viral infections, host defenses are unable to completely eradicate the virus, which may become reactivated when host defenses are compromised. Persistence of viruses has been observed in sensory ganglia (herpesviruses); tonsillar and adenoidal tissues (adenoviruses); brain tissues and lymph nodes (measles variant in SSPE); and lymphocytes (EB virus).

It has been suggested that persistence of viruses in the host contributes to the long-term immunity against reinfection, as seen with poliomyelitis and measles. Long-term cell-mediated responses against influenza virus, vaccinia, and mumps have been detected by in vitro transformation assays; memory may last for at least 20 years.

Viral Immunosuppression

As with bacteria, viruses induce various suppressive effects on host immune responses involving B cells, T cells, and macrophages. The examples of viral immunosuppression presented in Table 17-8 suggest ways in which viral infections may predispose individuals to other infections.

Viral Immunopathology

One of the more prevalent forms of viral-induced immunopathology is immune complex disease resulting from the deposition of soluble viral antigen-antibody complexes in various host tissues such as the kidney. Immune complexes have been detected in infections with LDV, LCM, Aleutian mink disease virus, respiratory syncytial virus, and murine leukemia virus.

Infections with lymphocytic choriomeningitis (LCM) virus in mice not only involve immune complex disease in chronic infections but also T cell–mediated destruction of LCM-infected tissues, which occurs if high numbers of cytotoxic T cells are present and if many viruses are also present in a vital organ such as the choriomeningeal plexus.

Immunity in Fungal Infections

Fungal infections range from superficial, localized lesions on the skin and mucosae to systemic infections involving major organs such as the lungs and kidney. Infections may be classified as deep-seated, intermediate, or superficial, depending upon the location of fungal lesions. Fungi causing deep-seated infections include *Coccidioides immitis* (valley fever agent) and *Histoplasma capsulatum,* both of which cause respiratory infections that are self-limiting or chronic, involving granuloma formation. Intermediate mycoses are often caused by *Candida* species, usually *Candida albicans,* which is an opportunistic fungus responsible for superficial or disseminated infections of the skin and mucosae. Superficial mycoses are caused by dermatophytes, which are keratinophilic. Very little is known about the mechanisms of pathogenesis in fungal infections. Possible mechanisms include inhibition of phagosome-lysosome fusion in macrophages, antiphagocytic capsules, and induction of delayed type hypersensitivity (DTH) reactions (Table 17–9).

Mechanisms of Immunity

Both humoral and cell-mediated responses occur against fungi, as determined by antibody formation and in vitro assays for CMI functions such as the MIF test, antigen-induced lymphocyte transformation and in vivo DTH reactions to fungal antigens. However, the relative importance of different immune mechanisms in fungal infections is unclear, largely because only a few mechanisms have been identified (Table 17–9).

The frequent occurrence of fungal infections in patients with CMI deficiencies suggests that CMI mechanisms are critical in antifungal defense. Very little experimental evidence exists demonstrating the protective role of CMI reactions in these infections. That T cells are crucial to host defense was demonstrated in a study of *Cryptococcus neoformans* infections in nude mice. The ability of some fungi to survive within nonimmune macrophages suggests that CMI responses may be valuable in protection.

A number of studies designed to delineate the roles of phagocytes, antibodies, and CMI responses have been carried out with *C. albicans* in experimentally induced infections in mice. Yeast (blastospore) forms are highly susceptible to monocyte and PMN killing by the myeloperoxidase-H_2O_2-halide system described

Table 17-9 : Host-Parasite Relationships in Some Fungal Infections

Mycoses/Fungi	Possible Mechanisms of Pathogenesis	Important Host Defense Mechanisms
Deep-seated mycoses		
Coccidioides immitis	Delayed hypersensitivity reactions	Cell-mediated immunity
	Inhibition of lysosome-phagosome fusion in alveolar macrophages	
Histoplasma capsulatum	Intracellular growth in nonimmune macrophages	Cell-mediated immunity
	Inhibition of lysosome-phagosome fusion in macrophages	
Cryptococcus neoformans	Antiphagocytic capsule	T cells in CMI
	Predilection of fungus for CNS	IgG opsonins (macrophages)
Intermediate mycoses		
Candida albicans	Cell wall toxins	Neutrophils and monocytes (MPO-H_2O_2-halide)
	Stimulation of T suppressor cells	Antibodies
	Pseudohyphae?	Macrophages
		Cell-mediated immunity?
Superficial mycoses		
Dermatophytes	Delayed hypersensitivity reactions	Plasma antifungal factors

previously. Rabbit alveolar and peritoneal macrophages are able to kill *C. albicans* by a different mechanism (macrophages lack peroxidase). The passive transfer of protection with immune serum and not with immune cells suggests that antibodies are important in anti-*Candida* defense. Cyclophosphamide-induced decrease in antibody levels increased susceptibility of mice to infection. On the other hand, nude mice were able to handle infections as well if not better than their heterozygous littermates; thus T cell responses may not be crucial in defense against this particular fungus.

Immunity in Parasitic Infections

The prevalence of protozoan and helminthic diseases throughout the world continually demands more useful information about mechanisms of immunity that may prove to be effective in preventing or controlling infections. The complex parasite morphological structures undergo various life-cycle changes, necessitating a number of different defense mechanisms to effectively restrict the multiplication or persistence of these organisms in the host. In addition, some parasites acquire host antigens, which

Table 17-10 : Possible Mechanisms of Immunity in Parasitic Infections

Organism	Possible Mechanisms of Immunity
Protozoa	
Giardia lamblia	T cell–mediated (nude mice are susceptible to infection)
Trichomonas vaginalis	Natural cytotoxic cell, macrophage?
Leishmania sp.	Cell-mediated
Trypanosoma gambiense *Trypanosoma cruzi*	Antibodies, T cells (nude mice are susceptible to infection)
Plasmodium sp.	Opsonizing or merozoite-blocking antibody
Toxoplasma gondii	Probably cell-mediated (parasite inhibits phagosome-lysosome fusion in macrophages)
Helminths—Trematodes	
Schistosoma mansoni	Interactions of eosinophils, Ab, complement Interactions of PMNs, Ab, complement Interactions of macrophages, IgG, IgE T cell–dependent responses
Helminths—Nematodes	
Nippostrongylus brasiliensis	IgG-mediated damage to worms Expulsion of worms lymphocyte-dependent (T)
Trichinella spiralis	Eosinophils and Ab destroy larvae

mask foreign parasite antigens; this has been observed with schistosomes, which incorporate human ABO blood group antigens into their surfaces.

Mechanisms of Immunity

Both humoral and cell-mediated responses occur to parasite antigens. However, perhaps because these parasites are so complex, development of specific immune responses is often slow, and when acquired immunity does develop, the host is often still unable to eradicate the parasites. With some organisms, such as *Trypanosoma gambiense* and *T. cruzi,* development of immunity in man is difficult to detect. Different strains and species of animals vary widely in their susceptibility and resistance to parasites. This is illustrated by trypanosomal infections in mice, which produce antibodies and T cell–dependent responses against these organisms, and which are protected by these responses. Concomitant immunity, in which reinfection immunity exists in the presence of parasites, has been observed in human malaria infections and in *Schistosoma mansoni* infections in mice. Other infections are completely resolved by host immune responses,

Fig. 17-7 : Possible host defense mechanisms against Schistosoma mansoni during different stages of the life-cycle of the parasite.

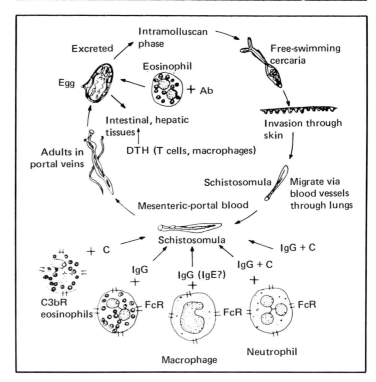

ending with elimination of parasites and development of reinfection immunity. Human cutaneous leishmaniasis is an example of this type of infection.

Some of the immune mechanisms shown to be effective in experimentally induced parasitic infections in animals (primarily rodents) are outlined in Table 17-10. Important factors that can modulate host responses include chronic antigenemia and circulating antigen-antibody complexes that may specifically block certain defense mechanisms. Information on effective mechanisms is scant, considering the magnitude of the health problems resulting from these infectious agents.

One particularly well-studied parasite is *Schistosoma mansoni,* a blood fluke that passes through several stages in its life cycle (Figure 17-7). A number of mechanisms effective against schistosomula (larvae) have been discovered, including (1) direct killing by IgG and complement; (2) enhanced killing when neutrophils are added to IgG and complement; (3) macrophage-mediated killing in the presence of specific IgG or IgE; (4) eosinophil-mediated killing in cooperation with complement; and (5) eosinophil-mediated killing in conjunction with IgG. Eosinophils and specific antibody are also effective in destroying schistosome eggs. The extrusion of eggs from the venules, their filtration into the surrounding tissues, and their expulsion into the intestinal lumen are events responsible for most of the pathological features in this disease (hemorrhages, pseudoabscesses around eggs trapped in perivascular tissues). Delayed hypersensitivity responses to egg antigens leads to granuloma formation. The nature of immune responses against *S. mansoni* illustrates the complexity of host-parasite relationships in helminthic infections.

Summary

1. Immunity in bacterial infections requires the functions of neutrophils and macrophages; phagocytes can kill bacteria by oxygen-dependent mechanisms (involving the MPO-H_2O_2-halide system or reduction products of oxygen) and by oxygen-independent mechanisms, such as the actions of cationic proteins.

2. Extracellular bacteria are usually susceptible to the bactericidal effects of phagocytes. Antibodies may assist phagocytosis by opsonization, especially in the presence of complement. Exotoxins produced by some extracellular bacteria are neutralized by antibody. Antibodies may also cause bacteriolysis in the presence of complement and lysozyme, or they may inhibit bacterial attachment to host epithelial cells.

3. Cell-mediated defenses, primarily involving immune T cell mediators that activate macrophages, are required for defense against facultative and obligate intracellular bacteria. The genetically determined resistance of some mice to *L. monocytogenes* may be expressed in terms of macrophage function.

4. Macrophages play an important role in limiting viral spread; resistance of macrophages to viral infections appears to be genetically determined in mice by a single mendelian dominant gene.

5. Antibody-mediated neutralization of viruses may involve the following mechanisms: viral aggregation, lysis in the presence of complement, enhancement of engulfment by phagocytes, inhibition of viral adsorption to host cells, and lysis of viral-infected cells in the presence of complement.

6. Cell-mediated defenses against viruses include cytotoxic T lymphocytes, sensitized T cell–macrophage interaction, ADCC reactions, and NK cell activity. Induction and activity of cytotoxic T lymphocytes is H-2 restricted.

7. Interferon released from virus-infected cells or antigen-stimulated lymphocytes directly or indirectly (through the production of antiviral protein) inhibits replication of infectious virus.

8. Immunity in fungal infections involves both cell-mediated and humoral mechanisms, depending upon the fungus. Mechanisms of fungal pathogenesis may involve DTH reactions, antiphagocytic capsules, cell wall toxins, and inhibition of phagosome-lysosome fusion in phagocytes.

9. Immunity in parasitic infections involves many aspects of host-parasite relationships. Effective protective immunity against parasites is often lacking, resulting in chronic infections.

10. Immune mechanisms against infectious agents are basically beneficial but may sometimes be harmful to the host. Immunopathology results from the formation and deposition of immune complexes on host tissues with resultant inflammation. Chronic granulomas may also cause damage to host tissues.

Bibliography and Selected Reading

General

Bach, J. F. (Ed.). *Immunology.* New York: Wiley, 1978.

Goren, M. B. Phagocyte lysosomes: Interactions with infectious agents, phagosomes, and experimental perturbations in function. *Annu. Rev. Microbiol.* 31:507, 1977.

Myrvik, Q. N., Pearsall, N. N., and Weiser, R. S. *Fundamentals of Medical Bacteriology and Mycology.* Philadelphia: Lea & Febiger, 1974.

Playfair, J. H. L. Effective and ineffective immune responses to parasites: Evidence from experimental models. *Curr. Top. Microbiol. Immunol.* 80:37, 1978.

Quie, P. G., Mills, E. L., and Holmes, B. Molecular events during phagocytosis by human neutrophils. *Prog. Hematol.* 10:193, 1977.

Schwab, J. H. Suppression of the immune response by microorganisms. *Bacteriological Rev., ASM.* 39:121, 1975.

van Oss, C. J. Phagocytosis as a Surface Phenomenon. *Annu. Rev. Microbiol.* 32:19, 1978.

Zukerman, S. H., and Douglas, S. D. Dynamics of the macrophage plasma membrane. *Annu. Rev. Microbiol.* 33:267, 1979.

Immunity in Bacterial Infections

Cheers, C., McKenzie, I. F. C., Pavlov, H., Waid, C., and York, J. Resistance and susceptibility of mice to bacterial infection: Course of listeriosis in resistant or susceptible mice. *Infect. Immun.* 19:763, 1978.

Fubara, E. S., and Freter, R. Protection against enteric bacterial infection by secretory IgA antibodies. *J. Immunol.* 111:395, 1973.

Martinez, R. J., and Carrol, S. F. Sequential metabolic expressions of the lethal process in human serum-treated *Escherichia coli:* Role of lysozyme. *Infect. Immun.* 28:735, 1980.

Mitsuyama, M., Takeya, K., Nomoto, K. and Shimotori, S. Three phases of phagocyte contribution to resistance against *Listeria monocytogenes. J. Gen. Microbiol.* 106:165, 1978.

Peterson, J. W., Hetjtmancik, K. E., Markel, D. E., Craig, J. P., and Kurosky, A. Antigenic specificity of neutralizing antibody to cholera toxin. *Infect. Immun.* 24:774, 1979.

Peterson, P. K., Wilkinson, B. J., Kim, Y., Schmeling, D., and Quie, P. G. Influence of encapsulation on staphylococcal opsonization and phagocytosis by human polymorphonuclear leukocytes. *Infect. Immun.* 19:943, 1978.

Skamene, E. and Kongshavn, P. A. L. Phenotypic expression of genetically controlled host resistance to *Listeria monocytogenes*. *Infect. Immun.* 25:345, 1979.

Immunity in Viral Infections

Burns, W. H. and Allison, A. C. Virus Infections and the Immune Responses They Elicit, p. 479–574. *In* M. Sela (Ed.). *The Antigens* Volume III. New York: Academic, 1975.

Ho, M. Role of specific cytotoxic lymphocytes in cellular immunity against murine cytomegalovirus. *Infect. Immun.* 27:767, 1980.

Merigan, T. C. Host defenses against viral disease. *N. Engl. J. Med.* 290:323, 1974.

Notkins, A. L. Viral infections: Mechanisms of immunologic defense and injury. *Hosp. Pract.* 9:65, 1974.

Piontek, G. E., Weltzin, R., and Tompkins W. A. F. Enhanced cytotoxicity of mouse natural killer cells for vaccinia and herpes virus-infected targets. *J. Reticuloendothel. Soc.* 27:175, 1980.

Pitha, P. M., Wivel, N. A., Fernie, B. F., and Harper, H. P. Effect of interferon on murine leukaemia virus infection. IV. Formation of non-fectious virus in chronically infected cells. *J. Gen. Virol.* 42:467, 1979.

Quinnan, G. V., Manichewitz, J. E., and Ennis, F. A. Cytotoxic T lymphocyte response to murine cytomegalovirus infection. *Nature* 273:541, 1978.

Zinkernagel, R. M., and Doherty, P. C. Restriction of *in vitro* T cell-mediated cytotoxicity in lymphocytic choriomeningitis within a syngeneic or semiallogeneic system. *Nature* (Lond.) 248:701, 1974.

Immunity in Fungal Infections

Graybill, J. R., and Drutz, D. J. Host defense in cryptococcosis II. Cryptococcosis in the nude mouse. *Cell. Immunol.* 40:263, 1978.

Kozel, T. R., and McGaw, T. G. Opsonization of *Cryptococcus neoformans* by human immunoglobulin G: Role of immunoglobulin G in phagocytosis by macrophages. *Infect. Immun.* 25:255, 1979.

Moser, S. A., and Domer, J. E. Effects of cyclophosphamide on murine candidiasis. *Infect. Immun.* 27:376, 1980.

Pearsall, N. N., Adams, B. L., and Bunni, R. Immunologic responses to *Candida albicans*. III. Effects of passive transfer of lymphoid cells or serum on murine candidiasis. *J. Immunol.* 120:1176, 1978.

Schuit, K. E. Phagocytosis and intracellular killing of pathogenic yeasts by human monocytes and neutrophils. *Infect. Immun.* 24:932, 1979.

Immunity in Parasitic Infections

Capron, M., Torpier, G. and Capron, A. *In vitro* killing of *S. mansoni* schistosomula by eosinophils from infected rats: Role of cytophilic antibodies. *J. Immunol.* 123:2220, 1979.

Heumann, A.-M., Stiffel, C., Monjour, L., Bucci, A., and Biozzi, G. Correlation between genetic regulation of antibody responsiveness and protective immunity induced by *Plasmodium berghei* vaccination. *Infect. Immun.* 24:829, 1979.

Landolfo, S., Martinotti, M. G., Martinetto, P., and Forni, G. Natural cell-mediated cytotoxicity against *Trichomonas vaginalis* in the mouse. I. Tissue, strain, age distribution, and some characteristics of the effector cells. *J. Immunol.* 124:508, 1980.

Quinn, T. C., and Syler, D. J. Mechanisms of action of hyperimmune serum in mediating protective immunity to rodent malaria (*Plasmodium berghei*). *J. Immunol.* 123:2245, 1979.

Reed, S. G. Adoptive transfer of resistance to acute *Trypanosoma cruzi* with T-lymphocyte enriched spleen cells. *Infect. Immun.* 28:404, 1980.

Index